PANCREATIC CANCER – CLINICAL MANAGEMENT

Edited by **Sanjay K. Srivastava**

Pancreatic Cancer – Clinical Management
Edited by Sanjay K. Srivastava

Published by InTech
Janeza Trdine 9, 51000 Rijeka, Croatia

Publishing Process Manager Martina Blecic

Technical Editor Teodora Smiljanic

Cover Designer InTech Design Team

Additional hard copies can be obtained from orders@intechopen.com

Pancreatic Cancer – Clinical Management, Edited by Sanjay K. Srivastava
p. cm.
ISBN 978-953-51-0394-3

For EU product safety concerns:
IN TECH d.o.o., Prolaz Marije Krucifikse Kozulić 3, 51000 Rijeka, Croatia,
info@intechopen.com or visit our website at intechopen.com.

Meet the editor

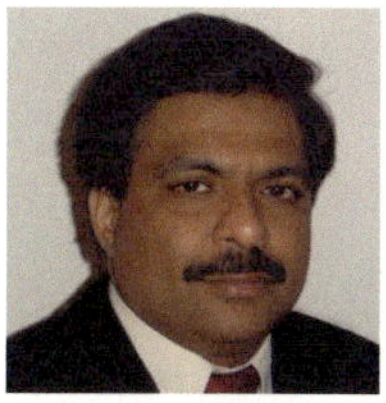

Dr. Sanjay K. Srivastava is a Professor of Biomedical Sciences at Texas Tech University Health Sciences Center (TTUHSC), Amarillo, Texas, specializing in cancer biology, cell signaling and nutritional chemoprevention. Dr. Srivastava served as an Assistant Professor in the Department of Pharmacology, University of Pittsburgh School of Medicine, and did his post-doc from University of Texas Medical Branch at Galveston, Texas. He received a M.S. in Biochemistry from Lucknow University and a Ph.D. in Biochemical Toxicology from Industrial Toxicology Research Center, India. Dr. Srivastava is funded by grants from the National Cancer Institute, NIH. He has authored/co-authored more than 100 research papers and book chapters and is in the editorial board of several journals. Dr. Srivastava has been the recipient of several awards including TTUHSC "President's Excellence in Research Award". His research has been featured by news agencies including BBC, MSNBC, CBS, ABC, Science News etc.

Contents

Dedicated to my mother Vidya Srivastava and father Dr. Balramji Srivastava,
who provided me constant love and support.

Preface

Pancreatic cancer is one of the most fatal human malignancies with extremely poor prognosis making it the fourth leading cause of cancer-related deaths in the United States. The molecular mechanisms of pancreatic carcinogenesis are not well understood. The major focus of these two books is towards the understanding of the basic biology of pancreatic carcinogenesis, identification of newer molecular targets and the development of adjuvant and neoadjuvant therapies.

Book 1 on pancreatic cancer provides the reader with an overall understanding of the biology of pancreatic cancer, hereditary, complex signaling pathways and alternative therapies. The book explains nutrigenomics and epigenetics mechanisms such as DNA methylation, which may explain the etiology or progression of pancreatic cancer. Apart from epigenetics, book summarizes the molecular control of oncogenic pathways such as K-Ras and KLF4. Since pancreatic cancer metastasizes to vital organs resulting in poor prognosis, special emphasis is given to the mechanism of tumor cell invasion and metastasis. Role of nitric oxide and Syk kinase in tumor metastasis is discussed in detail. Prevention strategies for pancreatic cancer are also described. The molecular mechanisms of the anti-cancer effects of curcumin, benzyl isothiocyante and vitamin D are discussed in detail. Furthermore, this book covers the basic mechanisms of resistance of pancreatic cancer to chemotherapy drugs such as gemcitabine and 5-flourouracil. The involvement of various survival pathways in chemo-drug resistance is discussed in depth. Major emphasis is given to the identification of newer therapeutic targets such as mesothalin, glycosylphosphatidylinositol, cell cycle regulatory proteins, glycans, galectins, p53, toll-like receptors, Grb7 and telomerase in pancreatic cancer for drug development.

Book 2 covers pancreatic cancer risk factors, treatment and clinical procedures. It provides an outline of pancreatic cancer genetic risk factors, signaling mechanisms, biomarkers and disorders and systems biology for the better understanding of disease. As pancreatic cancer suffers from lack of early diagnosis or prognosis markers, this book encompasses stem cell and genetic makers to identify the disease in early stages. The book uncovers the rationale and effectiveness of monotherapy and combination therapy in combating the devastating disease. As immunotherapy is emerging as an attractive approach to cease pancreatic cancer progression, the present book covers various aspects of immunotherapy including innate, adaptive, active, passive and bacterial approaches. The book also focuses on the disease management and clinical procedures. Book explains the role of pre-existing conditions such as diabetes and smoking in pancreatic cancer. Management of anesthesia during surgery and pain after surgery has been discussed. Book also takes the reader through the role of endoscopy and fine needle guided biopsies in diagnosing and observing the disease progression. As pancreatic cancer is recognized as a major risk factor for vein thromboembolism, this book reviews the basics of coagulation disorders and implication of expandable metallic stents in the management of portal vein stenosis of recurrent and resected pancreatic cancer. Emphasis is given to neuronal invasion of pancreatic tumors along with management of pancreatic neuroendocrine tumors.

We hope that this book will be helpful to the researchers, scientists and patients providing invaluable information of the basic, translational and clinical aspects of pancreatic cancer.

Sanjay K. Srivastava, Ph.D.
Department of Biomedical Sciences
Texas Tech University Health Sciences Center
Amarillo, Texas
USA

1

The Genetics of Pancreatic Cancer

Dagan Efrat[1,2] and Gershoni-Baruch Ruth[1,3]
[1]*Institute of Human Genetics, Rambam Health Care Campus, Haifa,*
[2]*Department of Nursing, the Faculty of Social Welfare and Health Sciences, University of Haifa,*
[3]*The Ruth and Bruce Rapoport Faculty of Medicine, Technion-Institute of Technology, Haifa, Israel*

1. Introduction

Globally, pancreatic cancer is considered a rare cause of cancer. More than 250,000 new cases, equivalent to 2.5% of all forms of cancer, were diagnosed in 2008 worldwide (Ferlay et al., 2008, 2010). Pancreatic adenocarcinoma currently represents the fourth most common cancer causing death in the United States and in most developed countries (Jemal et al., 2009, 2011). Despite advances in medical science, the overall prognosis of pancreatic cancer remains poor and five years survival is only 4% (Jemal et al., 2006). Those diagnosed early, with tumor limited to the pancreas, display a 25-30% five years survival following surgery (Ryu et al., 2010).

It has been suggested that it takes at least 10 years from tumor initiation to the development of the parental clone and another five years to the development of metastatic subclones, with patients dying within two years thereafter, on average (Costello & Neoptolemos, 2011). Given the limited treatment options there has been considerable focus on clinical and molecular harbingers of early disease. A mechanism for early detection and for early intervention remains to be elaborated. Current research is focused on the discovery and the development of diagnostic bio markers that can unveil pancreatic cancer in its early stages. Deciphering and understanding the genetics of sporadic and hereditary pancreatic cancer remains a fundamental milestone.

Based on family aggregation and family history of pancreatic disease, it is estimated that around 10% of cases diagnosed with pancreatic cancer host a hereditary germ line mutation (Lynch et al., 1996; Hruban et al., 1998). Furthermore, it has been observed that pancreatic cancer occurs in excess of expected frequencies, in several familial cancer syndromes, which are associated with specific germ-line mutations. The best characterized include hereditary breast-ovarian cancer syndrome ascribed to mutations in BRCA1/2 genes, especially BRCA2; familial pancreatic and breast cancer syndrome due to mutations in PALB2 gene; familial isolated pancreatic cancer caused by mutations in PALLD encoding palladin; and familial multiple mole melanoma with pancreatic cancer (FAMMM-PC) attributed to mutations in CDKN2A. Other hereditary cancer syndromes demonstrating increased hereditary risk for pancreatic cancer, yet with less significance, include hereditary non-polyposis colorectal syndrome - Lynch syndrome and Li-Fraumeni syndrome which is caused by mutations in p53 gene.

The identification of individuals at risk for pancreatic cancer would aid in targeting those who might benefit most from cancer surveillance strategies and early detection (Brentnall et al., 1999). This chapter describes the cutting edge data related to the genetics of sporadic and hereditary pancreatic cancer subdivided according to 'genes' function.

2. Oncogenes

2.1 KRAS gene (MIM 190070)

Recent studies have shown that the KRAS oncogene on chromosome 12p is activated by point mutations in approximately 90% of pancreatic cancers tumors, and these mutations involve codon 12 most commonly, and codons 13 and 61 thereafter (Caldas & Kern, 1995). The RAS protein produced by wild-type KRAS binds GTPase-activating protein and regulates cell-cycle progression. Mutations in KRAS constitute the earliest genetic abnormalities underlying the development of pancreatic neoplasms (Maitra et al., 2006; Feldmann et al., 2007). KRAS may thus be a promising bio marker for early detection of curable non-invasive pancreatic neoplasia (Maitra et al., 2006).

2.2 BRAF gene (MIM 164757)

The BRAF gene maps to chromosome 7q and takes part in the RAF–MAP signaling pathway, critical in mediating cancer causing signals in the RAS corridor (Calhoun et al., 2003). BRAF mutations have been described in about 15% of all human cancers, including pancreatic cancer (Davies et al., 2002). The BRAF gene is activated by oncogenic RAS, leading to cooperative mutual effects in cells responding to growth factor signals. BRAF and KRAS appear to be alternately mutated in pancreatic cancers; thus, pancreatic cancers with KRAS gene mutations do not harbor BRAF gene mutations and vice versa (Maitra et al., 2006).

2.3 PALLD gene (MIM 608092)

Palladin RNA is over-expressed in tissues from both precancerous dysplasia and pancreatic adenocarcinoma in familial and sporadic pancreatic disease. The mutated gene is assumingly, best detected in very early precancerous dysplastic tissue, heralding neoplastic transformation before the overarching of genetic instability, underlying cancer, has occurred. Palladin is a component of actin-containing microfilaments that control cell shape, adhesion and contraction and is associated with myocardial infarction and pancreatic cancer. Palladin is most probably a proto-oncogene (Pogue-Geile et al., 2006).

2.3.1 Familial pancreatic cancer associated PALLD gene (MIM 164757)

Few families with isolated pancreatic cancer of early onset and high penetrance have been identified (Lynch et al., 1990; Brentnall et al., 1999; Banke et al., 2000; Hruban et al., 2001;

Meckler et al., 2001). Genomewide linkage screen of a family, noted as 'family X', has shown significant linkage to chromosome 4q32-34 (Eberle et al., 2002). Pogue-Geile et al. (2006) later found a mutation, inducing a proline (hydrophobic) to serine (hydrophilic) amino acid change (P239S), in a highly conserved region of the gene encoding palladin (PALLD), segregating in all affected family members and absent in unaffected family members. Zogopoulous et al. (2007) identified this same mutation (P239S) in one of 84 (1.2%) patients with familial and early-onset pancreatic cancer and in one of 555 controls (0.002%). No evidence for palladin mutations in 48 individuals with familial pancreatic cancer was recorded by Klein et al. (2009). Further investigation is warranted in order to confirm the pathogenecity of mutations in PALLD.

2.4 Other oncogenes

AKT2 (MIM 164731) - It has been suggested that the AKT2 oncogene, on chromosome 19q, contributes to the malignant phenotype of a subset of human ductal pancreatic cancers. Cheng et al., (1996) demonstrated that the AKT2 oncogene is over expressed in approximately 10-15% of pancreatic carcinomas. AKT2 encodes a protein belonging to a subfamily of serine/threonine kinases.

AIB1 (MIM 601937) - AIB1 gene, on chromosome 20q, is amplified in as many as 60% of pancreatic cancers (Anzick et al., 1997; Calhoun et al., 2003; Aguirre et al., 2004). Altered AIB1 expression may contribute to the development of steroid-dependent cancers. It has also been reported that amplification of a localized region on the long arm of chromosome 8 is commonly seen in pancreatic cancers, and this amplification corresponds to the oncogenic transcription factor CMYC (MIM 190080) (Aguirre et al., 2004).

In addition to these genes, numbers of amplicons, amplified from DNA fragments, have been identified in pancreatic cancers by using gene chip technologies (Aguirre et al., 2004). Employing array comparative genomic hybridization (CGH) technology, a high resolution analysis of genome-wide copy number aberrations, permits to identify over expression of DNA fragments in tumor transformed pancreatic cells. Understanding the mechanisms underlying the development of pancreatic cancer may aid target early detection, gene-specific therapies and thereby improve prognosis.

3. Tumor suppressor genes

In pancreatic invasive adenocarcinoma, CDKN2A/INK4A, TP53, and DPC4/SMAD4/ MADH4 are commonly inactivated.

3.1 CDKN2A/INK4A gene (MIM 600160)

The CDKN2A gene on chromosome 9p21 encodes proteins that control two critical cell cycle regulatory pathways, the p53 (TP53) pathway and the retinoblastoma (RB1) pathway. Through the use of shared coding regions and alternative reading frames, the CDKN2A gene produces 2 major proteins: p16(INK4), which is a cyclin-dependent kinase inhibitor checkpoint, and p14(ARF), which binds the p53-stabilizing protein MDM2 (Robertson and Jones, 1999). P16 inhibits cyclin D1 by binding to the cyclin-dependent kinases Cdk4 and Cdk6 thereby causing G1-S cell-cycle arrest (Schutte et al., 1997). Loss of p16 function, consequent to several different mechanisms, including homozygous deletion, intragenic mutation and epigenetic silencing by gene promoter methylation, is seen in approximately 90% of pancreatic cancers (Caldas et al., 1994; Schutte et al., 1997; Ueki et al., 2000). As a bystander effect, homozygous deletions of the CDKN2A/INK4A gene can also delete both copies of the methylthio-adenosine phosphorylase (MTAP) gene, whose product is essential for the salvage pathway of purine synthesis. In about a third of pancreatic cancers co-deletion of the MTAP and CDKN2A/INK4A genes is observed (Hustinx et al., 2005).

This observation has a potential therapeutic significance, since chemotherapeutic regimes selectively targeted to cells demonstrating loss of Mtap function are currently available.

3.1.1 Familial Atypical Multiple Mole Melanoma – Pancreatic Cancer (FAMMM-PC) syndrome (MIM 606719)

The association between mutations in p16 (CDKN2A) and familial pancreatic cancer was previously noted by Caldas et al. (1994) and others (Liu et al., 1995; Whelan et al., 1995; Schutte et al., 1997). Further evidence for a plausible role of CDKN2A in pancreatic cancer was provided by Whelan et al. (1995) who described a kindred at risk for pancreatic cancers, melanomas, and additional types of tumors, co-segregating with a CDKN2A mutation. CDKN2A mutations were detected individuals with pancreatic cancer from melanoma families (Goldstein et al., 1995). Later, Lynch et al., 2002, coined the term hereditary FAMMM-PC syndrome to describe families with both melanoma and pancreatic cancers. Although rare, the life time risk of CDKN2A carriers, to develop pancreatic cancer and melanoma was calculated to be 58% and 39%, respectively (McWilliams et al., 2010). Basically, CDKN2A is a small gene, containing 3 coding exons. However, lack of founder mutations impedes the screening of families at risk in the clinical setting.

3.2 TP53 gene (MIM 191170)

The TP53 gene on chromosome 17p undergoes bi-allelic inactivation in approximately 50–75% of pancreatic cancers, almost always subject to the combination of an intragenic mutation and the loss of the second wild-type allele (Redston et al., 1994). The transcription factor p53 responds to diverse cellular stresses formulated to regulate target genes participating in G1-S cell cycle checkpoint, maintenance of G2-M arrest, cell cycle arrest, apoptosis, senescence and DNA repair (Redston et al., 1994). There is emerging evidence to suggest that loss of p53 function may contribute to the genomic instability observed in pancreatic cancers (Hingorani et al., 2005); and that TP53 gene mutations constitute late events in pancreatic cancer progression (Maitra et al., 2003).

3.2.1 Li- Fraumeni syndrome (MIM 151623)

Li-Fraumeni syndrome is a rare, clinically and genetically heterogeneous, inherited cancer syndrome caused by germline mutations in TP53. Li-Fraumeni syndrome is characterized by autosomal dominant inheritance and early onset of tumors, rather multiple tumors in one individual and multiple affected family members. In contrast to other inherited cancer syndromes, which are predominantly characterized by site-specific cancers, Li-Fraumeni syndrome presents with a variety of tumor types. The most common types are soft tissue sarcomas and osteosarcomas, breast cancer, brain tumors, leukemia, and adrenocortical carcinoma (Li et al., 1988). Several families with Li-Fraumeni syndrome presenting with pancreatic cancer were occasionally described (Lynch et al., 1985; Casey et al., 1993).

3.3 Deleted in pancreatic carcinoma 4 (DPC4) gene (MIM 600993)

About 90% of human somatic pancreatic carcinomas show allelic loss at 18q. Hahn et al. (1996) reported the identification of a putative tumor suppressor gene, namely, Deleted in Pancreatic Carcinoma 4 or DPC4 (also known as SMAD4/MADH4) on chromosome 18q21.1. Loss of Dpc4 protein function interferes with intracellular signaling cascades leading to decreased growth inhibition and uncontrolled proliferation. SMAD4 plays a pivotal role in signal transduction of the transforming growth factor beta superfamily cytokines by mediating transcriptional activation of target genes. Immunohistochemical labeling for Dpc4 protein expression mirrors DPC4/SMAD4/MADH4 gene status with rare exceptions, and like TP53, loss of Dpc4 expression is a late genetic event in pancreatic carcinoma and is observed in about 30% of progression lesions (Feldmann et al., 2007).

Genome-wide association studies (GWAS) have provided evidence that a person's risk of developing pancreatic cancer is influenced by multiple common disease alleles with small effects (Low et al., 2010; Petersen et al., 2010). Further research is required to evaluate the epidemiological input of these markers to the development of pancreatic cancer and their availability for early detection (Costello & Neoptolemos, 2011). Other tumor-suppressor genes are targeted at low frequency in pancreatic cancer. These genes provide a significant insight unto the molecular mechanism that underlines pancreatic cancers, and may serve as therapeutic targets in the early stages of pancreatic cancer.

4. Genome-maintenance genes

Several gene ensembles, that play a role in caring for genome stability, were found to be mutated in pancreatic cancer, more so, in familial rather than sporadic cancer, including familial pancreatic cancer. BRCA2 is with no doubt the prominent gene in this category.

4.1 BRCA1/2 genes (MIM 113705/600185)

BRCA1 - The gene product of BRCA1, functions in a number of cellular pathways that maintain genomic stability, including DNA damage-induced cell cycle checkpoint activation and arrest, DNA damage repair, protein ubiquitination, chromatin remodeling, as well as transcriptional regulation and apoptosis (see for example review by Wu et al., 2010). BRCA1 forms several distinct complexes through association with different adaptor proteins, and each complex assemble in a mutually exclusive manner (Wang et al., 2009).

BRCA2 – BRCA2 plays a key role in recombinational DNA repair, maintenance of genomic integrity and resistance to agents that damage DNA or collapse replication forks. The role of BRCA2 is best understood during DNA double-strand break repair (see for example Schlacher et al., 2011) as it co-localizes with PALB2 gene in nuclear foci, thereby promoting its stability in nuclear structures and enabling its recombinational repair and checkpoint functions (Xia et al., 2006).

Both BRCA1 and BRCA2 have transcriptional activation and seem to be mutually interrelated.

Traditionally BRCA1 and BRCA2 were classified as tumor suppressor genes. Nowadays, BRCA1 and BRCA2 are rather cataloged as 'caretaker' genes that act, amongst other, as nucleotide-excision-repair (NER) genes (Kinzler and Vogelstein, 1997). While, inactivated 'gatekeepers', namely, tumor suppressor genes, promote tumor initiation directly, the inactivation of caretaker genes leads to genetic instability resulting in increased mutations in other genes, including gatekeepers. Once a tumor is initiated by inactivation of a caretaker gene, it may progress rapidly due to an accelerated rate of mutations in other genes that directly control cell birth or death. Consistent with this hypothesis, mutations in BRCA1 and BRCA2 are rarely found in sporadic cancers, and the risk of cancer arising in people with BRCA somatic mutations is relatively low.

4.1.1 Hereditary breast-ovarian cancer syndrome

Since the late nineties of the 20th century, excess of pancreatic cancer cases was documented in families with hereditary breast-ovarian cancer syndrome, traditionally linked to BRCA1/2 genes. Several studies have shown high BRCA2 mutation carrier frequencies in pancreatic cancer patients, reaching 10-20%, more so in Jewish Ashkenazi compared to non-Jewish pancreatic cancer patients (Teng et al., 1996; Ozcelik et al., 1997; Slater et al., 2010), with greater penetrance for males over females (Risch et al., 2001; Murphy et al., 2002; McWilliams et al., 2005; Dagan, 2008; Dagan et al., 2010; Ferrone et al., 2009). BRCA1 mutations are less often associated with pancreatic cancer compared to BRCA2 mutations (Al-Sukhni et al., 2008; Dagan et al., 2010). Mutations within the OCCR-ovarian cancer-cluster region of the BRCA2 gene in exon 11 frequently cause either/or pancreatic cancer, ovarian cancer and other type of cancers (Risch et al., 2001; Thompson et al., 2001).

The distinction between gatekeepers and caretakers genes has important practical and theoretical ramifications. Tumors that have defective caretaker genes are expected to respond favorably to therapeutic agents that induce the type of genomic damage that is normally detected or repaired by the particular caretaker gene involved.

Poly (ADP-ribose) polymerase (PARP) inhibitors have raised recent excitement as to their deleterious effect on BRCA1 or BRCA2 associated ovarian, breast or pancreatic cancer cells. If either PARP or BRCA function remains intact, a cell will continue to survive. Thus, inhibiting PARP should not affect the non-cancerous cells that contain one functional copy of BRCA. Loss of both functions, however, is incompatible with life (Bryant et al., 2005; Helleday et al., 2005; Drew et al., 2011). With this in mind, this class of agents has the potential to potentiate cytotoxic therapy without increased side effects. Acting as sole agents, they are able to exterminate cancer cells with DNA repair defects. The genomic instability of tumor cells allows PARP inhibitors to selectively target tumor cells rather than normal cells. PARP proteins inhibitors have gained supremacy as ideal anticancer agents (Weil & Chen, 2011) and may promise better prognosis in pancreatic, ovarian and breast cancer due to hereditary mutations in BRCA1/2.

4.2 Partner and localizer of BRCA2 (PALB2) gene (MIM 610355)

PALB2 maps to chromosome 16p12 (Xia et al., 2006; Reid et al., 2007; Xia et al., 2007). Differential extraction showed that BRCA2 and PALB2 colocalize in S-phase foci and are associated with stable nuclear structures. As PALB2 is critical for the function of BRCA2 as regards DNA repair, it should be considered, in principle, as a caretaker gene. Like BRCA2, PALB2 participates in DNA damage response and both genes collectively cooperate allowing BRCA2 to escape the effects of proteasome-mediated degradation (Reid et al., 2007; Xia et al., 2007).

4.2.1 Familial pancreatic cancer associated PALB2

Germline mutations in PALB2 have been identified in approximately 1-2% of familial breast cancer and 3-4% of familial pancreatic cancer cases (Slater et al., 2010; Casadei et al., 2011; Hofstatter et al., 2011). Three pancreatic cancer patients out of 96, with a positive family history of pancreatic cancer were found to harbor a PALB2 germline deletion of 4 basepairs, that was absent in 1084 control samples (Jones et al., 2009; Rahman et al., 2007). PALB2 appears to be the second most commonly mutated gene implicated in hereditary pancreatic cancer after BRCA2 (Jones et al., 2009).

4.3 Hereditary non-polyposis colon syndrome – HNPCC (MIM 120435)

Pancreatic cancer was infrequently described in families with hereditary non-polyposis colon cancer (Lynch et al., 1985; Miyaki et al., 1997). HNPCC subdivided into Lynch I, primarily affecting the colon, Lynch II mainly targeting extra colonic organs including the pancreas and Muir-Torre syndrome. HNPCC is a genetically heterogeneous disease, with most mutations detected in MSH2 and MLH1 genes.

MSH2 (MIM 609309) - The microsatellite DNA instability that is associated with alteration in the MSH2 gene in hereditary nonpolyposis colon cancer and several forms of sporadic cancer is thought to arise from defective repair of DNA replication errors. MSH2 has a direct role in mutation avoidance and microsatellite stability in human cells (Fishel et al., 1994).

MLH1 (MIM 609310) – Similarly to MSH2, MLH1 gene encodes a protein involved in the identification and repair of DNA mismatch errors. The identification of germline mutations in *MLH1* and *MSH2* was rapidly followed by the discovery of other human genes that encode proteins involved in the mismatch repair (MMR) complex (see review by Lynch et al., 2009).

5. Synopsis

Pancreatic cancer is of the most lethal of all human malignancies caused by inherited and acquired (somatic) mutations. The poor prognosis of pancreatic cancer (Jemal et al., 2006) warrants early detection of asymptomatic individuals, at high risk, using imaging methods and molecular analyses and thereby providing them with a chance for better survival (Goggins et al., 2000). Understanding the complex genetic mechanisms underlying the development of pancreatic cancer, as depicted in this chapter, may conduit medical science in the path that will ultimately lead to early detection, tailored treatment and consequently better prognosis for this incurable disease.

Although, novel mechanisms, sprout on the horizon, could be exploited for early detection, as depicted by the KRAS detection technology, it seems that most pancreatic neoplasms in the general population will remain undetectable before invasive cancer develops. However, the recognition of early genetic somatic changes can advocate for presymptomatic chemo or surgical prevention schemes that may alleviate those with pre cancerous neoplasms before an invasive cancer had a chance to develop. This farfetched undertaking is already underway.

Although, pancreatic cancer is basically sporadic, about 10% of the patients harbor a germline mutation. It seems that BRCA2 is the major susceptibility gene contributing to hereditary pancreatic cancer, especially in populations segregating founder mutations, namely, Ashkenazi Jews, Icelandic (Thorlacius et al., 1996; Dagan, 2008; Dagan et al., 2010) and others. Beyond this, pancreatic cancer patients and family members at risk should follow the standard recommendations, as regards genetic counseling and diagnosis that befits hereditary breast-ovarian cancer. Thus, the follow-up surveillance schemes for BRCA1/2 mutation carriers have to focus, in addition to the standard recommendations, on early detection of pancreatic cancer.

Deciphering the precise functional role of genes, involved in the development of pancreatic cancer, may open new and exciting targets for chemotherapy. The recognition that BRCA1/2 and PARP proteins combine forces in maintaining genomic stability and DNA damage repair, as well as transcriptional regulation and apoptosis, has prompted the clinical development of PARP inhibitors. It has been recently shown that PARP inhibitors are selectively toxic to human cancer cell lines with BRCA1/2 mutations. Furthermore, these agents may have a therapeutic potential in tumors with defects in homologous recombinant DNA repair (HRR) system (Drew et al., 2010). Clinical trials of PARP inhibitors, especially with olaparib, in BRCA1/2 mutated cancer patients confirm their potential therapeutic effect. Further studies are required to address the many questions regarding safety and efficacy in the clinical setting (Fong et al., 2009).

6. References

Aguirre AJ, Brennan C, Bailey G Sinha R, Feng B, Leo C, Zhang Y, Zhang J, Gans JD, Bardeesy N, Cauwels C, Cordon-Cardo C, Redston MS, DePinho RA, Chin L (2004) High-resolution characterization of the pancreatic adenocarcinoma genome. Proc Natl Acad Sci USA. 101:9067–9072.

Al-Sukhni W, Rothenmund H, Eppel Borgida A, Zogopoulos G, O'Shea A-M, Pollett A, Gallinger S (2009) Germline BRCA1 mutations predispose to pancreatic adenocarcinoma. Hum Genet. 124:271-278.

Anzick SL, Kononen J, Walker RL, Azorsa DO, Tanner MM, Guan X-Y, Sauter G, Kallioniemi O-P, Trent JM, Meltzer PS (1997) AIB1, a steroid receptor coactivator amplified in breast and ovarian cancer. Science 277:965-968.

Banke MG, Mulvihill JJ, Aston CE (2000) Inheritance of pancreatic cancer in pancreatic cancer-prone families. Med Clin North Am. 84:677-690, x-xi.

Bryant HE, Schultz N, Thomas HD, Parker KM, Flower D, Lopez E, Kyle S, Meuth M, Curtin NJ, Helleday T (2005) Specific killing of BRCA2-deficient tumours with inhibitors of poly(ADP-ribose) polymerase. Nature 434:913-917.

Brentnall TA, Bronner MP, Byrd DR, Haggitt RC, Kimmey MB (1999) Early diagnosis and treatment of pancreatic dysplasia in patients with a family history of pancreatic cancer. Ann Intern Med. 131:247-255.

Caldas C, Hahn SA, da Costa LT, Redston MS, Schutte M, Seymour AB, Weinstein CL, Hruban RH, Yeo CJ, Kern SE (1994) Frequent somatic mutations and homozygous deletions of the p16 (MTS1) gene in pancreatic adenocarcinoma. Nat Genet. 8:27-32.

Caldas C, Kern SE (1995). K-ras mutation and pancreatic adenocarcinoma. Int J Pancreatol. 18:1-6.

Casadei S, Norquist BM, Walsh T, Stray SM, Mandell JB, Lee MK, Stamatoyannopoulos JA, King MC (2011) Contribution to Familial Breast Cancer of Inherited Mutations in the BRCA2-interacting Protein PALB2. Cancer Res. 71:2222-2229.

Calhoun ES, Jones JB, Ashfaq R Adsay V, Baker SJ, Valentine V, Hempen PM, Hilgers W, Yeo CJ, Hruban RH, Kern SE (2003) BRAF and FBXW7 (CDC4, FBW7, AGO, SEL10) mutations in distinct subsets of pancreatic cancer: potential therapeutic targets. Am J Pathol. 163:1255-1260.

Casey G, Yamanaka Y, Freiss H, Kobrin MS, Lopez ME, Buchler M, Beger HG, Korc M (1993) p53 mutations are common in pancreatic cancer and are absent in chronic pancreatitis. Cancer Lett. 69:151-160.

Cheng JQ, Ruggeri B, Klein WM, Sonoda G, Altomare DA, Watson DK, Testa JR (1996) Amplification of AKT2 in human pancreatic cells and inhibition of AKT2 expression and tumorigenicity by antisense RNA. Proc Natl Acad Sci U S A. 93:3636-3641.

Costello E, Neoptolemos JP (2011) New insights for early intervention and detection. Nat Rev Gastroenterol Hepatol. 8:71-73.

Dagan E (2008) Predominant Ashkenazi BRCA1/2 mutations in families with pancreatic cancer. Genet Test. 12:267-271.

Dagan E, Epelbaum R, Gershoni-Baruch R (2010) BRCA1/2 mutations in pancreatic cancer patients and their clinical characteristics. Am Soc Human Genet. 60th Annual Meeting. WA DC. Poster presentation No. 595.

Davies H, Bignell GR, Cox C, Stephens P, Edkins S, Clegg S, Teague J, Woffendin H, Garnett MJ, Bottomley W, Davis N, Dicks E, Ewing R, Floyd Y, Gray K, Hall S, Hawes R, Hughes J, Kosmidou V, Menzies A, Mould C, Parker A, Stevens C, Watt S, Hooper S, Wilson R, Jayatilake H, Gusterson BA, Cooper C, Shipley J, Hargrave D, Pritchard-Jones K, Maitland N, Chenevix-Trench G, Riggins GJ, Bigner DD, Palmieri G, Cossu A, Flanagan A, Nicholson A, Ho JW, Leung SY, Yuen ST, Weber BL, Seigler HF, Darrow TL, Paterson H, Marais R, Marshall CJ, Wooster R, Stratton MR, Futreal PA (2002) Mutations of the BRAF gene in human cancer. Nature 417:949-954.

Drew Y, Mulligan EA, Vong WT, Thomas HD, Kahn S, Kyle S, Mukhopadhyay A, Los G, Hostomsky Z, Plummer ER, Edmondson RJ, Curtin NJ (2011) Therapeutic potential of poly(ADP-ribose) polymerase inhibitor AG014699 in human cancers with mutated or methylated BRCA1 or BRCA2. J Natl Cancer Inst. 103:334-346.

Eberle MA, Pfützer R, Pogue-Geile KL, Bronner MP, Crispin D, Kimmey MB, Duerr RH, Kruglyak L, Whitcomb DC, Brentnall TA (2002) A new susceptibility locus for autosomal dominant pancreatic cancer maps to chromosome 4q32-34. Am J Hum Genet. 70:1044-1048.

Feldmann G, Beaty R, Hruban RH, Maitra A (2007). Molecular genetics of pancreatic intraepithelial neoplasia. J Hepatobiliary Pancreat Surg. 14:224-32.

Ferlay J, Shin HR, Bray F, Forman D, Mathers C, Parkin DM: GLOBOCAN 2008, Cancer Incidence and Mortality Worldwide: IARC CancerBase No. 10. Lyon, International Agency for Research on Cancer, 2010. http://globocan.iarc.fr.

Ferlay J, Shin HR, Bray F, Forman D, Mathers C, Parkin DM (2010) Estimates of worldwide burden of cancer in 2008: GLOBOCAN 2008. Int J Cancer 127:2893-2917.

Ferrone CR, Levine DA, Tang LH, Allen PJ, Jarnagin W, Brennan MF, Offit K, Robson ME (2009) BRCA germline mutations in Jewish patients with pancreatic adenocarcinoma. J Clin Oncol. 20:433-438.

Fishel R, Ewel A, Lee S, Lescoe MK, Griffith J (1994) Binding of mismatched microsatellite DNA sequences by the human MSH2 protein. Science 266:1403-1405.

Fong PC, Boss DS, Yap TA, Tutt A, Wu P, Mergui-Roelvink M, Mortimer P, Swaisland H, Lau A, O'Connor MJ, Ashworth A, Carmichael J, Kaye SB, Schellens JHM, de Bono JS (2009) Inhibition of poly(ADP-ribose) polymerase in tumors from BRCA mutation carriers. N Engl J Med. 361:123–134.

Goggins M, Canto M, Hruban R (2000) Can we screen high-risk individuals to detect early pancreatic carcinoma? J Surg Oncol. 74:243-248.

Goldstein AM, Fraser MC, Struewing JP, Hussussian CJ, Ranade K, Zametkin DP, Fontaine LS, Organic SM, Dracopoli NC, Clark WH Jr, Tucker MA (1995) Increased risk of pancreatic cancer in melanoma-prone kindreds with p16INK4 mutations. N Engl J Med. 333:970-974.

Hahn SA, Schutte M, Hoque TMS, Moskaluk CA, da Costa LT, Rozenblum E, Weinstein CL, Fischer A, Yeo CJ, Hruban RH, Kern SE (1996) DPC4, a candidate tumor suppressor gene at human chromosome 18q21.1. Science 271:350-354.

Helleday T, Bryant HE, Schultz N (2005) Poly(ADP-ribose) polymerase (PARP-1) in homologous recombination and as a target for cancer therapy. Cell Cycle 4:1176-1178.

Hingorani SR, Wang L, Multani AS, Combs C, Deramaudt TB, Hruban RH, Rustgi AK, Chang S, Tuveson DA (2005) Trp53R172H and KrasG12D cooperate to promote chromosomal instability and widely metastatic pancreatic ductal adenocarcinoma in mice. Cancer Cell 7:469–483.

Hofstatter EW, Domchek SM, Miron A, Garber J, Wang M, Componeschi K, Boghossian L, Miron PL, Nathanson KL, Tung N (2011) PALB2 mutations in familial breast and pancreatic cancer. Fam Cancer 10:225-231.

Hruban RH, Petersen GM, Ha PK, Kern SE (1998) Genetics of pancreatic cancer. From genes to families. Surg Oncol Clin N Am. 7:1-23.

Hruban RH, Canto MI, Yeo CJ (2001) Prevention of pancreatic cancer and strategies for management of familial pancreatic cancer. Dig Dis. 19:76-84.

Hustinx SR, Leoni LM, Yeo CJ, Brown PN, Goggins M, Kern SE, Hruban RH, Maitra A (2005) Concordant loss of MTAP and p16/CDKN2A expression in pancreatic intraepithelial neoplasia: evidence of homozygous deletion in a noninvasive precursor lesion. Mod Pathol. 18:959–63.

Jemal A, Siegel R, Ward E, Murray T, Xu J, Smigal C, Thun MJ (2006) Cancer statistics, 2006. CA Cancer J Clin. 56:106-130.

Jemal A, Siegel R, Ward E, Hao Y, Xu J, Thun MJ (2009) Cancer statistics, 2009. CA Cancer J Clin. 59:225-249.

Jemal A, Bray F, Center MM, Ferlay J, Ward E, Forman D (2011) Global Cancer Statistics. CA Cancer J Clin. 2011;61:69–90

Jones S, Hruban RH, Kamiyama M, Borges M, Zhang X, Parsons DW, Lin JC-H, Palmisano E, Brune K, Jaffee EM, Iacobuzio-Donahue CA, Maitra A, Parmigiani G, Kern SE, Velculescu VE, Kinzler KW, Vogelstein B, Eshleman JR, Goggins M, Klein AP (2009) Exomic sequencing identifies PALB2 as a pancreatic cancer susceptibility gene. Science 324: 217.

Kinzler KW, Vogelstein B (1997) Gatekeepers and caretakers. Nature 386:761-763.

Klein AP, Borges M, Griffith M, Brune K, Hong SM, Omura N, Hruban RH, Goggins M (2009) Absence of deleterious palladin mutations in patients with familial pancreatic cancer. Cancer Epidemiol Biomarkers Prev. 18:1328-1330.

Li FP, Fraumeni JR, Jr Mulvihill JJ, Blattner WA, Dreyfus MG, Tucker MA, Miller RW (1988) A cancer family syndrome in twenty-four kindreds. Cancer Res. 48:5358-5362.

Liu Q, Yan Y-X, McClure M, Nakagawa H, Fujimura F, Rustgi AK (1995) MTS-1 (CDKN2) tumor suppressor gene deletions are a frequent event in esophagus squamous cancer and pancreatic adenocarcinoma cell lines. Oncogene 10: 619-622.

Low SK, Kuchiba A, Zembutsu H, Saito A, Takahashi A, Kubo M, Daigo Y, Kamatani N, Chiku S, Totsuka H, Ohnami S, Hirose H, Shimada K, Okusaka T, Yoshida T, Nakamura Y, Sakamoto H (2010) Genome-wide association study of pancreatic cancer in Japanese population. PLoS ONE 5:e11824.

Lynch HT, Voorhees GJ, Lanspa SJ, McGreevy PS, Lynch JF (1985) Pancreatic carcinoma and hereditary nonpolyposis colorectal cancer: a family study. Brit J Cancer 52:271-273.

Lynch HT, Fitzsimmons ML, Smyrk TC, Lanspa SJ, Watson P, McClellan J, Lynch JF (1990) Familial pancreatic cancer: clinicopathologic study of 18 nuclear families. Am J Gastroenterol. 85:54-60.

Lynch HT, Smyrk T, Kern SE, Hruban RH, Lightdale CJ, Lemon SJ, Lynch JF, Fusaro LR, Fusaro RM, Ghadirian P (1996) Familial pancreatic cancer: a review. Semin Oncol. 23:251-275.

Lynch HT, Brand RE, Hogg D, Deters CA, Fusaro RM, Lynch JF, Liu L, Knezetic J, Lassam NJ, Goggins M, Kern S (2002) Phenotypic variation in eight extended CDKN2A germline mutation familial atypical multiple mole melanoma-pancreatic carcinoma-prone families: the familial atypical mole melanoma-pancreatic carcinoma syndrome. Cancer 94:84-96.

Lynch HT, Lynch PM, Lanspa SJ, Snyder CL, Lynch JF, Boland CR (2009) Review of the Lynch syndrome: history, molecular genetics, screening, differential diagnosis, and medicolegal ramifications. Clin Genet. 76:1-18.

Maitra A, Adsay NV, Argani P, Iacobuzio-Donahue C, De Marzo A, Cameron JL, Yeo CJ, Hruban RH (2003) Multicomponent analysis of the pancreatic adenocarcinoma progression model using a pancreatic intraepithelial neoplasia tissue microarray. Mod Pathol. 16:902–912.

Maitra A, Kern SE, Hruban RH (2006) Molecular pathogenesis of pancreatic cancer. Best Pract Res Clin Gastroenterol. 20:211-226.

McWilliams RR, Rabe KG, Olswold C, De Andrade M, Petersen GM (2005) Risk of malignancy in first-degree relatives of patients with pancreatic carcinoma. Cancer 104:388-394.

McWilliams RR, Wieben ED, Rabe KG, Pedersen KS, Wu Y, Sicotte H, Petersen GM (2010). Prevalence of CDKN2A mutations in pancreatic cancer patients: implications for genetic counseling. Eur J Hum Genet. Dec 8.

Meckler KA, Brentnall TA, Haggitt RC, Crispin D, Byrd DR, Kimmey MB, Bronner MP (2001) Familial fibrocystic pancreatic atrophy with endocrine cell hyperplasia and pancreatic carcinoma. Am J Surg Pathol. 25:1047-1053.

Miyaki M, Konishi M, Tanaka K, Kikuchi-Yanoshita R, Muraoka M, Yasuno M, Igari T, Koike M, Chiba M, Mori T (1997) Germline mutation of MSH6 as the cause of hereditary nonpolyposis colorectal cancer. Nature Genet. 17:271-272.

Murphy KM, Brune KA, Griffin C, Sollenberger JE, Petersen GM, Bansal R, Hruban RH, Kern SE (2002) Evaluation of candidate genes MAP2K4, MADH4, ACVR1B, and BRCA2 in familial pancreatic cancer: deleterious BRCA2 mutations in 17%. Cancer Res. 62: 3789-3793.

Ozcelik H, Schmocker B, Di Nicola N, Shi X-H, Langer B, Moore M, Taylor BR, Narod SA, Darlington G, Andrulis IL, Gallinger S, Redston M (1997) Germline BRCA2 6174delT mutations in Ashkenazi Jewish pancreatic cancer patients. Nature Genet. 16: 17-18.

Petersen GM et al. (2010) A genome-wide association study identifies pancreatic cancer susceptibility loci on chromosomes 13q22.1, 1q32.1 and 5p15.33. Nature Genet. 42:224–228.

Pogue-Geile KL, Chen R, Bronner MP, Crnogorac-Jurcevic T, Moyes KW, Dowen S, Otey CA, Crispin DA, George RD, Whitcomb DC, Brentnall TA (2006) Palladin mutation causes familial pancreatic cancer and suggests a new cancer mechanism. PLoS Med. 3: e516.

Rahman N, Seal S, Thompson D, Kelly P, Renwick A, Elliott A, Reid S, Spanova K, Barfoot R, Chagtai T, Jayatilake H, McGuffog L, Hanks S, Evans DG, Eccles D, The Breast Cancer Susceptibility Collaboration (UK), Easton DF, Stratton MR (2007) PALB2, which encodes a BRCA2-interacting protein, is a breast cancer susceptibility gene. Nature Genet. 39: 165-167.

Redston MS, Caldas C, Seymour AB Hruban RH, da Costa L, Yeo CJ, Kern SE (1994) p53 mutations in pancreatic carcinoma and evidence of common involvement of homocopolymer tracts in DNA microdeletions. Cancer Res. 54:3025–3033.

Reid S, Schindler D, Hanenberg H, Barker K, Hanks S, Kalb R, Neveling K, Kelly P, Seal S, Freund M, Wurm M, Batish SD, Lach FP, Yetgin S, Neitzel H, Ariffin H, Tischkowitz M, Mathew CG, Auerbach AD, Rahman N (2007) Biallelic mutations in PALB2 cause Fanconi anemia subtype FA-N and predispose to childhood cancer. Nature Genet. 39: 162-164.

Risch HA, McLaughlin JR, Cole DE, Rosen B, Bradley L, Kwan E, Jack E, Vesprini DJ, Kuperstein G, Abrahamson JL., Fan I, Wong B, Narod SA (2001) Prevalence and penetrance of germline BRCA1 and BRCA2 mutations in a population series of 649 women with ovarian cancer. Am J Hum Genet. 68:700-710.

Robertson KD, Jones PA (1999) Tissue-specific alternative splicing in the human INK4a/ARF cell cycle regulatory locus. Oncogene 18:3810-3820.

Ryu JK, Hong SM, Karikari CA, Hruban RH, Goggins MG, Maitra A (2010) Aberrant MicroRNA-155 expression is an early event in the multistep progression of pancreatic adenocarcinoma. Pancreatology 10:66-73.

Schlacher K, Christ N, Siaud N, Egashira A, Wu H, Jasin M (2011) Double-Strand Break Repair-Independent Role for BRCA2 in Blocking Stalled Replication Fork Degradation by MRE11. Cell 145:529-542.

Schutte M, Hruban RH, Geradts J, Maynard R, Hilgers W, Rabindran SK, Moskaluk CA, Hahn SA, Schwarte-Waldhoff I, Schmiegel W, Baylin SB, Kern SE, Herman JG (1997) Abrogation of theRb/p16 tumor-suppressive pathway in virtually all pancreatic carcinomas. Cancer Res. 57:3126–3130.

Slater EP, Langer P, Fendrich V, Habbe N, Chaloupka B, Matthäi E, Sina M, Hahn SA, Bartsch DK (2010) Prevalence of BRCA2 and CDKN2a mutations in German familial pancreatic cancer families. Fam Cancer 9:335-343.

Teng DH-F, Bogden R, Mitchell J, Baumgard M, Bell R, Berry S, David T, Ha PC, Kehrer R, Jammulapati S, Chen Q, Offit K, Skolnick MH, Tavtigian SV, Jhanwar S, Swedlund B, Wong AKC, Kamb A (1996) Low incidence of BRCA2 mutations in breast carcinoma and other cancers. Nature Genet. 13: 241-244.

Thompson D, Easton D, Breast Cancer Linkage Consortium (2001) Variation in cancer risks, by mutation position, in BRCA2 mutation carriers. Am J Hum Genet. 68:410-419.

Thorlacius S, Olafsdottir G, Tryggvadottir L, Neuhausen S, Jonasson JG, Tavtigian SV, Tulinius H, Ogmundsdottir HM, Eyfjord JE (1996) A single BRCA2 mutation in male and female breast cancer families from Iceland with varied cancer phenotypes. Nature Genet. 13:117-122.

Ueki T, Toyota M, Sohn T, Yeo CJ, Issa JP, Hruban RH, Goggins M (2000) Hypermethylation of multiple genes in pancreatic adenocarcinoma. Cancer Res. 60:1835–1839.

Wang B, Hurov K, Hofmann K, Elledge SJ (2009) NBA1, a new player in the Brca1 A complex, is required for DNA damage resistance and checkpoint control. Genes Dev. 23:729-739.

Weil MK, Chen AP (2011) PARP inhibitor treatment in ovarian and breast cancer. Curr Probl Cancer 35:7-50.

Whelan AJ, Bartsch D, Goodfellow PJ (1995) Brief report: a familial syndrome of pancreatic cancer and melanoma with a mutation in the CDKN2 tumor-suppressor gene. New Eng J Med. 333: 975-977.

Wu J, Lu LY, Yu X (2010) The role of BRCA1 in DNA damage response. Protein Cell 1:117-123.

Xia B, Sheng Q, Nakanishi K, Ohashi A, Wu J, Christ N, Liu X, Jasin M, Couch FJ, Livingston DM (2006) Control of BRCA2 cellular and clinical functions by a nuclear partner, PALB2. Molec Cell 22: 719-729.

Xia B, Dorsman JC, Ameziane N, de Vries Y, Rooimans MA, Sheng Q, Pals G, Errami A, Gluckman E, Llera J, Wang W, Livingston DM, Joenje H, de Winter J P (2007)

Fanconi anemia is associated with a defect in the BRCA2 partner PALB2. Nature Genet. 39: 159-161.

Zogopoulous G, Rothenmund H, Eppel A, Ash C, Akbari MR, Hedley D, Narod SA, Gallinger S (2007) The P239S palladin variant does not account for a significant fraction of hereditary or early onset pancreatic cancer. Hum Genet. 121: 635-637.

2

Systems and Network-Centric Understanding of Pancreatic Ductal Adenocarcinoma Signalling

Irfana Muqbil, Ramzi M. Mohammad,
Fazlul H. Sarkar and Asfar S. Azmi
Wayne State University,
USA

1. Introduction

Pancreatic ductal adenocarcinoma (PDAC) is a deadly disease that is intractable to currently available treatment modalities (Vincent et al. 2011). Failure of standard chemo-, radio- and neoadjuvant single pathway targeted therapies indicate that before newer treatment regimens are designed, one has to re-visit the basic understanding of the origins and complexity of PDAC. As such, PDAC is now appreciated to have not only a highly heterogeneous pathology but is also a disease characterized by dysregulation of multiple pathways governing fundamental cell processes (Kim and Simeone 2011). Such complexity has been suggested to be governed by molecular networks that execute metabolic or cytoskeletal processes, or their regulation by complex signal transduction originating from diverse genetic mutations (Figure 1). A major challenge, therefore, is to understand how to develop actionable modulation of this multivariate dysregulation, with respect to both how it arises from diverse genetic mutations and to how it may be ameliorated by prospective treatments in PDAC. Lack of understanding in both these areas is certainly a major underlying reason for failure of most of the available and clinically used drugs (Stathis and Moore 2010). The pharmaceutical industry handpicked drugs have been generally based on their specificity towards a particular protein and the subsequent targeted pathway (K-Ras, PI3K, MEK, EGFR, p53 etc) without considering the effect of modulating secondary and interacting pathways (Almhanna and Philip 2011; Philip 2011). However, as results from integrated network modeling and systems biology studies indicate, targeting one protein is not straightforward as each protein in a cellular system works in a complex interacting network comprised of a myriad interconnected pathways (Wist et al. 2009a). Silencing one protein/pathway can have multiple effects on different secondary pathways leading to secondary effects. For example, activation of salvage pathways (commonly observed in PDAC) can result in diminished drug response or in some cases acquired resistance. Therefore, in order to decode this complexity and to understand both the PDAC disease and identify drug targets, it requires a departure from a protein-centric to a more advanced network-centric view. This chapter deals with recent advancements on deciphering PDAC disease networks and drug response networks based on integrated systems and network biology-driven science. It is believed that such integrated and holistic approach will help in not only delineating the mechanism of resistance of this complex disease, it will also aid in the future design of targeted drug combinations that will improve the dismal cure rate.

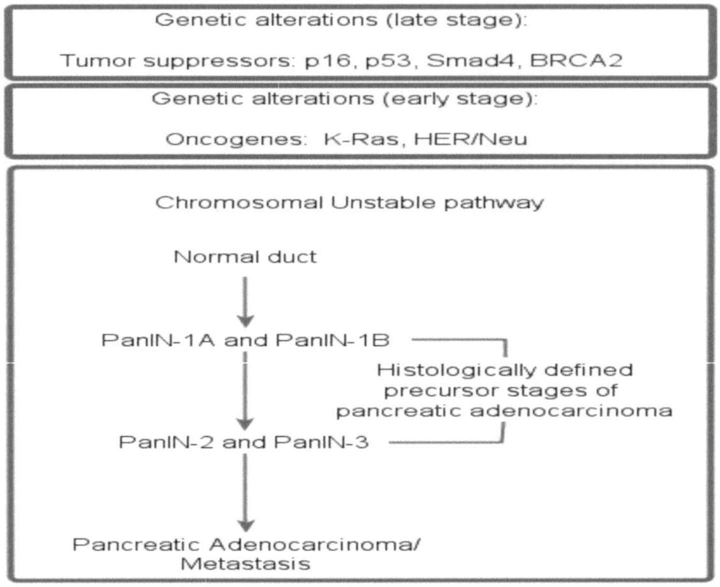

Fig. 1. Genetic alterations in PDAC are categorized into early state (oncogenes, K-Ras, Her2/Neu); Late Stage (tumor suppressors, p16, Smad4, BRCA2) and chromosomal instability pathways that accelerate progression from PanIN-1A lesions to metastatic PDAC.

2. Complex PDAC genetic network

PDAC is highly complex malignancy with myriad set of de-regulated mechanisms involved and affecting the tissue at different stages of the disease. Detailed molecular mechanisms of initiation, development and progression of PDAC have been thoroughly studied since the basic principles of the disease were revealed in the 1970s (Pour et al. 2003; Morosco et al. 1981; Morosco and Goeringer 1980). The most acceptable model is the classical one that describes morphological as well as molecular transformation from precursor lesions into invasive carcinoma (Hruban et al. 2000a; Hruban et al. 2000b). While the standard nomenclature and diagnostic criteria for classification of PDAC has primarily been based on grades of pancreatic intraepithelial neoplasia (PanIN) (Hruban et al. 2001), cumulatively it has been accepted that PDAC is a genetically and epigenetically complex disease that arises through a combination of events. It is increasingly being accepted that these complexities cannot be fully understood by traditional molecular biology techniques and integrated approaches may play pivotal role in the better understanding of PDAC as are discussed below.

2.1 Interaction of oncogenes and tumor suppressor genes in PDAC

PDAC origin and progression is broadly classified to be result of three major events (a) early stage genetic alterations in the proto-oncogenes mainly K-ras and Her-2/Neu; (b) late stage alterations in tumor suppressor genes such as p53, p16, Smad4 and BRCA2 and (c) chromosomal instability/precursor lesion in the normal duct (i.e. formation of PanIN-1a and PanIN-1B to Pan-IN-2 and Pan-IN3 (summarized in Figure 1).

These early and late genetic alterations have fundamental roles affecting key guardians of cellular signaling, which induces instability of entire molecular systems such as cell growth, division, apoptosis and migration. Mutation in proto-oncogenes gives rise to oncogenes that are often present in PDAC. These mutations cause the protein products of oncogenes to be permanently activated, resulting in uncontrolled cell proliferation. Oncogenic mutations exhibit a dominant characteristic and deficiency of one allele (i.e. heterozygous mutation) is sufficient for a lethal outcome. There are several key proto-oncogenes involved in PDAC, including KRAS, Her2/Neu, CTNNB1 (β-catenin), PIK3CA or AKT1. The most common oncogenic mutation types are point mutations, deletions, gene amplifications, and gene re-arrangements.

On the other hand, tumor suppressor genes code for proteins that act against cell proliferation. As a result of late event genetic alterations, their normal function may be reduced or even completely eliminated. Mutations in tumor suppressor genes have recessive characteristics and hence, the cell looses its function only when both alleles are affected. Commonly, described as a double hit model, one allele is initially mutated while the other is subsequently mutated or lost completely (Serra et al. 1997). In addition, there are numerous epigenetic controls of tumor suppressors that involve deactivation by hypermethylation (Herman et al. 1996). In PDAC, the frequently affected tumor suppressors include the guardian regulator TP53 (Barton et al. 1991), APC (Horii et al. 1992); SMAD4 (Bartsch et al. 1999) and TP16 (Caldas et al. 1994).

2.1.1 Complex de-regulatory signaling mechanisms in PDAC

Intense research over the last three decades have revealed that PDAC has a highly intricate web of de-regulatory signaling. In pancreatic duct cells, molecular biologist have identified some of the core signaling pathways that are aberrantly expressed that consequently leads to development of PDAC. Major cell surface receptor de-regulatory mechanisms include the c-MET/HGF (hepatocyte growth factor) signaling pathway which is a key factor in early progression of PDAC. This pathway is responsible for invasive growth of PDAC through activation of key oncogenes, angiogenesis and scattering (cell dissociation and metastasis). c-MET is a proto-oncogene that encodes an HGF receptor that has a primary function in embryonic development and wound healing (Chmielowiec et al. 2007). Even though c-MET mRNA is present at very small amounts in normal human exocrine pancreas, it is upregulated in a majority of PDAC. Interestingly overexpression of c-MET has been observed in regenerative tissue affected by acute pancreatitis (Otte et al. 2000), and has been linked to early events in PDAC carcinogenesis. HGF is a primary ligand of c-MET. Upon c-MET/HGF interaction, several different signaling pathways are activated, including the Ras, phosphoinositide 3-kinase (PI3K), JAK signal transducer and activator of transcription (STAT) and β-catenin (Wnt) pathways.

The second major cell surface signaling found altered in PDAC is the Ras/Raf/MAPK pathway. The Ras/Raf/mitogen-activated protein kinase (MAPK) pathway is one of the most elaborately studied signaling pathways in PDAC and other cancers (Molina and Adjei 2006). The role of Ras/Raf/MAPK signaling is critical for many carcinogeneic processes, including cell growth, division, cell differentiation, invasion and migration, wound healing repair, and angiogenic processes. The central regulator of this multivariate signal transduction from extracellular to intracellular environment is the Ras protein, which is localized at the inner side of the cellular membrane. Under normal physiological conditions, the hydrophobic Ras protein is in its inactive GDP-bound form. In the event of an extracellular signal coming through growth factor receptors, their is removal of GDP from Ras protein and its subsequent activation upon binding to GTP. Activated Ras complex triggers kinase activity of Raf kinase, which ultimately results in activation of an MAPK. MAPK kinase (MAPKK) in turn is an important regulator of DNA transcription and mRNA translation. Mutations that affect any of the Ras/Raf/MAPK members produce an increase in tumorigenicity through hyper-activation of DNA machinery and mRNA translation. Besides Raf and MAPK, there are other downstream effectors of Ras protein, including PI3K, thus providing crosstalk between multiple pathways.

Aside from Ras pathway, the PTEN/PI3K/AKT signaling axis is found altered in PDAC. This pathway is fundamentally based on regulated activation of AKT through its localization at the cell membrane (Carnero et al. 2008). PI3K and PTEN phosphatases are two important protein families involved in the membrane localization of AKT. PI3K phosphorylates certain membrane-bound lipids known as phosphoinositides producing three different phosphatidylinositol 3-phosphate (PIP), phosphatidylinositol (3,4)-bisphosphate (PIP_2), and phosphatidylinositol (3,4,5)-trisphosphate (PIP_3). The phosphorylated forms, PIP_3 and, to a lesser extent, PIP_2, attract important protein kinases to the cell membrane. The most prominent is AKT, a family of serine/threonine protein kinases that trigger a number of key cellular processes, including glucose metabolism, cell proliferation, and apoptosis, transcription, and cell migration (Maitra and Hruban 2005). AKT activity is strongly dependent on its proper localization on the cell membrane. The positioning of AKT at the membrane is achieved through its strong binding to PIP_3. In pancreatic carcinogenesis, AKT1 acts as an oncogene that upholds cell survival by overcoming cell cycle arrest, blocking apoptosis, and promoting angiogenesis. PTEN is a phosphatase that acts in opposition to PI3K. It has tumor suppression ability by converting PIP_3 back to PIP_2 and to PIP, hence disrupting membrane localization and reducing activity of AKT. In most cancers, expression levels of PI3Ks and AKT are high, while PTEN is often deactivated by mutation, or deleted completely. Through its key role in pancreatic carcinogenesis, PI3K/AKT/PTEN signaling is an important target for anticancer therapy.

The JAK/STAT signaling pathway also has an important role in regulation of DNA transcription by inducing chemical signals from cytokine receptors into the cell nucleus. The signal is phosphorylation dependent prompting activation and dimerization in a family of STAT proteins. Activated STAT dimers initiate DNA transcription inside the nucleus. It is known that inhibition of JAK/STAT signaling induces apoptosis in various human cancers, and is therefore, a primary focus for potential new drug candidates (Buettner et al. 2002). A recent study has reported reduced growth of pancreatic cancer cells *in vitro* when exposed to benzyl isothiocyanate, through suppression of STAT3 signaling and subsequent induction of apoptosis. This is suggested as a possible explanation of the anti-carcinogenic effect of cruciferous vegetables (such as broccoli, cauliflower, cabbage or horseradish) that are rich in isothiocyanates.

TGF-β is a ligand that binds to type II cytokine receptor dimer, which then interacts and activates type I cytokine receptor dimer, triggering phosphorylation of receptor-regulated SMADs (R-SMADs), mainly SMAD2 and SMAD3. In the phosphorylated form, the R-

SMADs form a complex with SMAD4, which localizes it in the nucleus and where it interacts with other factors to stimulate transcription of genes that are important for cell cycle arrest and migration. SMAD4 is therefore a key mediator for TGF-β signals. Due to its frequent absence in proliferating PDAC tissue, it is also known as DPC or "deleted in pancreatic cancer" (Schutte et al. 1995). Relatively high frequency of SMAD4 mutations and loss of heterozygosity at the DPC4 locus (18q21.1) strongly suggest that the protein is a primary tumor suppressor involved in PDAC carcinogenesis process. However, it should be noted that reinstating SMAD4 expression results in tumor growth suppression only *in vivo* and not *in vitro*. It has also been found that a SMAD4-independent pathways may be responsible for tumorigenic effect of TGF-β signaling (Levy and Hill 2005).

Wnt signaling is crucial to formation and maintenance of pancreas (Dessimoz and Grapin-Botton 2006; Dessimoz et al. 2005). During PDAC development, hyper-activation of Wnt triggers transcription of a number of genes that have a direct impact on cell proliferation, differentiation and migration (Cano et al. 2008; Rulifson et al. 2007). Activation of Wnt signaling is through interaction of a family of membrane-bound receptors known as Frizzleds with Wnt ligands. Once activated, the downstream signals may proceed through independent pathways. In a canonical pathway, signal transduction is mediated through stabilization and translocation of β-catenin from the cytosol into the nucleus followed by its interaction with T-cell factor that in turn activates transcription of target genes. The localization of high expression levels of β-catenin in the nucleus has been experimentally confirmed in various high grade PanIN lesions, as well as in advanced PDAC (Al-Aynati et al. 2004). In non-canonical, β-catenin-independent pathways, other signaling mediators are involved, that block the β-catenin assisted transcription. The nuclear localization of β-catenin and high expression levels of WNT5a, a gene involved in non-canonical Wnt pathways, suggests involvement of both pathways in PDAC progression.

The cell cycle control genes have profound importance in PDAC and CDKN2A is one of key factors in its negative control. The CDKN2A has two promoters and alternative splicing sites that give rise to two alternative protein products: cyclin-dependent kinase inhibitor p16INK4a and p53-activator p14ARF. Although both proteins are active in negative control of the cell cycle, only the function of p16INK4a is frequently lost in PDAC due to point mutations, deletions or hypermethylation . p16INK4a protein (also known as p16) inhibits key elements of cell cycle progression at the G1 checkpoint. p16 inactivation is an early event in pancreatic carcinogenesis, and low levels of p16 expression are associated with larger tumors, risk of early metastases and poor survival. The network interactions of de-regulatory signaling pathways in PDAC are depicted in Figure 2.

In summary, the above comprehensive set of studies accumulated over the years clearly show that PDAC is a highly complex disease. Traditional molecular biology focuses on studying these alterations in a single protein-centric manner honing on individual pathways. There are unanswered questions regarding the interaction between these de-regulatory signaling mechanisms that may be related to the cause of such dismal outcomes in PDAC. This is indeed the case as pharmaceutical companies handpick drugs to target individual protein and not multiple pathways. Even if a drug blocks one signaling molecule in the tumor, another salvage pathway becomes activated leading to diminished efficacy of the drugs. Therefore, we are of the view that an integrated holistic approach is needed to to first understand the interactions between individual pathways that will aid in the design of single or combination regimens for the elimination of PDAC.

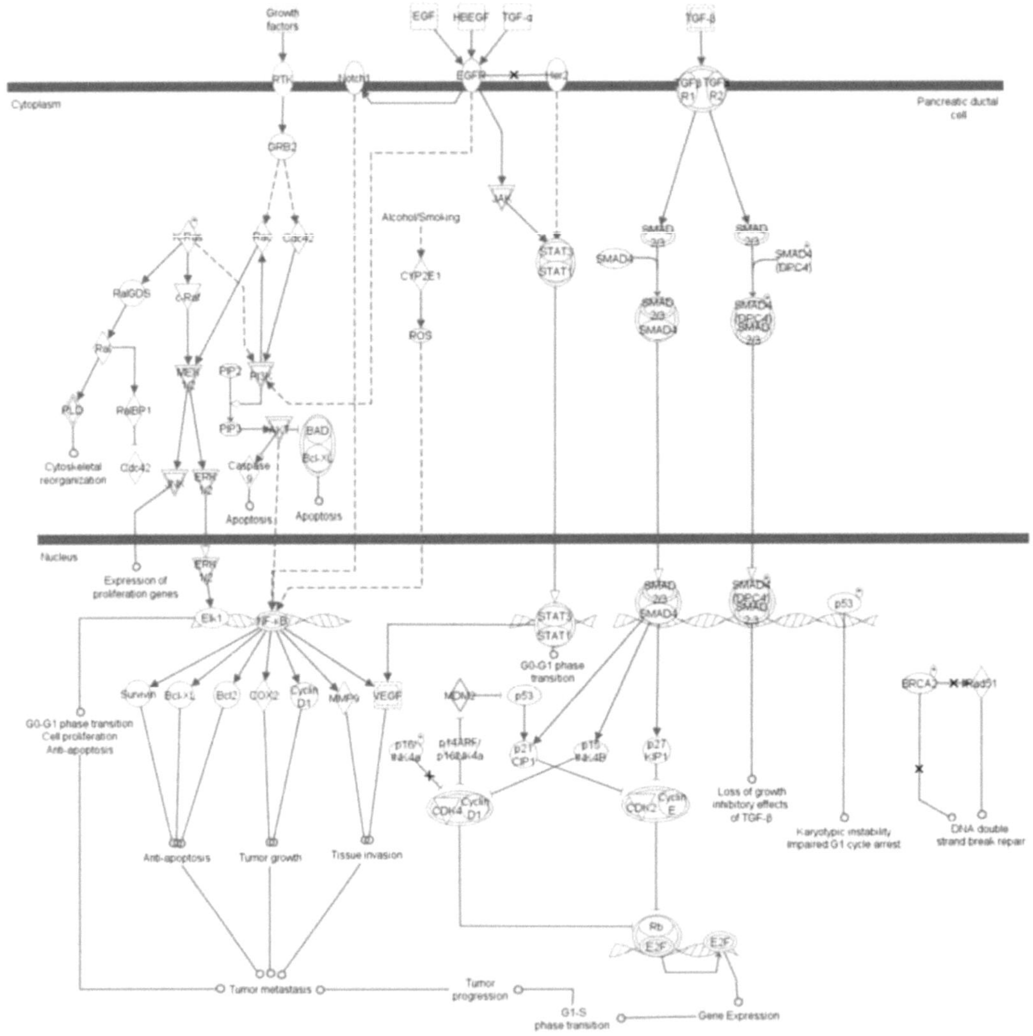

Fig. 2. Complex de-regulatory network of PDAC obtained from Ingenuity Pathway Analysis Database.

3. Systems biology and its use in understanding the complexity of PDAC

Applicability of systems biology is slowly being realized in the clinic (Faratian et al. 2009). Currently, combining information on patient history with high throughput bioinformatics such as genotyping, transcriptomics and comparative genomic hybridization, sequencing, and proteomics, followed by molecular network analysis, one can predict biomarkers and targets and that would ultimately benefit in designing personalized medicine (Figure 3 depicting integration of multiple high-throughput technologies for better approach and treatment to a disease).

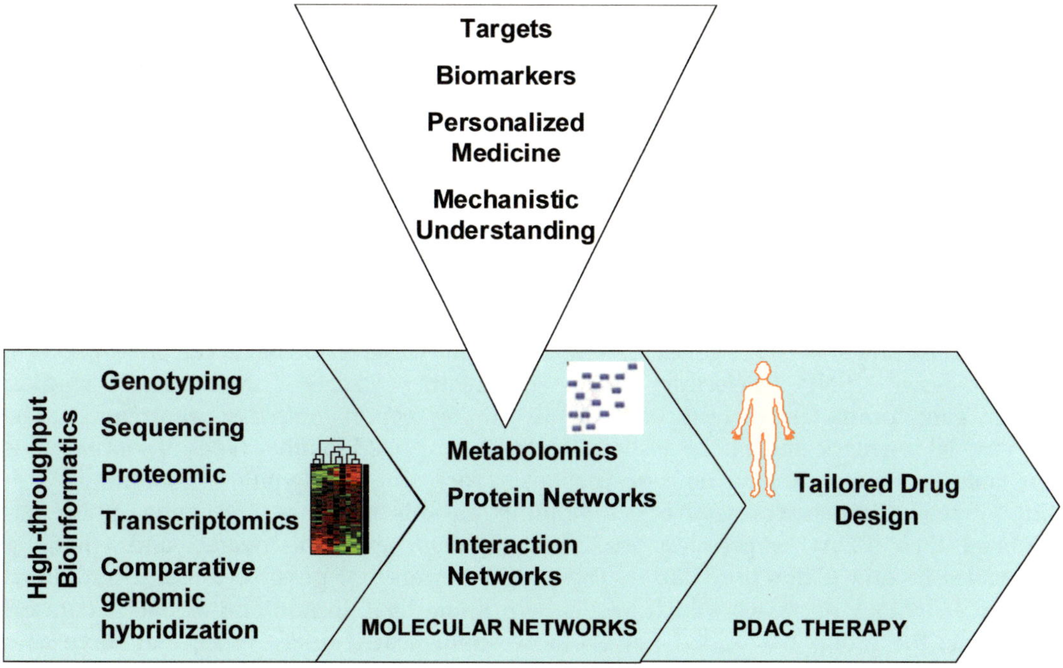

Fig. 3. Systems Biology is a potent tool for designing personalized medicine, predicting biomarkers and targets and mechanistic understanding of complex diseases.

This type of association study can be applied to both affected and healthy cohorts, or in relation to particular phenotypes, such as disease susceptibility (for example, diabetes) (Saxena et al. 2007), or to study individual responses to drugs. As a result, genetic variations have been identified through comprehensive re-sequencing studies of cancer-related mutations in colon and breast tumors, leading to the identification of around 80 DNA alterations in a typical cancer (Wood et al. 2007). This technology has been applied to understand PDAC genetics, pathway interactions and in identifying PDAC stem cells and are discussed below.

3.1 Systems understanding of PDAC expression datasets

As a proof of concept, the first study on the use of proteomic profiling was published by Lohr and group and they showed how integrated technologies could be utilized in obtaining PDAC biomarkers (Lohr et al. 2006). In this study, it was postulated that this type of proteomic approach was extremely necessary in the rationale for the design of drugs for this deadly malignancy. Later, a number of investigations have demonstrated that indeed this technology can be applied to unwind the complex web of interacting pathways in PDAC. For example, in an elegant study, Chelala and colleagues provided pancreatic expression database that was a generic model for organization, integration and mining of complex pancreatic cancer datasets (Chelala et al. 2007). The database holds 32 datasets comprising 7636 gene expression measurements extracted from 20 different published gene or protein expression studies from various PDAC types, pancreatic precursor lesions (PanINs) and chronic pancreatitis. The pancreatic data are stored in a data management system based on the BioMart technology alongside the human genome gene and protein annotations, sequence, homologue, SNP and antibody data. Interrogation of the database can be achieved through both a web-based query interface and through web services using combined criteria from pancreatic (disease stages, regulation, differential expression, expression, platform technology, publication) and/or public data (antibodies, genomic region, gene-related accessions, ontology, expression patterns, multi-species comparisons, protein data, SNPs). This database enables connections between otherwise disparate data sources and allows relatively simple navigation between all data types and annotations. The database structure and content provides a powerful and high-speed data-mining tool for cancer research. It can be used for target discovery i.e. of biomarkers from body fluids, identification and analysis of genes associated with the progression of cancer, cross-platform meta-analysis, SNP selection for pancreatic cancer association studies, cancer gene promoter analysis as well as mining cancer ontology information. The data model is generic and can be easily extended and applied to other types of cancer and is available online with no restrictions for the scientific community at http://www.pancreasexpression.org/. Building on this database, the same group has updated their PDAC expression studies combining newly discovered and emerging molecules in 2011 (Cutts et al. 2011). These studies were not possible through traditional molecular biology approach which has its own limitations. In addition to the 32 datasets discovery, the group has added newer, more sophisticated query types that serve as a prototype for possible questions of interest that might be addressed towards greater understanding of PDAC (Chelala et al. 2009).

3.1.1 Integrated systems biology in identification of PDAC biomarkers

Comprehensive progress has been made on the use of systems biology in identification of biomarkers for PDAC. In a recent study, PDAC cell line related conditioned media and pancreatic juice were both mined for identification of putative diagnostic leads (Makawita et al. 2011). The proteome of the condition media were identified using strong cation exchange chromatography, followed by LC-MS/MS on an LTQ-Orbitrap mass spectrometer from six pancreatic cancer cell lines (BxPc3, MIA-PaCa2, PANC1, CAPAN1, CFPAC1 and SU.86.86), one normal human pancreatic ductal epithelial cell line, HPDE, and two pools of six pancreatic juice samples from ductal adenocarcinoma patients. These studies identified 1261 and 2171 proteins with two or more peptides, in each of the cell lines, while an average of 521 proteins were identified in the pancreatic juice pools. In total, 3,479 non-redundant proteins were identified with high confidence, of which ~40% were extracellular or cell membrane-bound based on genome ontology classifications. Three strategies were employed for identification of candidate biomarkers (1) examination of differential protein expression between the cancer and normal cell lines using label-free protein quantification, (2) integrative analysis, focusing on the overlap of proteins between the multiple biological fluids, and (3) tissue specificity analysis through mining of publically available databases. However, further validation of these proteins is warranted, as is the investigation of the remaining group of candidate biomarkers in PDAC. In another study on PDAC, secreted serum biomarker identification the profiling pancreatic cancer-secreted proteome using 15N amino acids and serum-free media was performed (Xiao et al. 2010). In this study the effect of oxythiamine chloride on PDAC cell secreteome was studied. The authors further improved on the existing biomarker discovery technology (i.e. coupling of proteomics and in vitro labeling of proteins in cells (SILAC) to enhance the efficacy of biomarker discovery. The authors concluded that labeling protein with ^{15}N amino acids in conjunction with depleted serum allows the identification of actively secreted proteins from pancreatic cancer cells, and the rate of production of a secreted protein may be used as an independent biomarker of the presence of tumor.

3.1.2 Integrated analysis of pathways collectively targeted by co-expressed microRNAs in PDAC

Apart from investigations on signaling pathway de-regulation, multiple recent studies have found aberrant expression profiles of small non-coding RNAs (microRNAs) in PDAC. While several target genes have been experimentally identified for some microRNAs in various tumors, the global pattern of cellular functions and pathways affected by co-expressed microRNAs in PDAC remained elusive. Here too systems biology has found application in identification through computational approach and global analysis of the major biological processes and signaling pathways that are most likely to be affected collectively by co-expressed microRNAs in cancer cells. In a recent study, using five datasets of aberrantly expressed microRNAs in pancreatic and other cancers (breast cancer, colon cancer, lung cancer and lymphoma) and combinatorial target prediction algorithm miRgate and a two-step data reduction procedure Gene Ontology categories were determined (Gusev 2008; Gusev et al. 2007). These studies demonstrated biological functions, disease categories, toxicological categories and signaling pathways that are: targeted by multiple microRNAs; statistically significantly enriched with target genes; and known to be affected in PDAC. The analysis of predicted miRNA targets suggests that co-expressed miRNAs collectively provide systemic compensatory response to the abnormal phenotypic changes in cancer cells by targeting a broad range of functional categories and signaling pathways known to be affected in PDAC. The analysis revealed that E2F1 is a predicted microRNA target as well as caspase3 that were also validated experimentally as a target of multiple miRNAs in PDAC. Such a systems biology based approach provides new avenues for biological interpretation of miRNA profiling data and generation of experimentally testable hypotheses regarding collective regulatory functions of miRNA in PDAC for the design of effective therapies.

3.1.3 Proteomic profiling in identification of PDAC stems cells

PDAC tumors are heterogenous in nature and harbor many different types of cells. In recent years it has been realized that PDAC and other tumors carry a sub-population of cells with stem cell characteristics that are resistant to chemotherapeutic treatment modalities. However, this concept is still controversial since these cells have yet to be comprehensively identified and characterized. PDAC stem cells (CSCs) are such a group of cells that only constitute 0.2-0.8% of the total tumor cells but have been found to be the origin of carcinogenesis and metastasis. However, the extremely low availability of pancreatic tissue

CSCs (around 10 000 cells per xenograft tumor or patient sample) has limited the utilization of currently available molecular biology techniques. Global proteome profiling of pancreatic CSCs from xenograft tumors in mice using integrated systems biology is a promising way to unveil the molecular machinery underlying the signaling pathways in these CSCs. Using a capillary scale shotgun technique by coupling offline capillary isoelectric focusing (cIEF) with nano reversed phase liquid chromatography (RPLC) followed by spectral counting peptide quantification, Lubman and group investigated the proteomic profile of PDAC stems cells (Dai et al. 2010). In comparison with a non-tumorigenic tumor cell sample, among 1159 distinct proteins identified with FDR and less than 0.2%, 169 differentially expressed proteins are identified after multiple testing corrections where 24% of the proteins are up-regulated in the CSCs group. Ingenuity Pathway analysis of these differential expression signatures further indicated that a significant involvement of signaling pathways related to cell proliferation, inflammation, and metastasis were indentified. This was the first study to represents the proteome profiling study on PDAC stem cells from xenografted tumors in mice.

4. Systems biology can aid understanding of the drug mechanism of action in PDAC

Although partially successful in PDAC, new adjuvant targeted therapies (k-ras, EGFR, VEGF, src etc) have been met with more failure than success. The major reason for the low response is related to incomplete understanding and validation of the specific molecular targets at the gene level. The complexities of genetic and epigenetic changes in PDAC, coupled with redundancies and cross-talk in signaling pathways may explain the failure of single-pathway targeted therapies. This can be envisioned from the fact that of the 25,000 genes representing the human genome, about 1,800 are involved in the etiology of numerous diseases including cancer (Wist et al. 2009b). Currently available FDA approved drugs (~ 1200 in the market) have been designed to target approximately 400 genes (**Drugome**). However, targeting this drugome by individually analyzing each gene is an impossible task because the functional product of each gene or (Proteome) is under multiple control, including splice variants and post translational modifications, giving rise to >40,000 functionally distinct proteins. In addition, such studies, thus far have been hindered by lack of suitable rapid technology. Therefore, novel and high-throughput data acquisition technologies coupled with integrated systems network modeling are urgently required to identify target genes in a tumor-specific manner. Such technologies are crucial for identifying and understanding the mechanisms of potential target candidates in complex diseases like PDAC.

4.1 Systems pharmacology view of drug action

Most of the known targeted drugs currently being used in the clinic were initially designed to affect a single gene. Unfortunately, contrary to the original idea, even the most specific drugs eventually target more than one gene (in most cases, >10 secondary targets). The use of systems pharmacology categorizes these off-targets into two types i) off-targets (resulting in side effects [often toxic]) and ii) secondary targets resulting in partial synergy] (Figure 4) (Berger and Iyengar 2009). These secondary targets exist within a complex network which can mediate the response to the drugs leading to both therapeutic and adverse effects. Understanding these beneficial secondary targets specially observed in potent synergistic combinations will provide fundamental information for the design of the most potent drug combination for individualized/personalized treatments.

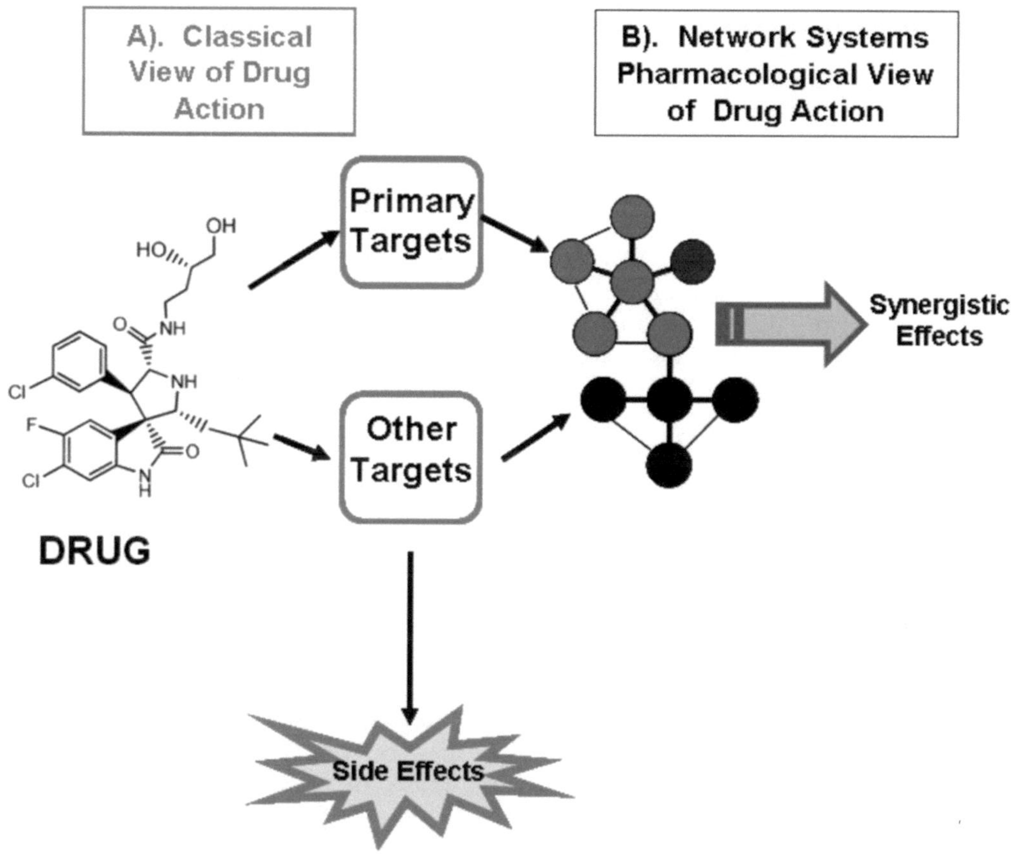

Fig. 4. Traditional vs Network view of drug mechanism of action. Network view differs in understanding the mechanism of action of drugs. Classic view pools all secondary effects as off targets that are considered to cause side effects and toxicity. Network pharmacology categorizes secondary targets into off targets and interacting secondary targets which can mediate the response to the drugs to both the therapeutic or adverse effects. Adopted from Azmi et al., 2011b

Such an understanding requires mechanistic studies in the laboratory to be coupled with robust, state of the art computational tools to obtain irrevocably strong proof for the integration of pathways involved in the observed synergy. One such approach involves the use of network modeling which provides mathematically and statistically robust information regarding the involvement of effector genes in the efficacy or synergy between two drugs. These network models can also predict key secondary targets of such interaction, thus, also providing information on novel previously unrecognized targets and pathways which could be useful for future therapeutic interventions in the treatment of different cancers where, at present, information is gravely lacking, such as in PDAC.

4.1.1 Validation of the systems approach for predicting potent drug combination in PDAC

Our laboratory has been working on a specific small molecule inhibitor of MDM2 (MI-219) and indentifying, in greater detail, its mechanism of action in PDAC (Azmi et al. 2010b). MI-219 is currently in Phase I clinical trial (Brown et al. 2009). Our initial studies were restricted to evaluating its efficacy against wt-p53 tumors. However, we have recently found that MDM2 inhibitor, when combined with chemotherapy such as oxaliplatin, synergistically enhanced apoptosis in wt-p53 cancers and most importantly, 50% of tumor bearing mice treated with this combination remained tumor free without recurrence for 120 days (Azmi et al. 2010a). We used this model to validate a systems approach in predicting potent drug combinations in PDAC and to obtain critical information into understanding the mechanism for this synergy. Therefore, our study included integrated microarray gene expression profiling (IGEMP) and pathway network modeling (PNM) (Azmi et al. 2011a). The systems analysis data for MI-219-oxaliplatin combination treated wt-p53 capan-2 cells revealed that indeed synergy is at the gene level. Principle component analysis showed that one can differentiate the gene signatures between single treatment versus combination. The emergence of certain unique synergy-related genes indicated their potential as key players supporting the overall response of MI-219-oxaliplatin in positively regulating the p53 re-activation (Azmi et al. 2010c; Azmi et al. 2011b). Presented with this vast amount of information regarding the mechanism involved in the response to MI-219-oxaliplatin synergy, we believe it validates the applicability of this technology for use in identifying the relevant pathways involved in both cure and resistance. Ultimately, results of these studies will significantly aid in the design of clinically successful drug combinations for PDAC, which will benefit the overall survival of patients.

4.1.2 Systems identification of biomarker of response with implications for PDAC therapy

Our intended goal in using IGEMP and PNM analysis was to demonstrate the synergy between MI-219-oxaliplatin at the gene level and to demonstrate the local network of p53 and crucial neighboring network that augment p53 re-activation mediated events. Systems network modeling, although a powerful technological tool has not yet been fully explored for use in PDAC (the most genetically complex cancer). We had previously identified several genes responsible for cross-talk within the local network of p53 which included NFkB, cadherin anti-tumor module, the tumor suppressor EGR1 and MDM2 negative regulator CREBBP. Our more in-depth analysis using these integrated approach, revealed the prominent role of HNF4A (hepatocyte nuclear factor 4 alpha) that modulates a totally distinct yet p53-linked set of proteins driving apoptosis (Azmi et al. 2010c). The identification of HNF4A as a key player was certainly revealing since it has not been well defined in PDAC cells used in this study (Capan-2 (wt-p53)). However, a search of the literature indicated that this gene is highly expresses in pancreatic tumors compared to their normal counterpart. HNF4A is known to interact with the p53 positive regulator CREBBP (Yoshida et al. 1997) and thus, confirmed its role in augmenting apoptotic effects in this synergic combination. Therefore, not only does systems biology provide information on the networks involved in drug efficacy, it can also provide information on biomarkers of therapeutic response that can be utilized for evaluation of drug response during actual clinical trials in PDAC patients.

5. Conclusion

PDAC is a complex disease that arises from a complex set of genetic mutations and pathway alterations. Traditional sciences have not been very successful in clearly delineating the interaction between these multiple pathways and this could be the primary reason for the observed failure of chemo- and targeted therapies. All of these genetic alterations can now be "re-discovered" using next-generation integrated systems technology. As described above, integrated sciences have revealed that these signaling pathways cross talk with one another and can regulate cell growth, proliferation, survival, angiogenesis and metastasis in PDAC. In addition, these high-throughput technologies can achieve many different goals such as cataloging the driver mutations, exploring functional role of cancer genes, proteins and interaction networks, identifying microRNAs, understanding protein–DNA interactions, and comprehensive analyses of transcriptomes and interactomes. Furthermore, these technologies can be utilized to identify, understand and differentiate sub population of CSCs in PDAC heterogeneous tumor mass. Systems biology has the power to catalog complex events leading to origin, progression, recurrence and resistance of PDAC and can greatly assist in understanding how cancer genomes operate as part of the whole biological system. Now, high-quality clinical treatment and outcomes (death or survival) data from biobanks, and extensive genetics and genomics data for some PDAC and other tumors, including breast, colorectal, and lung are available. How all these clinical and genetics data could be integrated into reverse engineering-based network modeling to approach the extremely complex genotype–phenotype map of different tumors is currently being explored. These studies will pave way for the discovery of new molecular innovations, both predictive markers and therapies, towards personalized treatment of PDAC. Therefore systems biology can aid in the overall understanding of PDAC.

6. Acknowledgment

We thank Dr. Frances W.J. Beck for critically evaluating this manuscript. All members of Dr. Fazlul H. Sarkar's team who could not be added in this chapter are acknowledged.

7. References

Al-Aynati MM, Radulovich N, Riddell RH and Tsao MS. (2004). *Clin Cancer Res,* 10, 1235-1240.

Almhanna K and Philip PA. (2011). *Curr Treat Options Oncol,* 12, 111-125.

Azmi AS, Aboukameel A, Banerjee S, Wang Z, Mohammad M, Wu J, Wang S, Yang D, Philip PA, Sarkar FH and Mohammad RM. (2010a). *Eur J Cancer.*

Azmi AS, Banerjee S, Ali S, Wang Z, Bao B, Beck FW, Maitah M, Choi M, Shields TF, Philip PA, Sarkar FH and Mohammad RM. (2011a). *Oncotarget.*

Azmi AS, Beck FW, Sarkar FH and Mohammad RM. (2011b). *Curr Pharm Des,* 17, 640-652.

Azmi AS, Philip PA, Aboukameel A, Wang Z, Banerjee S, Zafar SF, Goustin AS, Almhanna K, Yang D, Sarkar FH and Mohammad RM. (2010b). *Curr Cancer Drug Targets,* 10, 319-331.

Azmi AS, Wang Z, Philip PA, Mohammad RM and Sarkar FH. (2010c). *Mol Cancer Ther,* 9, 3137-3144.

Barton CM, Staddon SL, Hughes CM, Hall PA, O'Sullivan C, Kloppel G, Theis B, Russell RC, Neoptolemos J, Williamson RC and . (1991). *Br J Cancer,* 64, 1076-1082.

Bartsch D, Hahn SA, Danichevski KD, Ramaswamy A, Bastian D, Galehdari H, Barth P, Schmiegel W, Simon B and Rothmund M. (1999). *Oncogene,* 18, 2367-2371.

Berger SI and Iyengar R. (2009). *Bioinformatics,* 25, 2466-2472.

Brown CJ, Lain S, Verma CS, Fersht AR and Lane DP. (2009). *Nat Rev Cancer,* 9, 862-873.

Buettner R, Mora LB and Jove R. (2002). *Clin Cancer Res,* 8, 945-954.

Caldas C, Hahn SA, da Costa LT, Redston MS, Schutte M, Seymour AB, Weinstein CL, Hruban RH, Yeo CJ and Kern SE. (1994). *Nat Genet,* 8, 27-32.

Cano DA, Rulifson IC, Heiser PW, Swigart LB, Pelengaris S, German M, Evan GI, Bluestone JA and Hebrok M. (2008). *Diabetes,* 57, 958-966.

Carnero A, Blanco-Aparicio C, Renner O, Link W and Leal JF. (2008). *Curr Cancer Drug Targets,* 8, 187-198.

Chelala C, Hahn SA, Whiteman HJ, Barry S, Hariharan D, Radon TP, Lemoine NR and Crnogorac-Jurcevic T. (2007). *BMC Genomics,* 8, 439.

Chelala C, Lemoine NR, Hahn SA and Crnogorac-Jurcevic T. (2009). *Pancreatology,* 9, 340-343.

Chmielowiec J, Borowiak M, Morkel M, Stradal T, Munz B, Werner S, Wehland J, Birchmeier C and Birchmeier W. (2007). *J Cell Biol,* 177, 151-162.

Cutts RJ, Gadaleta E, Hahn SA, Crnogorac-Jurcevic T, Lemoine NR and Chelala C. (2011). *Nucleic Acids Res,* 39, D1023-D1028.

Dai L, Li C, Shedden KA, Lee CJ, Li C, Quoc H, Simeone DM and Lubman DM. (2010). *J Proteome Res,* 9, 3394-3402.

Dessimoz J, Bonnard C, Huelsken J and Grapin-Botton A. (2005). *Curr Biol,* 15, 1677-1683.

Dessimoz J and Grapin-Botton A. (2006). *Cell Cycle,* 5, 7-10.

Faratian D, Clyde RG, Crawford JW and Harrison DJ. (2009). *Nat Rev Clin Oncol,* 6, 455-464.

Gusev Y. (2008). *Methods,* 44, 61-72.

Gusev Y, Schmittgen TD, Lerner M, Postier R and Brackett D. (2007). *BMC Bioinformatics,* 8 Suppl 7, S16.

Herman JG, Jen J, Merlo A and Baylin SB. (1996). *Cancer Res,* 56, 722-727.

Horii A, Nakatsuru S, Miyoshi Y, Ichii S, Nagase H, Ando H, Yanagisawa A, Tsuchiya E, Kato Y and Nakamura Y. (1992). *Cancer Res,* 52, 6696-6698.
Hruban RH, Adsay NV, bores-Saavedra J, Compton C, Garrett ES, Goodman SN, Kern SE, Klimstra DS, Kloppel G, Longnecker DS, Luttges J and Offerhaus GJ. (2001). *Am J Surg Pathol,* 25, 579-586.
Hruban RH, Goggins M, Parsons J and Kern SE. (2000a). *Clin Cancer Res,* 6, 2969-2972.
Hruban RH, Wilentz RE and Kern SE. (2000b). *Am J Pathol,* 156, 1821-1825.
Kim EJ and Simeone DM. (2011). *Curr Opin Gastroenterol.*
Levy L and Hill CS. (2005). *Mol Cell Biol,* 25, 8108-8125.
Lohr JM, Faissner R, Findeisen P and Neumaier M. (2006). *Internist (Berl),* 47 Suppl 1, S40-S48.
Maitra A and Hruban RH. (2005). *Cancer Cell,* 8, 171-172.
Makawita S, Smith C, Batruch I, Zheng Y, Ruckert F, Grutzmann R, Pilarsky C, Gallinger S and Diamandis EP. (2011). *Mol Cell Proteomics.*
Molina JR and Adjei AA. (2006). *J Thorac Oncol,* 1, 7-9.
Morosco GJ and Goeringer GC. (1980). *Med Hypotheses,* 6, 971-985.
Morosco GJ, Nightingale TE, Frasinel C and Goeringer GC. (1981). *J Toxicol Environ Health,* 8, 89-94.
Otte JM, Kiehne K, Schmitz F, Folsch UR and Herzig KH. (2000). *Scand J Gastroenterol,* 35, 90-95.
Philip PA. (2011). *Lancet Oncol,* 12, 206-207.
Pour PM, Pandey KK and Batra SK. (2003). *Mol Cancer,* 2, 13.
Rulifson IC, Karnik SK, Heiser PW, ten BD, Chen H, Gu X, Taketo MM, Nusse R, Hebrok M and Kim SK. (2007). *Proc Natl Acad Sci U S A,* 104, 6247-6252.
Saxena R, Voight BF, Lyssenko V, Burtt NP, de Bakker PI, Chen H, Roix JJ, Kathiresan S, Hirschhorn JN, Daly MJ, Hughes TE, Groop L, Altshuler D, Almgren P, Florez JC, Meyer J, Ardlie K, Bengtsson BK, Isomaa B, Lettre G, Lindblad U, Lyon HN, Melander O, Newton-Cheh C, Nilsson P, Orho-Melander M, Rastam L, Speliotes EK, Taskinen MR, Tuomi T, Guiducci C, Berglund A, Carlson J, Gianniny L, Hackett R, Hall L, Holmkvist J, Laurila E, Sjogren M, Sterner M, Surti A, Svensson M, Svensson M, Tewhey R, Blumenstiel B, Parkin M, Defelice M, Barry R, Brodeur W, Camarata J, Chia N, Fava M, Gibbons J, Handsaker B, Healy C, Nguyen K, Gates C, Sougnez C, Gage D, Nizzari M, Gabriel SB, Chirn GW, Ma Q, Parikh H, Richardson D, Ricke D and Purcell S. (2007). *Science,* 316, 1331-1336.
Schutte M, Rozenblum E, Moskaluk CA, Guan X, Hoque AT, Hahn SA, da Costa LT, de Jong PJ and Kern SE. (1995). *Cancer Res,* 55, 4570-4574.
Serra E, Puig S, Otero D, Gaona A, Kruyer H, Ars E, Estivill X and Lazaro C. (1997). *Am J Hum Genet,* 61, 512-519.
Stathis A and Moore MJ. (2010). *Nat Rev Clin Oncol,* 7, 163-172.
Vincent A, Herman J, Schulick R, Hruban RH and Goggins M. (2011). *Lancet.*
Wist AD, Berger SI and Iyengar R. (2009a). *Genome Med,* 1, 11.
Wood LD, Parsons DW, Jones S, Lin J, Sjoblom T, Leary RJ, Shen D, Boca SM, Barber T, Ptak J, Silliman N, Szabo S, Dezso Z, Ustyanksky V, Nikolskaya T, Nikolsky Y, Karchin R, Wilson PA, Kaminker JS, Zhang Z, Croshaw R, Willis J, Dawson D, Shipitsin M, Willson JK, Sukumar S, Polyak K, Park BH, Pethiyagoda CL, Pant PV, Ballinger DG, Sparks AB, Hartigan J, Smith DR, Suh E, Papadopoulos N, Buckhaults P,

Markowitz SD, Parmigiani G, Kinzler KW, Velculescu VE and Vogelstein B. (2007). *Science,* 318, 1108-1113.

Xiao J, Lee WN, Zhao Y, Cao R, Go VL, Recker RR, Wang Q and Xiao GG. (2010). *Pancreas,* 39, e17-e23.

Yoshida E, Aratani S, Itou H, Miyagishi M, Takiguchi M, Osumu T, Murakami K and Fukamizu A. (1997). *Biochem Biophys Res Commun,* 241, 664-669.

3

Novel Biomarkers in Pancreatic Cancer

Simona O. Dima[1], Cristiana Tanase[2], Radu Albulescu[2], Anca Botezatu[3] and Irinel Popescu[1]
[1]*Center of General Surgery and Liver Transplantation, Fundeni Clinical Institute of Digestive Disease and Liver Transplantation, Bucharest,*
[2]*Biochemistry and Proteomics Department, "Victor Babes" National Institute of Pathology, Bucharest,*
[3]*Viral Genetic Engineering Laboratory, Romanian Academy 'Stefan S. Nicolau' Virology Institute, Bucharest, Romania*

1. Introduction

Pancreatic ductal adenocarcinoma(PDAC) cancer is one of the most aggressive human cancers, and the fifth most frequent cause of cancer-related mortality in Western society. Pancreatic cancer is well known for high metastatic potential, early local invasion and poor outcome. The overall 5-year survival rate is less than 5%, respectively 10-30% for R0 resection (Huang et al., 2010). Less than 10% of newly diagnosed pancreatic cancers could be detected in early-stage (Takayama et al., 2010).

Clinical research in the field of cancer biomarkers is essential in understanding the biology and the heterogeneity of cancer disease. The factors involved in early PDAC development remain unknown. The detection of pancreatic cancer at early stages, the prediction of the potential resectability, or response to therapy are the current major challenges in improving the clinical outcome of PDAC. Therefore, predictive markers of responsiveness to adjuvant therapy would allow patients selection to appropriate treatment (Duffy et al., 2007). The aim of the postoperative surveillance following curative surgery for PDAC is to detect recurrences or metastases as early as possible.

Currently, there are only few studies that have identified cancer biomarkers with clinical significance.

Molecular biological factors are important tools for early diagnosis, prognosis, not only for therapeutic strategy but also for novel and more efficient therapeutic agents' identification. On the other hand a biomarker must be easily quantified, in order to minimize the invasiveness of therapeutically interventions. Recent finding in the molecular biology field of pancreatic cancer have assisted in translational research, giving hope for individualized therapy and better disease management.

2. Identification of new potential tumor tissue biomarkers

Much effort goes into finding new accurate prognostic, diagnostic single or combined tumor biomarkers. Nowadays, the research in this field is focused not only on finding biomarkers that could discriminate between pathological pancreas conditions (disease related biomarkers), but also to evaluate the aggressiveness grade of PDAC and to determine the therapy response (drug related biomarkers).

Presently, screening for pancreatic cancer is based on state-of-the-art imaging or even invasive diagnostic methods (Balasenthil et al., 2011). Serum and other body fluids, such as urine, pancreatic juice represents sources available by less invasive methods for biomarkers screening.

Several techniques like immunohistochemistry, fluorescence and chromogenic *in situ* hybridization, expression profiling- performed by microarray or quantitative real-time reverse transcriptase-polymerase chain reaction (qRT-PCR), and mutation analysis are used in identification of new biomarkers. Among these techniques, immunohistochemical tests remain the most widely used in routine practice and, importantly, in the assessment of biomarkers in translational research.

In a recent study, *Wacher et. al* investigated the expression level of an oncofetal protein, insulin-like growth factor II messenger ribonucleic acid-binding protein 3 (IMP3), which represent a marker for tumor aggressiveness in many different tumors (Wachter et al., 2011; Ozdemir et al., 2011).

The investigation was conducted on tissue biopsies from PDAC, chronic sclerosing pancreatitis, PDAC metastases cases in order to determine IMP3 expression. For IMP3 expression evaluation large tissue sections were used in the immunohistochemical analysis. The results obtained showed that PDAC were positive for IMP3 expression in a high percentage (88.4%) of cases, whereas normal or inflammatory pancreatic tissue was weakly positive (23.1%). A strong IMP3 expression was found in PDAC metastases (94.4%). The sensitivity and specificity of IMP3 expression test to discriminate between PDAC and chronic sclerosing pancreatitis using core needle biopsies were found to be 88.4% and 94.6%, respectively. The authors consider that IMP3 might be an easy to use and potentially new immunohistochemical marker for the diagnosis of PDAC in core needle biopsies (Asioli et al., 2010; Walter et al., 2009).

Another prognostic biomarker in PDAC which characterize the tumor aggressiveness recently studied was vimentin. Vimentin protein is a marker of mesenchymal differentiation, being correlated especially with aggressive carcinomas. In a high percentage primary pancreatic adenocarcinomas contain neoplastic cells that express vimentin, and the presence of this protein was correlated with poor histological differentiation and predicts a shorter postsurgical survival (Li et al., 2009; Handra-Luca et al., 2011).

Several technical strategies (SDS-PAGE, mass spectrometry, immunoblot) are used to find candidate biomarkers for the presurgical management of malignant and premalignant pancreatic conditions. Pancreatic cystic neoplasms represent 10–15% of primary cystic masses of the pancreas and are detected with an increasing frequency due to the use of advanced imaging modalities in clinical practice. On the other hand, the diagnosis of pancreatic cystic neoplasms remains a challenge because available diagnostic techniques are not so specific. The analysis of pancreatic cyst fluids obtained from various cystic lesions showed that specific histological lesions are associated with distinct protein patterns. Two important factors, olfactomedin-4 (antiapoptotic protein that promotes tumor growth) and mucin-18 (melanoma cell adhesion molecule) were proposed as biomarkers of pancreatic cancer (Cuoghi et al., 2011).

CD99 (cell surface glycoprotein involved in leukocyte migration), a useful diagnostic marker for Ewing sarcoma/primitive neuroectodermal tumor (Rocchi et al., 2010) was proposed for differentiation of solid-pseudopapillary neoplasm from other pancreatic tumor. The tissues positivity for CD99 was investigated in a recent study (Guo et al., 2011) using immunohistochemical staining technique. The solid-pseudopapillary neoplasm cells tumors exhibited paranuclear dot-like immunoreactivity for CD99. In contrast, in pancreatic neuroendocrine tumors a small percent of PDAC stained positive for CD99 at cytoplasmatic and membrane level. Pancreatic solid-pseudopapillary neoplasm exhibits a unique dot-like staining pattern for CD99 and could provide a definitive diagnosis of solid-pseudopapillary neoplasm and differentiation from other pancreatic tumors.

Immunohistochemical analysis of pancreatic cancer tissue provided also several candidate biomarkers for survival estimation. CDCP1 (CUB domain containing protein 1) determines anchorage- independent growth and migration of cancer cells. A higher expression level of this factor is correlated with the overall survival of pancreatic cancer patients (Miyazava et al., 2010). L1-CAM (L1-cell adhesion molecule) expression was also correlated with perineural invasion of pancreatic cancer cells and poor survival (Ben at al., 2010). Higher expression of B7-H3, a co-stimulatory immune molecule, plays a critical role in the T cell-mediated immune response and presents a positive correlation with pancreatic cancer prognosis.

KOC (K homology domain containing protein) gene encodes a protein that contains several KH domains, which are important in RNA binding and are known to be involved in RNA synthesis and metabolism. This protein was found to be overexpressed in pancreatic cancer. Immunohystochemical analysis showed strong staining for KOC protein in invasive pancreatic tissue carcinomas versus normal pancreatic tissue. It was proposed to be a molecular marker with a high sensitivity and specificity in discriminating PDAC from benign ductal epithelium (Toll et al., 2009).

3. Genome candidate biomarkers

Most of the adenocarcinomas develop gradually from precursor lesions PanINs (Pancreatic intraepithelial neoplasias). These events are accompanied by genetic modifications. Most genetic abnormalities reported in pancreatic cancer are represented by deletions and duplications of specific chromosomal loci, mutations/deletions of oncogenes and tumor-suppresor genes (KRAS, CDKN1A/p16, TP53, MADH4/SMAD4/DPC4 and BRCA2) [www.cancer-genetics.org].

3.1 Gene expression studies and potential factors involved in pancreas oncogenesis

Quantification of target mRNA gene levels represents a new tool for genome function analysis. High-throughput technologies like gene expression profiling using microarray and sequencing become important investigation methods for normal physiological and pathological processes. Therefore, studies based on quantification of gene expression levels revealed new potential factors involved in pancreas oncogenesis. Using Affymetrix and cDNA microarrays, nearly 1,100 molecules have been reported to be overexpressed in PanIN and IPMN lesions. A large majority of these molecules showed elevated mRNA levels expression in PDAC and in precursor lesions. Molecules such as S100P, MMP7, MUC4, FSCN1, and MUC5AC are found to be overexpressed in all type of lesions PanIN, IPMN and PDAC (Harsha et al., 2009).

Badea et al. using microarray study identificated a number of genes whose over-expression appears to be inversely correlated with patient survival: keratin 7, laminin gamma 2, stratifin, platelet phosphofructokinase, annexin A2, MAP4K4 and OACT2 (MBOAT2), which are specifically upregulated in the neoplastic epithelium (Badea et al., 2008).

The attention was focused especially on the calcium-binding protein- S100P. This protein was found to be expressed in pancreatic precursor lesions PanIN 2 or PanIN 3 and in pancreatic tumor creating the possibility to use the quantification of its expression level for earlier detection (Dowen et al., 2005). Expression levels of *S100P* mRNA were found to be higher in pancreatic juice from patients with pancreatic cancer and IPMN (Ohucida et al., 2006). On the other hand, three members of S100A family (S100A2, S100A4, and S100A6) were found to be associated with poor prognostic. S100A family members were involved in cell cycle regulation and cell invasion (Tanase et al., 2010).

The STAT3 transcription factor was found to be constitutively activated in PDAC. This is an important factor in stem cell self-renewal process, cancer cell survival, and inflammation. A close correlation between the levels of tyrosine-phosphorylated STAT3 and of the gp130 receptor was found. An upregulation of the IL6/LIF-gp130 pathway was also showed to be involved in STAT3 activation in pancreatic cancer (Corcoran et al., 2011). The same study asserts that STAT3 is required for the development of the precursor pancreatic lesions, acinar-to-ductal metaplasia (ADM) and PanIN, therefore evaluation of gp130 and phospho-STAT3 expression may be an effective biomarker.

3.2 Angiogenesis factors

With the increasing use of antiangiogenic agents for the treatment of cancers, is necessary the identification of candidate biomarkers for evaluation of the response and resistance. Is also, important to identify new biomarkers and to eliminate the risk for antiangiogenic therapies failure (Duda et al., 2010).

EGF (Epidermal Growth Factor), VEGF (Vascular Endothelial, Growth Factor) , heparanase, thrombospondin, cathepsins were the most important angiogenic factor specific for pancreatic cancer involved in cell growth promoting. The overexpression of EGF and his receptor EGFR were linked to tumor staging, but no clear data regarding the overall survival are available at this moment (Heidemann et al.,2006).

Another important factor that acts on angiogenesis process is VEGF. His effects in PDAC are increased by interaction with MMP-9, a cellular matrix remodeling factor. The therapy against both MMP-9 and VEGF in pancreatic cancer resulted in a significant decrease in PDAC growth and microvessel density versus a single target treatment (Tanase-Pistol et al.,2008).

Heparanases are endoglycosidases that cleave the heparan sulfate side chain of heparan sulfate proteoglycans (major membrane components) inducing extracellular matrix remodelling. On the other hand, heparanase increased growth factor bFGF (fibroblast growth factor) release, stimulating the angiogenesis process (Rohloff et al., 2002)

Thrombospondin (TSP-1) expression level was linked to a good prognostic for PDAC development. TSP-1 protein was found abundantly in stroma surrounding tumor cells and its expression is inversely correlated with microvessel density(Tobita et al., 2002).

The role of cathepsins in pancreatic cancer development and progression is still controversed. Cathepsin b (CTSB) and cathepsin l CTSL was found to be overexpressd in PDAC. A correlation between CTSB expression level and perineural invasion concludes the role of cathepsins in local tumor invasion (Niedergethmann et al., 2000).

3.3 ZIP3 (Zinc/iron regulated transporter-related protein 3) a possible tumor suppressor

Zinc is the most abundant trace element in cells. For example, about 25% of the total zinc present is found within the cell nuclei, being a component of chromatin. Zinc is an important factor in cellular processes, including cell division and proliferation, immune function, and defense against free radicals; zinc deficiency may be associated with an increased risk of cancer (Christudoss et al.,2011; Prasad et al., 2002). Zinc is found in over 300 enzymes, including copper/zinc superoxide dismutase, which is an important antioxidant enzyme, involved in cellular protection components from oxidation and damage.

In a current study, *Costello et al.* found a major loss of zinc in ductal and acinar epithelium in adenocarcinoma compared to the normal epithelium (Costello et al., 2011). The decrease in zinc quantity is a characteristic not only for pancreatic cancer, but also for precursor lesions. The mentioned group showed that the gene expression of ZIP3 (basilar membrane zinc uptake transporter) is present in normal ductal/acinar epithelium and absent in adenocarcinoma. The decreased expression of ZIP3 determines the loss of zinc in early and progressing malignancy. RREB1 transcription factor was found to be down regulated along with ZIP3 and might be the silencing cause of ZIP3 gene. Zinc treatment exhibited cytotoxic effect on Panc1 cell line. ZIP3 and RREB-1 expression level changes represent early events in the development of adenocarcinoma suggesting that ZIP3 might be a tumor suppressor gene.

3.4 Other important factors

FAP (fibroblast activation protein) is involved in the control of fibroblast growth or epithelial-mesenchymal interactions during development, tissue repair, and epithelial carcinogenesis. It is highly expressed in PDAC and is considered to be related to a poor prognostic. Targeting FAP factors are considered to be a promising and a new therapeuthical road (Cohen et al., 2008).

Maspin (SerpinB5- mammary serine protease inhibitor) is a tumor suppressor gene. Maspin induces apoptosis in neoplastic cells and expression of maspin are suppressed as the carcinoma progresses in breast and prostatic carcinoma (Jiang et al., 2002). The pattern of maspin gene expression is dependent of the disease stage. For example, highly expression was observed in intraductal papillary mucinous neoplasms, mucinous cystic neoplasms. and in carcinomas, whereas in adenomas is lower.It was also observed a significant decrease in maspin expression when intraductal papillary mucinous neoplasms progresses to invasion. However, the group with high maspin expression presented microinvasion, whereas low expression maspin group showed extensive invasion (Kashima et al., 2008). These results conclude that maspine could be a good prognostic factor for invasion.

4. Cancer stem cell biomarkers

Stem cell markers are a promising group of new biomarkers. Solid tumors contain small proportions of cells that are capable of proliferation, self-renewal, and differentiation into various cell types. These types of cells (cancer stem cells) are characterized by treatment resistance, especially to ionizing radiation. Therefore, it is a very challenging situation in order to identify these cells, to understand the mechanisms of resistance, and to evaluate the patient therapy outcome regarding the response to treatment. Identifying the markers that characterize cancer stem cells is the main research and a specific pattern regarding cell surface markers is emerging. In breast cancer, stem cells presented a characteristic antigenic pattern, whereas in high-grade gliomas, expression of CD133 on the cell surface selects a population of treatment resistant cells (Woodward & Sulman, 2008).

In pancreatic cancer, several surface markers have been identified for a subpopulation of the tumor cells with stem cell characteristics. These cancer stem cells were identified by expression of the cell surface markers CD44, CD24, and ESA (Li et al., 2007). When injected in the pancreas of immunocompromised mice these human cells are able to self-renew and generate differentiated progeny, to recapitulate the phenotype of the tumor from which they were derived.

Another subpopulation of cancer stem cells highly tumorigenic was isolated from patients with PDAC. These cell types were CD133+ and were able to induce tumor formation in athymic mice. This subpopulation of migrating cancer stem cells are characterized also by expression of the CXCR4 receptor and are involved in tumor metastasis Hermann et al., 2007.

Another candidate cell marker investigated was aldehyde dehydrogenase 1A1 (ALDH1A1), which has been identified to label cancer stem cells in breast cancer (Ginestier et al., 2007), colon cancer (Huang et al., 2009), lung cancer (Jiang et al., 2009) and head and neck squamous cancer (Chen et al., 2009). ALDH1 is a member of the aldehyde dehydrogenase gene (ALDH) superfamily playing an important role in the metabolism of endogenous and exogenous aldehydes. This NAD(P)(+)-dependent enzyme is also involved in the formation of molecules that are important in cellular processes, like retinoic acid (acting like modulator of gene regulation and cell differentiation), betaine and gamma-aminobutyric acid and exhibits additional, non-enzymatic functions, being able to bind to some hormones (Yoshida et al., 1998). The ALDH1 gene expression is ubiquitous in many human tissues; the protein is found localized mainly in the cellular cytoplasm.

It was also shown that ALDH1 has the capacity to detoxify aldophosphamide, conferring chemoresistance against cyclophosphamide to overexpressing cell (Hilton, 1984). Data regarding the effect of ALDH1A1 overexpression are controversial. Increased expression of

ALDH1 in ovarian cancer correlates with a favourable prognostic. In contrast, pancreatic cancer increased expression of ALDH1A1 was correlated with poor survival (Rasheed et al., 2010).

ALDH1+ breast tumors are negative for estrogen receptor and progesterone receptor overexpression, but present a high level of Ki67 expression (a nuclear protein that is associated with cellular proliferation) (Morimoto et al., 2009). Therefore, *Kahlert et al.* showed that a high expression of ALDH1A1 is significantly correlated with the proliferation rate of pancreatic tumour cells (Kahlert et al., 2011).

5. Drug-related biomarkers

Most of the pancreatic cancer patients have inoperable disease due to distant metastases or locally advanced tumor and the main therapeutic decision in this case is systemic chemotherapy or chemoradiation. Therefore, understanding the mechanisms that govern drug-related resistance and the factors involved in this process are a mandatory condition for therapeutic management success.

5.1 Metabolic prognosis factors for gemcitabine resistance

Patients with advanced or metastatic pancreatic cancer are treated with gemcitabine as a first line chemotherapeutic agent. Gemcitabine is a 2',2'-difluoro-2-deoxycytidine analogue that inhibits DNA replication and repair. Gemcitabine possesses radiosensitizing properties and its administration must be combined with radiotherapy. The sensitivity to gemcitabine and its efficiency were correlated with several factors. One of the factors that correlate with gemcitabine sensitivity is hENT1 (human equilibrative nucleoside transporter 1) (Nakano et al., 2007).

Pancreatic cancer cells that highly express hENT1 are sensitive to gemcitabine by uptaking this therapeutic agent in cancer cells. The absence hENT1 expression in metastatic pancreatic adenocarcinoma pacients treated with gemcitabine was associated with a poor prognostic compared with patients whom tumor cancer cells presented hENT1 expression (Hamada & Shimosegawa, 2011).

At the cellular level, gemcitabine is phosphorylated to its active metabolites by dCK (deoxycytidine kinase). Another group reported that not only hENT1 higher expression is a possible prognostic factor, but also dCK expression level and its activity correlates with gemcitabine activity (Ashida et al., 2009). High dCK enzyme activity was linked with gemcitabine sensitivity in experimental models (Kroep et al., 2002) and biopsy samples analysis (Sebastiani et al., 2006).

Gemcitabine inactivation is performed through an enzymatic deamination process. There are three important enzymes involved in gemcitabine deamination (deoxycytidylate deaminase-DCD, cytidine deaminase-CDA and 5'-nucleotidase -5'-NT). The increased activity of such enzymes could induce the resistance to gemcitabine (Kroep et al., 2002; Giovannetti et al., 2006; Nakano et al., 2007) Gemcitabine resistance mechanism is also realized by high expression of RRM1 and RRM2, which are the two subunits (large and small) of ribonucleotide reductase. This enzyme regulates the rate of DNA synthesis, and is also known to convert ribonucleotides to deoxyribonucleotides. Gemcitabine exerts its cytotoxicity by inhibiting ribonucleotide reductase (Davidson et al., 2004; Bergman et al., 2005; Nakahira et al., 2006)

6. Epigenetic biomarkers

Cancer initiation and progression is traditionally characterized as a genetic alteration, but recent years crystallized in a new direction regarding epigenetic mechanisms involvement in oncogenesis. Epigenetic mechanisms are essential for normal development and for maintaining of a tissue specific pattern of gene expression. Epigenetic modifications lead to an abnormal genetic expression and further to malign transformation. The research in epigenetic field has demonstrated the involvement of an intensive reprogramming of epigenetic machinery (DNA methylation, histone modifications, microRNA expression). The reverse nature of epigenetic abnormalities permitted the development of epigenetic therapy field.

6.1 Gene promoter methylation status and pancreatic oncogenesis

The most known epigenetic modification in oncogenesis is DNA hypermethylation. This event is accompanied by genetic silencing. Identification and characterization of epigenetically silenced genes is important in order to understand the roles of such epigenetic modification in oncogenesis and to discover new tumor markers. It was reported that in pancreas cancer some tumor suppressor genes presented aberrant CpG islands hypermethylation at gene promoter level.

The first tumor suppressor gene identified to be specific for pancreatic cancer was p16/CDKN1A (Schutte et al., 1997). Subsequently, new hypermethylated genes were associated with pancreatic cancer (hMLH1, E-cadherin, ppENK, CDKN1C, SPARC, TFPI-2, GATA4,5, BNIP3, TSLC1, HHIP, MUC2, reprimo, CXCR4 si SOCS1) (Omura et al., 2009).

Several important epigenetically silenced factors have been identified (hsa-miR-9-1, ZNF415, CNTNAP2 si ELOVL4) (Omura et al 2009; Grady et al.,2008; Lehmann et al,.2008; Fabbri et al., 2007; Moriss et al., 2004).

Using methylated CpG island amplification (MCA) and representational difference analysis (RDA), Ueki *et al* group identified that gene preproenkephalin (*ppENK*) presented a hypermethylated promoter in most pancreatic cancers (Ueki et al., 2001). *ppENK* encodes an opioid peptide which presents growth-suppressor properties.

It was showed that CDKN1C/p57KIP2 gene presented a decrease expression in intraductal papillary mucinous neoplasm. The gene encodes for cyclin-dependent kinase inhibitor, and is a negative regulator of cell proliferation (Sato et al., 2005). Partial methylation of the *CDKN1C* promoter was found in pancreatic cancer cell lines and pancreas cancer.

SPARC (secreted protein acidic and rich in cysteine, or osteonectin/BM40) is a matrix-associated protein; calcium binding, that inhibits cell-cycle progression, and influences the synthesis of extracellular matrix. The gene codifying this protein was found aberrantly methylated in pancreatic cancer by. SPARC is a factor involved in many processes like cell migration, proliferation, matrix cell adhesion (Sato et al., 2003, Gao et al., 2010).

Tissue factor pathway inhibitor 2 (TFPI-2) is a Kunitz-type serine proteinase inhibitor, which has been identified as a putative tumor-suppressor gene. Aberrant methylation of *TFPI-2* was found in pancreatic cancer xenografts and primary pancreatic adenocarcinomas. Re-expression of the *TFPI-2* gene led in the proliferation, migration and invasion of cancer cells (Sato et al., 2005).

GATA gene family members were also epigenetic silenced in pancreatic cancer. For example, *GATA-5* was frequently methylated in pancreatic cancers, whereas *GATA-4* was hypomethylated (Fu et al., 2007).

Another gene commonly silenced epigenetically in pancreatic cancer is BNIP3. The protein encoded by this gene contains a BH3 domain and a transmembrane domain associated with pro-apoptotic function. BNIP3 gene silencing induced a drug resistance mechanism in pancreatic cancer cells, as a potential drug resistance mechanism (Okami et al., 2004)

Shimizu et al. using a novel method called "microarray coupled with methyl-CpG targeted transcriptional activation" (MeTA-array for short), identified 16 genes hypermethylated in three representative pancreatic cancer cell lines, AsPC-1, MIA PaCa-2 and PANC-1. Among these 16 genes several presented higher methylation level (CSMD2, SLC32A1, TMEM204 and TRH). CSMD2, SLC32A1 and TRH genes presented also a hypermethylated pattern in primary pancreatic cancers (Shimizu et al., 2011).

In contrast, a great number of genes are overexpressed in pancreatic cancer. These genes presented hypomethylation of the promoter in pancreatic cancer versus normal pancreatic tissue.

DNA hypomethylation of promoter CpGs were identified in genes with overexpression pattern including claudin4, lipocalin2, 14-3-3sigma/ stratifin, trefoil factor 2, S100A4, mesothelin, PSCA, S100P and maspin (Sato et al., 2003).

6.2 Histone modifications hallmarks for oncogenesis process

Covalent histone modifications are important regulatory elements in many biological processes. These modifications control the chromatin status by electrostatic interaction changes and non-histonic protein recruitement. Histones suffer specific N-terminal end post-translational changes represented by acethylation, methylation, phosphorylation, sumoylation, ubiquitination and ADP-ribosylation. These modifications alter DNA-histones interaction having a major impact on chromatin structure (Strahl et al., 2000).

Certain histone modifications influence gene transcription level. The interplay between histone modifications led to 'histone code hypothesis'. For example, lysine acetylation neutralizes the charge between DNA and histone tails and correlates with a more transcription permissive status of chromatin (Jenuwein et al., 2001).

Hypermethylated CpG islands of silenced tumor-suppressor genes are correlated with deacetylation of histones H3 and H4, methylation of H3 lysine 9 (H3K9), H3 lysine 27 (H3K27), and H4 lysine 20 (H4K20), and demethylation of H3 lysine 4 (Rosenfeld et al., 2009; Barski et al., 2007). Methylation of histone H3 lysine 4 (H3K4) and H3 lysine 36 is associated with relaxed chromatin status (Benevolenskaya et al., 2007). Histone modifications recruit effector proteins. Acetylated lysines are recognized by bromodomains within nucleosome remodeling complexes, methylated H3K4 and the helicase Chd1 chromodomain recruits activating complexes of chromatin (Daniel et al., 2005). In contrast, methylated H3K9 and

H3K27 interacts with heterochromatin protein 1 (HP 1) and Polycomb-group (PcG) proteins leading to chromatin compaction (Fischle et al., 2003). PcG proteins function as transcriptional repressors, but the molecular mechanisms of Polycomb repressive complex (PRC)-mediated repression is not clear (Sparmann et al., 2006). PcG proteins recruits DNMTs (DNA methyl transferase) involved in the hypermethylation of tumor suppressor genes (Vire et al., 2006).

Only few studies have examined genes that are regulated by histone modifications in pancreatic cancers. For example, mucin family gene underwent histone alterations in pancreatic cancers in association with gene overexpression. The 5′ region of MUC1 gene transcriptional start site is enriched in tri/dimethylated H3K9 and methylated DNA in non-tumor cells (Yamada et al., 2008). Transcriptional start site of MUC2 is highly enriched in di- and tri-methylated H3K4, acetylated H3K9, and acetylated H3K27 in pancreatic cancer cells. Vincent *et al* demonstrated that *MUC4* transcription activity is affected by many factors (DNMT3A, DNMT3B, HDAC1 and HDAC3, DNA methylation, histone modification (Vincent et al., 2008).

7. Model organisms studies provide potential biomarkers in pancreas oncogenesis

Model organisms are widely used to explore potential causes and treatments for human disease. This strategy is made possible by the conservation of metabolic and developmental pathways and genetic material over the course of evolution.

It is known that Enolase 1 (α-enolase or non-neuronal enolase –NNE), is an isoenzyme of enolase, which catalyze the conversion of 2-phosphoglycerate into phosphoenolpyruvate.

Several studies have shown that enolase 1 plays an important role in in tumorigenesis, cancer invasion and metastasis. Proteomic studies reported that expression of enolase 1 is increased in cancers, such as hepatocellular carcinoma (Takashima et al. 2008, Hamaguchi et al., 2008) , non-small lung cancer (He et al., 2007), esophageal adenocarcinoma (Zhao et al., 2007), prostate cancer (van den Bemd et al., 2006), colon cancer (Katayama et al., 2006), oral epithelial and squamous cell carcinoma (Ito et al., 2007).

In pancreatic cancer Mikuriya et al using two-dimensional electrophoresis and liquid chromatography-mass spectrometry/mass spectrometry showed that the expression levels of glycolytic enzymes, including enolase 1, increased in the cancerous pancreatic tissues patients compared with the paired non-cancerous tissues (Mikuriya et al., 2007).

In order to evaluate Enolase 1 expression changes, Lei et al. used chemical induced carcinogenesis in rats. Implantation of 7,12-dimethylbenzanthracene in rat pancreas leads to pancreatic cancer and PanINs. Alpha-enolase was specifically overexpressed in tumors compared with normal and pancreatic tissues (Lei et al., 2011).

The group found several proteins overexpressed in this carcinogenesis model, along with enolase 1 (Tumor protein translationally controlled 1, Expressed in non-metastatic cells 2, Pancreatic elastase 3B , Necdin, Hbp23, Chromodomain helicase DNA-binding protein, Albumin+retinoid X receptor-interacting protein, Heterogeneous nuclear ribonucleoprotein A2/B1-hnRNP A2/B1).

The hnRNP A2/B1 protein plays an important role in the biogenesis and transport of mRNA. Abnormal expression of this protein leads to alteration of normal transcription. In concordance with this study a previous work found high levels of hnRNP A2/B1 expression in a limited number of human pancreatic adenocarcinomas from smokers and two pancreatic tumor cell lines, HPAF-11 and SU 86 (Shen et al., 2004). In contrast, carboxyl ester lipase (CEL pancreatic exocrine enzyme) expression level progressively decreased with DMBA-induced disease severity.

DMBA implantation into the rat pancreas is an effective method to induce PanINs and pancreas cancer in order to determine which the first change in proteins expression pattern is, and to identify markers for pancreas lesions progression.

8. Novel biomarkers for the non-invasive diagnosis of pancreatic cancer

Actually, diagnostic methods for pancreatic cancer include invasive procedures (tissue sampling by endoscopy), involving risks and causing complications. The necessity for less invasive diagnostic methods is increasing; therefore the development of non-invasive biomarkers in pancreatic cancer is mandatory.

8.1 Plasma biomarkers

The major directions of proteomic range from basic research to discovery, validation and use of clinical applications. Protein profiling methods include high resolution two-dimensional gels, two-dimensional differential in-gel electrophoresis, LC-MS and LC-MS/MS using accurate mass tags, and protein identifications using mass spectrometry methods. These methods were used in many studies for identification of prognostic and/or predictive biomarkers that may help stratify patients.

The only clinically available serum biomarker for PDAC is CA 19-9, which is useful for the follow-up of pancreatic cancer patients receiving treatment, but has not been recommended for cancer screening (Goggins et al., 2000; Locker et al., 2006). The American Society of Clinical Oncology (ASCO) 2006 guidelines for the use of tumor markers do not recommend CA19-9 as a screening test for pancreatic cancer (Rosty et al., 2002; Liang et al., 2009). Several other serum markers have been proposed for pancreatic cancer.

Recent papers published new promising biomarkers, which can potentially detect early stage pancreatic cancer (Chen et al., 2011).

Roberts *et al.* analyzed serum samples from patients with locally advanced or metastatic adenocarcinoma of the pancreas. Patient group was selected based on length of survival and type of therapy, and serum was subjected to liquid chromatography coupled to tandem mass spectrometry analysis (LC-MS-MS) (Roberts et al., 2011). The proteins presenting important changes in expression levels were validated by enzyme-linked immunosorbent assay (ELISA). After the data were analyzed, the authors selected 1 putative prognostic protein, alpha 1-antichymotrypsin (AACT), and 2 putative predictive proteins, histidine-rich glycoprotein (HRG) and complement factor H (CFH). AACT was found to be negatively correlated with overall survival, whereas CFH was found to have no predictive value as prognostic factor for overall survival. AACT may be a useful prognostic marker in patients with advanced stage pancreatic carcinoma, although additional validation studies are needed.

Another study involving quantification in patient serum of tumor cell metabolites, or secreted factor was conducted by He *et al.* . This study focused on DJ-1 oncoprotein secreted by cancer cells (He et al., 2011). The study group involved patients diagnosed with pancreatic cancer and chronic pancreatitis, along with healthy subjects. DJ-1 serum level and the conventional tumor marker carbohydrate antigen 19-9 (CA 19-9) were measured in order to establish the diagnostic and prognostic value of DJ-1. Serum DJ-1 level was increased in patients with pancreas cancer compared with chronic pancreatitis and healthy individuals. Serum DJ-1 levels were higher than CA 19-9, and combined the two biomarkers provided a sensitivity of 87.5%. After resection DJ-1 levels decreased and patient with lower value of this factor had a better prognosis. This study provides a potential clinical biomarker, easy to quantify from serum, in order to establish a rapid diagnosis and to evaluate prognosis in patients with pancreas cancer.

8.2 Pancreatic juice biomarkers

Analysis of protein expression profiles of pancreatic juice samples harvested from the pancreatic duct has the potential to identify markers that could serve for diagnosis triage of benign from malignant pancreatic lesions and to discriminate between different stages of PDAC.

The research performed by *Vareed et al.* has shown that 56 proteins were found to be elevated in pancreatic juice of PDAC patients compared to benign controls (Vareed et al., 2011).

Protein profiles studies revealed an unique presence of proteins associated with Parkinson's disease namely: aSyn and PARK7 (Bonifati et al., 2003; Singleton et al., 2003).

Increased expression of aSyn has been also identified in melanoma (Matsuo et al., 2010), while its isoform gamma-synuclein (cSyn) has been shown to be elevated in tumors of breast, uterine, colorectal and pancreas (Ye et al., 2009; Hibi et al., 2009; Ahmad et al., 2007; Li et al., 2004; Gupta et al., 2003; Jia et al., 1999; Morgan et al., 2009). Moreover, due to the structural omology between cSyn and aSyn, these factors potentiate invasion in these tumors.

Interestingly, tissue arrays demonstrated a strong staining for aSyn in tumors, and this protein expressed in a subset of PDAC patients was identified in its aggregated form similar to Lewy Bodies seen in Parkinson's disease (Polymeropoulus et al., 1997). Another interesting coincidence is the presence of increased levels of Parkinson's disease associated protein PARK7 (DJ1) (van Duijin et al., 2001) in pancreatic ductal juice of adenocarcinomas. The mechanism by which the protein PARK-7 exerts its oncogenic effect remains unclear. It is presumed the involvement of p38 mitogen activated-protein kinase signaling (Mo et al., 2010).

On the other hand PDAC-associated secretory proteome analysis also revealed increased levels of several metabolic enzymes. The most important metabolic factor was Purine NucleosidePhosphorylase (NP), enzyme involved in salvage pathway of purines, which is operational during inflammation and neoplastic progression, (Bantia et al., 2010). NP activity has been reported to be high in cancer sera (Roberts et al., 2004) and NP expression has also been used to determine the clinical severity of various types of cancers, in combination with another factor adenosine deaminase (ADA) (Mesarosova et al., 1993).

This strong association between NP with inflammation determined to evaluate the expression and activity of this protein in PDAC, specifically in patients with antecedent inflammatory conditions like chronic pancreatitis, and pancreatic intraepithelial neoplasia (PanIN) (Rebours et al., 2010). Therefore, this correlation makes NP levels quantification to be a useful marker for surveillance progression from inflammation to PDAC.

8.3 Saliva biomarkers

Saliva is a body fluid that can be easily obtained without using a special technique. Recent reports suggested the possible utility of saliva in quantification of specific factors to discriminate between pancreatic cancer patients and patients with normal or chronic pancreatitis.

Using transcriptome profiles, Zhang *et al.* group could differentiate pancreatic cancer patients from healthy subject with a sensitivity of 90.0% and a specificity of 95.0%. The group found 12 mRNA biomarkers specific for pancreatic cancer patients. Seven genes were found to be up-regulated (*MBD3L2, KRAS, STIM2, DMXL2ACRV1, DMD, CABLES1*), whereas five genes presented a decreased expression *TK2, GLTSCR2, CDKL3, DPM1, TPT1* (Zhang et al., 2010).

A similar approach has been made by another group, which evaluated metabolites in saliva using mass spectrometry. Pancreatic cancer cases were successfully detected based on the pancreatic cancer-specific signature (Sugimoto et al., 2010). The levels of ornithine and putrescine were higher in patients with breast or pancreatic cancer, and were markedly higher in patients with oral cancer. The level of tryptophan is also increased in oral and pancreatic cancer, in contrast to arginine level which is decreased several cancers including breast, colonic and pancreatic cancer, which might be due to increased uptake of arginine by tumor tissues with high arginase activity.

8.4 Non- coding RNA as new era biomarkers

A new and important atractive tool is represented by small non-coding RNA. These are regulators of various biological processes like gene expression and are involved in cancer progression. One of the most important players is microRNAs which control many cellular functions, such as migration, invasion and stem cell functions. Abnormal microRNA gene expression was found in many cancers, including pancreatic cancer (Rachangani et al., 2010, Eis et al., 2005, Calin et al., 2005, Yanaihara et al., 2006).

MicroRNA molecules are present in various body fluids (blood, urine, cerebrospinal fluid, pancreatic juice, billiary secretion). Moreover, several microRNAs from sera seemed to be identical for many cancer types. Very important is the fact that miRNAs from sera are stable and exhibit resistance to RN-ase activity, intermittent frosting and defrosting, high temperature values and extreme pH (Mitchell et al., 2008; Albulescu et al., 2011).

Using microarray technology it was established that several microRNAs are highly expressed in pancreatic cancer (miR-21, miR-17-5p,miR-191,miR-29b-2,miR-223 miR-128b, miR-199a-1, miR-24-1, miR-24-2,miR-146, miR-181b-1, miR-20a,miR-107,miR-32 , miR-92-2, miR-214,miR-30c, miR-25, miR-221, miR-106) (Volinia et al., 2006). More recently, was established that microRNAs, miR-200a and miR-200b are highly expressed in pancreatic cancer cell lines, and their expression levels were significantly increased in the sera from pancreatic cancer patients, suggesting that microRNA itself could be a biomarker for pancreatic cancer (Li et al., 2010). The attention was also focused on two pancreas specific miRNAs miR-216 and miR-217. The expression of those miRNAs is decreased or even absent in PADC and in cell lines (Sood et al., 2006). Only miR-217 and miR-196a are able to discriminate between normal pancreas, chronic pancreatitis and tumor PDAC (Szafranska et al., 2008). Furthermore, miR-196a expression is likely specific to PDAC cells and is positively associated with the progression of PDAC.

miR-21 and miR-155 are overexpressed in pancreatic tumor, as compared to tissues from normal pancreas and chronic pancreatitis. Both miR-21 and miR-155 have been suggested to have a proto-oncogene role being overexpressed in several cancers (breast cancer, lung cancer, Burkitt lymphoma, B-cell lymphoma) (Metzler et al., 2004;Yin et al., 2008)

Several studies demonstrated that miR-155 transcription is regulated by transforming growthfactor β -TGF β/Smad, nuclear factor-κB and activator protein-1 family transcription factors through direct interaction with the miR-155/BIC bidirectional promoter. These studies suggests that overexpression of miR-155 in cancer is due to transcriptional activation, involving other cellular deregulated mechanisms (Kong et al., 2008).

9. Conclusions

Asymptomatic pancreatic cancer is hard to detect, but possibly curable. Recent research identified novel biomarkers of pancreatic cancer, but screening for early pancreatic cancer is still challenging. Future work should be addressed to the development of diagnostic techniques with a higher sensitivity to detect even asymptomatic cases. Currently no clinically useful interventions to screen for patients with PDAC are available.

10. Acknowledgements

The authors are grateful for the funding support offered by POSDRU/89/1.5/S/60746 Grant.

11. References

Ahmad, M., Attoub, S., Singh, M.N., Martin, F.L. & El-Agnaf, O.M. (2007). Gammasynuclein and the progression of cancer. *FASEB J*, 21: 3419–3430.

Albulescu, R., Tănase, C. & Neagu, M. (2011). Tissular and soluble microRNAs for diagnostic improvement and therapy in digestive tract cancers. *Expert Review of Molecular Diagnostics*, 11(1): 101-120.

Ashida, R., Nakata, B., Shigekawa, M., Mizuno, N., Sawaki, A., Hirakawa, K., Arakawa, T., Yamao, K. (2009) Gemcitabine sensitivity-related mRNA expression in endoscopic ultrasound-guided fine-needle aspiration biopsy of unresectable pancreatic cancer. *J Exp Clin Cancer Re*, 28: 83.

Asioli, S., Erickson, L.A., Righi, A., Jin, L., Volante, M., Jenkins, S., Papotti, M., Bussolati, G. & Lloyd, R.V. (2010). Poorly differentiated carcinoma of the thyroid: validation of the Turin proposal and analysis of IMP3 expression. *Mod Pathol.*, 23(9):1269-78.

Badea, L., Herlea, V., Dima, S.O., Dumitrascu, T. & Popescu, I. (2008) Combined gene expression analysis of whole-tissue and microdissected pancreatic ductal adenocarcinoma identifies genes specifically overexpressed in tumor epithelia , 55(88):2016-27.

Balasenthil, S., Chen, N. & Lott, S.T. (2011) A migration signature and plasma biomarker panel for pancreatic adenocarcinoma. *Cancer Prev Res (Phila)*, 4:137-149.

Bantia, S., Parker, C., Upshaw, R., Cunningham, A. & Kotian P.(2010). Potent orally bioavailable purine nucleoside phosphorylase inhibitor BCX-4208 induces apoptosis in B- and T-lymphocytes–a novel treatment approach for autoimmune diseases, organ transplantation and hematologic malignancies. *Int Immunopharmacol.*, 10(7):784-90.

Barski, A., Cuddapah, S., Cui, K., Roh, T.Y., Schones, D.E., Wang, Z., Wei, G., Chepelev, I. & Zhao, K. (2007). High-resolution profiling of histone methylations in the human genome". *Cell*, 129(4): 823–37.

Beer, D.G., Lubman, D.M. (2007). Comparative proteomics analysis of Barrett metaplasia and esophageal adenocarcinoma using two-dimensional liquid mass mapping. *Mol Cell Proteomics*, 6, 987-999

Ben, Q.W., Wang, J.C., Liu, J., Zhu, Y., Yuan, F., Yao, W.Y. & Yuan, Y.Z. (2010) Positive expression of L1-CAM is associated with perineural invasion and poor outcome in pancreatic ductal adenocarcinoma. *Ann Surg Oncol*, 17: 2213–2221.

Benevolenskaya, E.V. (2007). Histone H3K4 demethylases are essential in development and differentiation. *Biochem. Cell Biol.*, 85 (4): 435–43.

Bergman, A.M., Eijk, P.P., Ruiz van Haperen, V.W., Smid, K., Veerman, G., Hubeek, I., van den Ijssel, P., Ylstra, B. & Peters, G.J. (2005) In vivo induction of resistance to gemcitabine results in increased expression of ribonucleotide reductase subunit M1 as the major determinant. *Cancer Res*, 65:9510-9516.

Bonifati, V., Rizzu, P., Squitieri, F., Krieger, E. & Vanacore, N. (2003). DJ-1(PARK7), a novel gene for autosomal recessive, early onset parkinsonism.*Neurol Sci*, 24: 159–160.

Calin, G.A., Querzoli, P., Negrini, M. & Croce, C.M. (2005). MicroRNA gene expression deregulation in human breast cancer. *CancerRes*; 65: 7065-7070.

Chen, Y.C., Bunger, S., Laubert, T., Roblick, U.J. & Habermann, J.K. (2011). Serum biomarkers for improved diagnostic of pancreatic cancer: a current overview. *J Cancer Res Clin Oncol*; 137:375-389.

Chen, Y.W., Hsu, H.S., Tseng, L.M., Huang, P.I., Lu, K.H., Chen, D.T., Tai, L.K., Yung, M.C., Chang, B., Liu, G., Xue, F., Rosen, D.G., Xiao, L., Wang, X. & Liu, J. (2009) ALDH1 expression correlates with favorable prognosis in ovarian cancers. *Mod Pathol*, 22(6):817-823.

Christudoss, P., Selvakumar, R., Fleming, J.J. & Gopalakrishnan, G. (2011) Zinc status of patients with benign prostatic hyperplasia and prostate carcinoma. *Indian J Urol*, 27(1):14-8.

Cohen, S.J., Alpaugh, R.K., Palazzo, I., Meropol, N.J., Rogatko, A. & Xu Z. (2008) Fibroblast activation protein and its relationship to clinical outcome in pancreatic adenocarcinoma. *Pancreas*, 37(2):154–158.

Corcoran, R.B., Contino, G., Deshpande, V., Tzatsos, A., Conrad, C., Benes, C.H., Levy, D.E., Settleman, J., Engelman, J.A. & Bardeesy, N. (2011) STAT3 Plays a Critical Role in KRAS-Induced Pancreatic Tumorigenesis. *Cancer Res*; 71(14): 1-10.

Costello, L.C., Levy, B.A., Desouki, M.M., Zou, J., Bagasra, O., Johnson, L.A., Hanna, N.& Franklin, R.B. (2011). Decreased zinc and down regulation of ZIP3 zinc uptake transporter in the development of pancreatic adenocarcinoma. *Cancer Biol Ther.* 12(4).

Cuoghi, A., Farina, A., Z'graggen, K., Dumonceau, J.M., Tomasi, A., Hochstrasser, D.F., Genevay, M., Lescuyer, P. & Frossard, J.L. (2011) Role of proteomics to differentiate between benign and potentially malignant pancreatic cysts. *J Proteome Res,* 10(5):2664-70.

Daniel, J.A., Pray-Grant, M.G., Grant, P.A. (2005) Effector proteins for methylated histones: an expanding family. *Cell Cycle,* 4:919–926.

Davidson, J.D., Ma, L., Flagella, M., Geeganage, S., Gelbert, L.M. & Slapak, C.A. (2004) An increase in the expression of ribonucleotide reductase large subunit 1 is associated with gemcitabine resistance in non-small cell lung cancer cell lines. *Cancer Res,* 64:3761-3766.

Dowen, S.E., Crnogorac-Jurcevic, T., Gangeswaran, R., Hansen, M., Eloranta, J.J., Bhakta, V., Brentnall, T.A., Luttges, J., Kloppel, G. & Lemoine, N.R. (2005) Expression of S100P and its novel binding partner S100PBPR in early pancreatic cancer. *Am J Pathol,* 166: 81–92.

Duda, D.G., Ancukiewicz, M. & Rakesh, K. (2010) Jain Biomarkers of Antiangiogenic Therapy: How Do We Move From Candidate Biomarkers to Valid Biomarkers? *JCO,* 28(2): 183-185.

Duffy, MJ. 2007 Role of tumor markers in patients with solid cancers: A critical review. *Eur J Intern Med,* 18:175-184.

Eis, P.S., Tam, W., Sun, L., Chadburn, A., Li, Z., Gomez, M.F., Lund, E., & Dahlberg, J.E. (2005). Accumulation of miR-155 and BIC RNA in human B cell lymphomas. *Proc Natl Acad Sci USA* ,102:3627-3632.

Fabbri, M., Garzon, R., Cimmino, A., Liu, Z., Zanesi, N., Callegari, E., Liu, S., Alder, H., Costinean, S., Fernandez-Cymering, C., Volinia, S., Guler, G., Morrison, C.D., Chan, K.K., Marcucci, G., Calin, G.A., Huebner, K., & Croce, C.M. (2007). MicroRNA-29 family reverts aberrant methylation in lung cancer by targeting DNA methyltransferases 3A and 3B. *Proc Natl Acad Sci USA,* 104: 15805-15810.

Fischle, W., Wang, Y., Jacobs, S.A., Kim, Y., Allis, C.D.& Khorasanizadeh, S.(2003) Molecular basis for the discrimination of repressive methyl-lysine marks in histone H3 by Polycomb and HP1 chromodomains. *Genes Dev,* 17:1870–1881.

Fu, B., Guo, M., Wang, S., Campagna, D., Luo, M., Herman, J.G.& Iacobuzio-Donahue, C.A. (2007). Evaluation of GATA-4 and GATA-5 methylation profiles in human pancreatic cancers indicate promoter methylation patterns distinct from other human tumor types. *Cancer Biol Ther.*, 6(10):1546-52.

Gao, J., Song, J., Huang, H., Li, Z., Du, Y., Cao, J., Li, M., Lv, S., Lin, H. & Gong, Y. (2010). Methylation of the SPARC gene promoter and its clinical implication in pancreatic cancer. *J Exp Clin Cancer Res.*, 26;29:28.

Ginestier, C., Hur, M.H., Charafe-Jauffret, E., Monville, F., Dutcher, J., Brown, M., Jacquemier, J., Viens, P., Kleer, C.G., Liu, S., et al. (2007). ALDH1 is a marker of normal and malignant human mammary stem cells and a predictor of poorclinical outcome. *Cell Stem Cell* , 1(5):555-567.

Giovannetti, E., Del Tacca, M., Mey, V., Funel, N., Nannizzi, S., Ricci, S, Orlandini, C., Boggi, U., Campani, D., Del Chiaro, M., Iannopollo, M., Bevilacqua, G., Mosca, F. & Danesi, R. (2006). Transcription analysis of human equilibrative nucleoside transpoter-1 predicts survival in pancreas cancer patients treated with gemcitabine. *Cancer Res* , 66:3928-3935.

Goggins, M., Canto, M. & Hruban, R. (2000) Can we screen high-risk individuals to detect early pancreatic carcinoma? *J Surg Oncol,* 74:243-248.

Grady, W.M., Parkin, R.K., Mitchell, P.S., Lee, J.H., Kim, Y.H., Tsuchiya, K.D., Washington, M.K., Paraskeva, C., Willson, J.K., Kaz, A.M., Kroh, E.M., Allen, A., Fritz, B.R., Markowitz, S.D & Tewari, M.(2008). Epigenetic silencing of the intronic microRNA hsa-miR-342 and its host gene EVL in colorectal cancer. *Oncogene* ,27: 3880-3888.

Guo, Y., Yuan, F., Deng, H., Wang, H.F., Jin, X.L., & Xiao, J.C.(2011). Paranuclear dot-like immunostaining for CD99: a unique staining pattern for diagnosing solid-pseudopapillary neoplasm of the pancreas. *Am J Surg Pathol,* 35(6):799-806.

Gupta, A., Inaba, S., Wong, O.K., Fang, G.,& Liu, J. (2003). Breast cancer-specific gene 1 interacts with the mitotic checkpoint kinase BubR1. *Oncogene,* 22: 7593–7599.

Hamada, S. & Shimosegawa, T. (2011). Biomarkers of Pancreatic Cancer. *Pancreatology,* 11(suppl 2):14–19.

Hamaguchi, T., Iizuka, N., Tsunedomi, R., Hamamoto, Y., Miyamoto, T., Iida, M., Tokuhisa, Y., Sakamoto, K., Takashima, M., Tamesa, T., & Oka, M. (2008). Glycolysis module activated by hypoxiainducible factor 1alpha is related to the aggressive phenotype of hepatocellular carcinoma. *Int J Oncol,* 33: 725-731.

Handra-Luca, A., Hong, S.M., Walter, K., Wolfgang, C., Hruban, R., & Goggins, M. (2011). Tumour epithelial vimentin expression and outcome of pancreatic ductal adenocarcinomas. *Br J Cancer,* 104(8):1296-302.

Harsha, H.C., Kandasamy, K., Ranganathan, P., Rani, S., Ramabadran, S., Gollapudi, S., Balakrishnan, L., Dwivedi, S.B., Telikicherla, D., Selvan, L.D., Goel, R., Mathivanan, S., Marimuthu, A., Kashyap, M., Vizza, R.F., Mayer, R.J., Decaprio, J.A., Srivastava, S., Hanash, S.M., Hruban, R.H., & Pandey, A. (2009). A compendium of potential biomarkers of pancreatic cancer. *PLoS Med,* 6(4):e1000046.

He, L., Thomson, J.M., Hemann, M.T., Hernando-Monge, E., Mu, D.,Goodson, S., Powers, S., Cordon-Cardo, C., Lowe, S.W., Hannon, G.J., & Hammond, S.M.(2005). A microRNA polycistron as a potential human oncogene. *Nature,* 435: 828-833.

He, P., Naka, T., Serada, S., Fujimoto, M., Tanaka, T., Hashimoto, S., Shima, Y., Yamadori, T., Suzuki, H., Hirashima, T., Matsui, K., Shiono, H., Okumura, M., Nishida, T.,Tachibana, I., Norioka, N., Norioka, S., & Kawase, I. (2007). Proteomics-based Identification of alpha-enolase as a tumor antigen in non-small lung cancer.*Cancer Sci,* 98: 1234-1240

He, X.Y., Liu, B.Y., Yao, W.Y., Zhao, X.J., Zheng, Z., Li, J.F., Yu, B.Q., & Yuan, Y.Z. (2011). Serum DJ-1 as a diagnostic marker and prognostic factor for pancreatic cancer. *J Dig Dis,* 12(2):131-7.

Heidemann, J., Binion, D.G., Domschke, W., & Kucharzik, T. (2006). Antiangiogenic therapy in human gastrointestinal malignancies. *Gut,* 55:1497–1511.

Hermann, P.C., Huber, S.L., Herrler, T., Aicher, A., Ellwart, J.W., Guba, M., Bruns, C.J., & Heeschen, C. (2007). Distinct populations of cancer stem cells determine tumor growth and metastatic activity in human pancreatic cancer. *Cell Stem Cell*, 1(3):313-323.

Hibi, T., Mori, T., Fukuma, M., Yamazaki, K., & Hashiguchi, A. (2009). Synucleingamma is closely involved in perineural invasion and distant metastasis in mouse models and is a novel prognostic factor in pancreatic cancer. *Clin Cancer Res*, 15: 2864–2871.

Hilton, J. (1984). Role of aldehyde dehydrogenase in cyclophosphamide-resistantL1210 leukemia. *Cancer Res*, 44(11):5156-5160.

Huang, E.H., Hynes, M.J., Zhang, T., Ginestier, C., Dontu, G., Appelman, H., Fields, J.Z., Wicha, M.S., & Boman, B.M. (2009). Aldehyde dehydrogenase 1 is a marker for normal and malignant human colonic stem cells (SC) and tracks SC overpopulation during colon tumorigenesis. *Cancer Res*, 69(8):3382-3389.

Huang, H., Dong, X.,& Kang, M.X.(2010). Novel blood biomarkers of pancreatic cancer-associated diabetes mellitus identified by peripheral blood-based gene expression profiles. *Am J Gastroenterol*, 105:1661-1669 .

Ito, S., Honma, T., Ishida, K., Wada, N., Sasaoka, S., Hosoda, M., & Nohno, T. (2007). Differential expression of the human alpha-enolase gene in oral epithelium and squamous cell carcinoma. *Cancer Sci*, 98: 499-505.

Jenuwein, T., & Allis, C.D. (2001). "Translating the histone code". *Science* ,293 (5532): 1074–80.

Jia, T., Liu, Y.E., Liu, J., & Shi, Y.E. (1999). Stimulation of breast cancer invasion and metastasis by synuclein gamma. *Cancer Res* , 59: 742–747.

Jiang, F., Qiu, Q., Khanna, A., Todd, N.W., Deepak, J., Xing, L., Wang, H., Liu, Z., Su, Y., & Stass, S.A. (2009). Aldehyde dehydrogenase 1 is a tumor stem cellassociated marker in lung cancer. *Mol Cancer Res* , 7(3):330-338.

Jiang, N., Meng, Y., Zhang, S., Mensah-Osman, E., & Sheng, S. (2002). Maspin sensitizes breast carcinoma cells to induced apoptosis. *Oncogene*, 21:4089-4098.

Kahlert, C., Bergmann, F., Beck, J., Welsch, T., Mogler, C., Herpel, E., Dutta, S., Niemietz, T., Koch, M., & Weitz, J. (2011). Low expression of aldehyde deyhdrogenase 1A1 (ALDH1A1) is a prognostic marker for poor survival in pancreatic cancer .*BMC Cancer*, 27;11:275.

Kashima, K., Ohike, N., Mukai, S., Sato, M., Takahashi, M., & Morohoshi, T.(2008). Expression of the tumor suppressor gene maspin and its significance in intraductal papillary mucinous neoplasms of the pancreas. *Hepatobiliary Pancreat. Dis. Int*, 7 (1) 86–90.

Katayama, M., Nakano, H., Ishiuchi, A., Wu, W., Oshima, R., Sakurai, J., Nishikawa, H., Yamaguchi, S., & Otsubo, T. (2006). Protein pattern difference in the colon cancer cell lines examined by two-dimensional differential in-gel electrophoresis and mass spectrometry. *Surg Today*, 36: 1085-1093.

Kong, W., Yang, H., He, L., Zhao, J.J., Coppola, D., Dalton, W.S., & Cheng, J.Q. (2008). MicroRNA-155 is regulated by the transforming growth factor beta/Smad pathway and contributes to epithelial cell plasticity by targeting RhoA. *Mol Cell Biol*, 28: 6773-6784.

Kroep, J.R., Loves, W.J.P., Wilt, C.L., Alvarez, E., Talianidis, I., Boven, E., Braakhuis, B.J., van Groeningen, C.J., Pinedo, H.M., & Peters, G.J. (2002). Pretreatment deoxycytidine kinase levels predict in vivo gemcitabine sensitivity. *Mol Cancer Ther,* 1:371-376.

Lehmann, U., Hasemeier, B., Christgen, M., Muller, M., Romermann, D., Langer, F., & Kreipe, H. (2008). Epigenetic inactivation of microRNA gene hsa-mir-9-1 in human breast cancer. *J Pathol* , 214:17-24.

Lei, W., Hai-Lin, L., Ya, L., & Ping Y. (2011). Proteomic analysis of pancreatic intraepithelial neoplasia and pancreatic carcinoma in rat models. *World J Gastroenterol,* 17(11): 1434-1441.

Li, A., Omura, N., Hong, S.M., Vincent, A., Walter, K., Griffith, M., Borges, M.,& Goggins, M.(2010). Pancreatic cancers epigenetically silence SIP1and hypomethylate and overexpress miR- 200a/200b in association with elevated circulating miR-200a and miR-200b levels.*Cancer Res,* 70: 5226–5237.

Li, C., Heidt, D.G., Dalerba, P., Burant, C.F., Zhang, L., Adsay, V., Wicha, M., Clarke, M.F., Simeone, D.M.(2007). Identification of pancreatic cancer stem cells. *Cancer Res,* 67(3):1030-1037.

Li, D., Yan, D., Tang, H., Zhou, C., Fan, J., Li, S., Wang, X., Xia, J., Huang, F., Qiu, G., & Peng, Z. (2009). IMP3 is a novel prognostic marker that correlates with colon cancer progression and pathogenesis. *Ann Surg Oncol,* 16(12):3499-506.

Li, Z., Sclabas, G.M., Peng, B., Hess, K.R., & Abbruzzese, J.L. (2004). Overexpression of synuclein-gamma in pancreatic adenocarcinoma. *Cancer,* 101: 58–65.

Liang, J.J., Kimchi, E.T., Staveley-O'Carroll, K.F. & Tan, D. (2009) Diagnostic and prognostic biomarkers in pancreatic carcinoma. *Int J Clin Exp Pathol,* 2:1-10

Locker, G.Y., Hamilton, S., Harris, J., Jessup, J.M., Kemeny, N., Macdonald, J.S., Somerfield, M.R., Hayes, D.F., Bast, R.C. Jr.; ASCO (2006) ASCO update of recommendations for the use of tumor markers in gastrointestinal cancer. *J Clin Oncol,* 24:5313-5327.

Matsuo, Y. & Kamitani, T. (2010) Parkinson's disease-related protein, alpha-synuclein, in malignant melanoma. *PLoS One,* 5(5):e1048.

Mesarosova, A., Hrivnakova, A.& Babusikova, O. (1993) Acute myeloid leukemia:correlation between purine metabolism enzyme activities and membrane immunophenotype. *Neoplasma,* 40: 341–345.

Metzler, M., Wilda, M., Busch, K., Viehmann, S. & Borkhardt, A.(2004) High expression of precursor microRNA-155/BIC RNA in children with Burkitt lymphoma. *Genes Chromosomes Cancer,* 39: 167-169.

Mikuriya, K., Kuramitsu, Y., Ryozawa, S., Fujimoto, M., Mori, S., Oka, M., Hamano, K., Okita, K., Sakaida, I. & Nakamura, K. (2007) Expression of glycolytic enzymes is increased in pancreatic cancerous tissues as evidenced by proteomic profiling by two-dimensional electrophoresis and liquid chromatography-mass spectrometry/mass spectrometry. *Int J Oncol,* 30: 849-855.

Mitchell, P.S., Parkin, R.K., Kroh, E.M., Fritz, B.R., Wyman, S.K., Pogosova-Agadjanyan, E.L., Peterson, A., Noteboom, J., O'Briant, K.C., Allen, A., Lin, D.W., Urban, N., Drescher, C.W., Knudsen, B.S., Stirewalt, D.L., Gentleman, R., Vessella, R.L., Nelson, P.S., Martin, D.B. &Tewari, M. (2008) Circulating microRNAs as stable blood-based markers for cancer detection. *Proc Natl Acad Sci USA;* 105: 10513–10518.

Miyazawa, Y., Uekita, T., Hiraoka, N., Fujii, S., Kosuge, T., Kanai, Y., Nojima, Y. & Sakai, R.(2010) CUB domain-containing protein 1, a prognostic factor for human pancreatic cancers, promotes cell migration and extracellular matrix degradation. *Cancer Res*, 70: 5136– 5146.

Mo, J.S., Jung, J., Yoon, J.H., Hong, J.A. & Kim, M.Y. (2010)DJ-1 modulates the p38 mitogen-activated protein kinase pathway through physical interaction with apoptosis signal-regulating kinase 1. *J Cell Biochem.*, 110(1):229-37.

Morgan, J., Hoekstra, A.V., Chapman-Davis, E., Hardt, J.L. & Kim, J.J. (2009). Synuclein-gamma (SNCG) may be a novel prognostic biomarker in uterine papillary serous carcinoma. *Gynecol Oncol*, 114: 293–298.

Morimoto, K., Kim, S.J., Tanei, T., Shimazu, K., Tanji, Y., Taguchi, T., Tamaki, Y., Terada, N. & Noguchi, S. (2009). Stem cell marker aldehyde dehydrogenase 1-positive breast cancers are characterized by negative estrogen receptor, positive human epidermal growth factor receptor type 2, and high Ki67 expression. *Cancer Sci*, 100(6):1062-1068.

Morris, K.V., Chan, S.W., Jacobsen, S.E. & Looney, D.J. (2004). Small interfering RNA-induced transcriptional gene silencing in human cells. *Science*, 305:1289-1292.

Nakahira, S., Nakamori, S., Tsujie, M., Takahashi, Y., Okami, J., Yoshioka, S., Yamasaki, M., Marubashi, S., Takemasa, I., Miyamoto, A., Takeda, Y., Nagano, H., Dono, K., Umeshita, K., Sakon, M. & Monden, M. (2006). Involvement of ribonucleotide reductase M1 subunit overexpression in gemcitabine resistance of human pancreatic cancer. *Int J Cancer.*, 120(6):1355-1363.

Nakano Y, Tanno S, Koizumi K, Nishikawa T, Nakamura K, Minoguchi M, Izawa, T Mizukami, Y., Okumura, T. & Kohgo, Y. (2007) Gemcitabine chemoresistance and molecular markers associated with gemcitabine transport and metabolism in human pancreatic cancer cells. *Br J Cancer* 2007, 96:457-463

Niedergethmann, M., Hildenbrand, R., Wolf, G., Verbeke, C.S., Richter, A. & Post, S. (2000). Angiogenesis and cathepsin expression are prognostic factors in pancreatic adenocarcinoma after curative resection. *Int. J. Pancreatol.* 28:31–39.

Ohuchida, K., Mizumoto, K., Egami, T., Yamaguchi, H., Fujii, K., Konomi, H., Nagai, E., Yamaguchi, K., Tsuneyoshi, M.& Tanaka, M. (2006). S100P is an early developmental marker of pancreatic carcinogenesis. *Clin Cancer Res*, 12:5411–5416.

Okami, J., Simeone, D.M. & Logsdon, C.D. (2004). Silencing of the hypoxia-inducible cell death protein BNIP3 in pancreatic cancer. *Cancer Res.*, Aug 1;64(15):5338-46

Omura N, Li CP, Li A, Hong SM, Walter K, Jimeno A, Hidalgo M and Goggins M. (2008) Genome wide profiling of methylated promoters in pancreatic adenocarcinoma. *Cancer Biol Ther*;7:1146-1156.

Ozdemir, N.O., Türk, N.S. & Düzcan, E. (2011). IMP3 expression in urothelial carcinomas of the urinary bladder. *Turk Patoloji Derg.*, 27(1):31-7.

Polymeropoulos, M.H., Lavedan, C., Leroy, E., Ide, S.E. & Dehejia, A. (1997). Mutation in the alpha-synuclein gene identified in families with Parkinson's disease. *Science*, 276: 2045–2047.

Prasad,A.S. & Kucuk O. (2002). Zinc in Cancer Prevention. *Cancer Metastasis Reviews*, 21(3-4): 291-295.

Rachagani, S., Kumar, S. & Batra, S.K. (2010). MicroRNA in pancreatic cancer: pathological, diagnostic and therapeutic implications. *Cancer Lett*, 292: 8–16.

Rasheed, Z.A., Yang, J., Wang, Q., Kowalski, J., Freed, I., Murter, C., Hong, S.M., Koorstra, J.B., Rajeshkumar, N.V. & He, X. (2010). Prognostic significance of tumorigenic cells with mesenchymal features in pancreatic adenocarcinoma. *J Natl Cancer Inst* 102(5):340-351.

Rebours, V., Levy, P., Mosnier, J.F., Scoazec, J.Y. & Soubeyrand, M.S. (2010) Pathology analysis reveals that dysplastic pancreatic ductal lesions are frequent in patients with hereditary pancreatitis. *Clin Gastroenterol Hepatol.* 8(2):206-12.

Roberts, A.S., Campa, M.J., Gottlin, E.B., Jiang, C., Owzar, K., Kindler, H.L., Venook, A.P., Goldberg, R.M., O'Reilly, E.M. & Patz, E.F. (2011). Identification of potential prognostic biomarkers in patients with untreated, advanced pancreatic cancer from a phase 3 trial (cancer and leukemia group B 80303). *Cancer*, early on-line.

Roberts, E.L., Newton, R.P. & Axford, A.T. (2004). Plasma purine nucleoside phosphorylase in cancer patients. *Clin Chim Acta,* 344: 109–114.

Rocchi, A., Manara, M.C., Sciandra, M., Zambelli, D., Nardi, F., Nicoletti, G., Garofalo, C., Meschini, S., Astolfi A., Colombo, M.P., Lessnick, S.L., Picci, P. & Scotlandi, K. (2010). CD99 inhibits neural differentiation of human Ewing sarcoma cells and thereby contributes to oncogenesis. *J Clin Invest.*, 120(3):668-80.

Rohloff, J., Zinke, J., Schoppmeyer, K., Tannapfel, A., Witzigmann, H. & Mossner, J. (2002). Heparanase expression is a prognostic indicator for postoperative survival in pancreatic adenocarcinoma. *Br. J. Cancer*, 22:1270–1275.

Rosenfeld, J.A., Wang, Z., Schones, D.E., Zhao, K., DeSalle, R. & Zhang, M.Q. (2009). Determination of enriched histone modifications in non-genic portions of the human genome. *BMC Genomics*, 10: 143.

Rosty, C. & Goggins, M. (2002). Early detection of pancreatic carcinoma. *Hematol Oncol Clin North Am*, 16:37-52.

Sato, N., Fukushima, N., Maehara, N., Matsubayashi, H., Koopmann, J., Su, G.H., Hruban, R.H., Goggins & M. (2003). SPARC/osteonectin is a frequent target for aberrant methylation in pancreatic adenocarcinoma and a mediator of tumor-stromal interactions. *Oncogene*. 22(32):5021-30.

Sato, N., Maitra, A., Fukushima, N., van Heek, N.T., Matsubayashi, H., Iacobuzio-Donahue, C.A., Rosty, C. & Goggins, M. (2003). Frequent hypomethylation of multiple genes overexpressed in pancreatic ductal adenocarcinoma. *Cancer Res.*, 63(14):4158-66.

Sato, N., Matsubayashi, H., Abe, T., Fukushima, N. & Goggins, M. (2005). Epigenetic down-regulation of CDKN1C/p57KIP2 in pancreatic ductal neoplasms identified by gene expression profiling. *Clin Cancer Res.*, 11(13):4681-8.

Sato, N., Parker, A.R., Fukushima, N., Miyagi, Y., Iacobuzio-Donahue, C.A., Eshleman, J.R., Goggins, M. (2005). Epigenetic inactivation of TFPI-2 as a common mechanism associated with growth and invasion of pancreatic ductal adenocarcinoma. *Oncogene.*, 24(5):850-8.

Schutte, M., Hruban, R.H., Geradts, J., Maynard, R., Hilgers, W., Rabindran, S.K., Moskaluk, C.A., Hahn, S.A., Schwarte-Waldhoff, I., Schmiegel, W., Baylin, S.B., Kern, S.E. & Herman, J.G. (1997). Abrogation of the Rb/p16 tumor-suppressive pathway in virtually all pancreatic carcinomas. *Cancer Res*; 57:3126-3130.

Sebastiani, V., Ricci, F., Rubio-Viquiera, B., Kulesza, P., Yeo, C.J., Hidalgo, M., Klein, A., Laheru, D. & Iacobuzio-Donahue, C.A. (2006). Immunohistochemical and genetic evaluation of deoxycytidine kinase in pancreatic cancer: relationship to molecular mechanisms of gemcitabine resistance and survival. *Clin Cancer Res*, 12:2492-2497.

Shen, J., Person, M.D., Zhu, J., Abbruzzese, J.L. & Li, D. (2004). Protein expression profiles in pancreatic adenocarcinoma compared with normal pancreatic tissue and tissue affected by pancreatitis as detected by two-dimensional gel electrophoresis and mass spectrometry. *Cancer Res*, 64: 9018-9026.

Shimizu, H., Horii, A., Sunamura, M., Motoi, F., Egawa, S., Unno, M., Fukushige, S. Identification of epigenetically silenced genes in human pancreatic cancer by a novel method "microarray coupled with methyl-CpG targeted transcriptional activation" (MeTA-array) (2011) .*Biochem Biophys Res Commun.*, early on line.

Singleton, A.B., Farrer, M., Johnson, J., Singleton, A., & Hague, S. (2003) alpha- Synuclein locus triplication causes Parkinson's disease. *Science*, 302: 841.

Sood, P., Krek, A., Zavolan, M., Macino, G. & Rajewsky, N. (2006). Cell type-specific signatures of microRNAs on target mRNA expression. *Proc Natl Acad Sci USA*, 103: 2746-2751.

Sparmann, A. & van Lohuizen, M. (2006). Polycomb silencers control cell fate, development and cancer. *Nat Rev Cancer*.6:846–856.

Strahl, B.D.& Allis, C.D. (2000). The language of covalent histone modifications. *Nature* 403 (6765): 41–5.

Sugimoto, M., Wong, D.T., Hirayama, A, Soga, T. & Tomita, M. (2010) Capillary electrophoresis mass spectrometry-based saliva metabolomics identified oral, breast and pancreatic cancer specific profiles. *Metabolomics*; 6: 78–95.

Szafranska, A.E., Doleshal, M., Edmunds, H.S., Gordon, S., Luttges, J., Munding, J.B., Barth, R.J.Jr., Gutmann, E.J., Suriawinata, A.A., Marc Pipas, J., Tannapfel, A., Korc, M., Hahn, S.A., Labourier, E. & Tsongalis, G.J. (2008). Analysis of microRNAs in pancreatic fine needle aspirates can classify benign and malignant tissues. *Clin Chem*. 54: 1716-1724.

Takayama, R., Nakagawa, H., Sawaki, A. Takayama R, Nakagawa H, Sawaki A, Mizuno N, Kawai H, Tajika M, Yatabe Y, Matsuo K, Uehara R, Ono K, Nakamura Y, &Yamao K (2010). Serum tumor antigen REG4 as a diagnostic biomarker in pancreatic ductal adenocarcinoma. *J Gastroenterol* , 45, 52-59

Tanase C.P., Neagu, M., Albulescu, R., Hinescu, M.E.(2010). Advances in pancreatic cancer detection. *Adv Clin Chem.*, 51:145-80.

Tănase, C.P., Raducan, E., Dima, S. O., Albulescu, L., Alina, I., Marius, P., Cruceru, L. M., Codorean, E., Neagu, T.M. & Popescu I. (2008). Assessment of soluble angiogenic markers in pancreatic cancer. *Biomarkers in Medicine*, 2(5):447-455.

Tobita, K., Kijima, H., Dowaki, S., Oida, Y., Kashiwagi, H. & Ishii, M. (2002). Thrombospondin-1 expression as a prognostic predictor of pancreatic ductal carcinoma, *Int. J. Oncol.*, 21, 1189–1195

Toll, A.D., Witkiewicz,A.K. & Bibbo, M. (2009). Expression of K homology domain containing protein (KOC) in pancreatic cytology with corresponding histology, *Acta Cytol.*, 53, (2), 123–129

Ueki, T, Toyota, M., Skinner, H., Walter, K.M., Yeo, C.J., Issa, J.P., Hruban, R.H. & Goggins, M. (2001). Identification and characterization of differentially methylated CpG islands in pancreatic carcinoma. *Cancer Res.*, 61(23), 8540-8546.

van den Bemd, G.J., Krijgsveld. J, Luider. T.M., van Rijswijk, A.L., Demmers, J.A. & Jenster, G. (2006). Mass spectrometric identificationof human prostate cancer-derived proteins in serum of xenograft-bearing mice. *Mol Cell Proteomics,* 5,1830-1839.

van Duijn CM, Dekker MC, Bonifati V, Galjaard RJ, Houwing-Duistermaat JJ, Snijders PJ, Testers L, Breedveld GJ, Horstink M, Sandkuijl LA, van Swieten JC, Oostra BA & Heutink P. (2001) Park7, a novel locus for autosomal recessive early-onset parkinsonism, on chromosome 1p36. *Am J Hum Genet,* 69, 629–634,

Vareed, S.K., Bhat, V.B., Thompson, C., Vasu, V.T., Fermin, D., Choi, H., Creighton, C.J., Gayatri, S., Lan, L., Putluri, N., Thangjam, G.S., Kaur, P., Shabahang, M., Giri, J.G., Nesvizhskii, A.I., Asea, A.A., Cashikar, A.G., Rao, A., McLoughlin, J. & Sreekumar, A. (2011). Metabolites of purine nucleoside phosphorylase (NP) in serum have the potential to delineate pancreatic adenocarcinoma. *PLoS One.*, 23, 6(3),e17177.

Vincent, A., Ducourouble, M.P. & Van Seuningen, I. (2008). Epigenetic regulation of the human mucin gene MUC4 in epithelial cancer cell lines involves both DNA methylation and histone modifications mediated by DNA methyltransferases and histone deacetylases. *Faseb J.* 22, 3035–3045.

Vire, E., Brenner, C., Deplus, R., Blanchon, L., Fraga, M., Didelot, C., Morey, L., Van Eynde, A., Bernard, D., Vanderwinden, J.M., Bollen, M., Esteller, M., Di Croce, L., de Launoit, Y. & Fuks, F. (2006). The Polycomb group protein EZH2 directly controls DNA methylation. *Nature.* , 439, 871–874.

Volinia, S., Calin, G.A., Liu, C.G., Ambs, S., Cimmino, A., Petrocca, F., Visone, R., Iorio, M., Roldo, C., Ferracin, M., Prueitt, R.L., Yanaihara, N., Lanza, G., Scarpa, A., Vecchione, A., Negrini, M., Harris, C.C. & Croce, C.M. (2006). A microRNA expression signature of human solid tumors defines cancer gene targets. *Proc Natl Acad Sci U S A.* 103(7), 2257-2261.

Wachter, D.L., Schlabrakowski, A., Hoegel, J., Kristiansen, G., Hartmann, A. & Riener, M.O. (2011). Diagnostic value of immunohistochemical IMP3 expression in core needle biopsies of pancreatic ductal adenocarcinoma. Am J Surg Pathol., 35(6), 873-877.

Walter, O., Prasad, M., Lu, S., Quinlan, R.M., Edmiston, K.L., & Khan, A. I. (2009). MP3 is a novel biomarker for triple negative invasive mammary carcinoma associated with a more aggressive phenotype. Hum Pathol. , 40(11), 1528-1533

Woodward, W.A. & Sulman E.P.(2008). Cancer stem cells: markers or biomarkers? *Cancer and Metastasis Reviews,* 27(3): 459-470.

Yamada, N., Nishida, Y., Tsutsumida, H., Hamada, T., Goto, M., Higashi, M., Nomoto, M. & Yonezawa, S. (2008) MUC1 expression is regulated by DNA methylation and histone H3 lysine 9 modification in cancer cells. *Cancer Res,*.68:2708–2716

Yanaihara, N., Caplen, N., Bowman, E., Seike, M., Kumamoto, K., Yi, M., Stephens, R.M., Okamoto, A., Yokota, J., Tanaka, T., Calin, G.A., Liu, C.G., Croce, C.M. & Harris, C.C. (2006).Unique microRNA molecular profiles in lung cancer diagnosis and prognosis. *Cancer Cell.*, 9, 189-198

Ye, Q., Feng, B., Peng, Y.F., Chen, X.H., Cai, Q., Yu, B.Q., Li, L.H., Qiu, M.Y., Liu, B.Y. & Zheng, M.H. (2009). Expression of gammasynuclein in colorectal cancer tissues and its role on colorectal cancer cell line HCT116. *World J Gastroenterol.,* 15: 5035-5043.

Yin, Q., Wang, X., McBride, J., Fewell, C. & Flemington, E. (2008). B-cell receptor activation induces BIC/miR-155 expression through a conserved AP-1 element. *J Biol Chem* , 283, 2654-2662

Yoshida, A., Rzhetsky, A., Hsu, L.C. &Chang, C. (1998). Human aldehyde dehydrogenase gene family. Eur J Biochem , 251(3), 549-557

Zhang, L., Farrell, J.J., Zhou, H., Elashoff, D., Akin, D., Park, N.H., Chia, D., Wong, D.T.(2010). Salivary transcriptomic biomarkers for detection of resectable pancreatic cancer. *Gastroenterology,* 138:949–957.

Zhao, J., Chang, A.C., Li ,C., Shedden, K.A., Thomas DG, Misek, D.E., Manoharan, A.P., Giordano, T.J., Beer, D.G., Lubman, D.M. (2007). Comparative proteomics analysis of Barrett metaplasia and esophageal adenocarcinoma using two-dimensional liquid mass mapping. *Mol Cell Proteomics*, 6, 987-999

4

Medical Therapy of Pancreatic Cancer: Current Status and Future Targets

Edward Livshin[1] and Michael Michael[2]
[1]*Division of Cancer Medicine, Peter MacCallum Cancer Centre, Victoria,*
[2]*Division of Cancer Medicine, Upper GI Oncology Service, Peter MacCallum Cancer Centre, University of Melbourne, Victoria, Australia*

1. Introduction

Pancreatic cancer is a major cause of cancer-related mortality relative to its incidence. In the US alone, it is estimated that there were 43,140 new cases in 2010 with 36,800 deaths making it the fourth leading cause of cancer-related mortality.[1]

Typically patients come to clinical attention at an advanced stage of their disease with only 10-15% having potentially operable disease. Surgery is the only established method shown to cure pancreatic adenocarcinoma, yet the rate of cure amongst patients with resectable disease still remains low. Improvements in survival with the addition of chemotherapy or radiotherapy have only been relatively modest.

The medical management of pancreatic cancer in the adjuvant and advanced settings will be reviewed. The current standard of care in both settings is gemcitabine, with modest improvements in survival provided by the addition of erlotinib in the advanced setting. Despite arguably poor evidence for added survival benefit from combination cytotoxic regimens or other biological agents in the advanced setting, recent evidence for considering this in select patients will be discussed, along with a recent non-gemcitabine containing combination cytotoxic approach (FOLFIRINOX), that has challenged the traditional paradigm.

Some of the important molecular signaling pathways involved in pancreatic cancer growth, invasion, angiogenesis, metastasis, and drug resistance will also be summarised. It is hoped that in future, survival outcomes may be improved by better targeting of these pathways in the individual patient, aided by appropriate predictive and prognostic biomarkers.

2. Chemotherapy and chemoradiotherapy in resected pancreatic cancer

There is an established survival advantage with adjuvant systemic therapy in pancreatic cancer. Adjuvant systemic therapy can be delivered either solely, or in combination with radiotherapy following pancreatic resection, however the role of the latter is more controversial, and will be briefly summarised. *A further discussion of radiotherapy and its role in the neoadjuvant and adjuvant setting is discussed elsewhere.*

2.1 Adjuvant chemoradiotherapy compared with surgery alone

A Gastrointestinal Study Group (GITSG) trial assessed the role of concurrent post-operative radiotherapy and radiosensitising bolus 5-fluorouracil (5-FU) compared with surgery alone.[2]

Patients were randomised to a split-course of radiotherapy in combination with bolus 5-FU compared with post-operative observation alone. Chemotherapy was given at 500mg/m^2 per day over the first three days of each course of radiotherapy. Patients were given 20 Gray (Gy) in 10 fractions followed by a 14 day break, then a further course of radiotherapy up to a dose of 40Gy. Although demonstrating a median overall survival of 21 months vs. 11 months (p=0.035) favouring the chemoradiotherapy group, criticisms include small patient numbers (43 patients), a slow patient accrual of 8 years, and selection bias where only a more prognostically favourable group of patients with microscopically clear (R0 resection) margins, were included in the study. A later GITSG analysis[3] of an additional 30 patients - all treated with adjuvant combined therapy - showed a median overall survival of 18 months.

The larger European Organization of Research and Treatment of Cancer (EORTC) 40891 study[4] however only showed a non-statistically significant trend towards an improved overall survival with chemoradiotherapy in a subgroup of 114 out of 218 patients with carcinoma of the pancreatic head. The median overall survival was 17.1 months vs. 12.6 months in the observation alone arm (p = 0.099). 5-FU delivery here was given as bolus daily doses at 25mg/kg up to 1,500mg/day, days 1-7 of each course of radiotherapy. There were two courses of radiotherapy given up to a total of 40Gy. EORTC 40891 included patients with T1 or T2 disease, and allowed patients with node-positive (N1) disease. 45% however had T1-3 periampullary disease. Shortcomings included the lack of maintenance chemotherapy, a significant (20%) of patients not proceeding with combination therapy and the large percentage of patients with periampullary cancers affecting the interpretation of outcome in pancreatic cancer.

The largest body of evidence has come from The European Study Group for Pancreatic Cancer (ESPAC) publishing the results the ESPAC-1 trial in 2004.[5] This study employing a 2x2 factorial design allowed a comparison between adjuvant radiotherapy or no radiotherapy, chemotherapy or no chemotherapy, and chemoradiotherapy vs. chemotherapy alone. Chemoradiotherapy was given as two courses of 20Gy separated by 14 days, combined with bolus 5-FU (500mg/m^2) given for three days during each course. Following this, patients continued with a maintenance course of chemotherapy with 5FU/leucovorin (LV). Chemotherapy was given as bolus 5-FU (425mg/m^2) with LV (20mg/m^2) days 1-5 every 28 days, for a total of six cycles. 53% of patients had nodal involvement and 19% had involved margins. Patients who received chemotherapy compared with those who did not, survived a median of 20.6 months vs. 15.5 months (HR 0.71; 95% CI, 0.55-0.92 p=0.009). Patients who received chemoradiotherapy survived a median of only 15.9 months vs. 17.9 months in those who did not receive chemoradiotherapy (HR 1.28 ; 95% CI, 0.99-1.66 p=0.05). Notably, 2 and 5 year survival rates of patients who received chemotherapy alone improved from 30 to 40% and 8 to 12% when compared to those who did not receive chemotherapy. Therefore in this analysis, patients did not benefit from a combined modality approach, and in fact their outcome appeared to be worse. Based on the results of ESPAC-1 it was difficult to justify the role of adjuvant chemoradiotherapy over chemotherapy with bolus 5-FU alone.

The question of incorporating infusional 5-FU and gemcitabine into adjuvant radiotherapy has been addressed in the Radiation Therapy Oncology Group (RTOG) 9704 trial.[6] This was a phase III trial of 442 patients with pathological T1-4 and nodal stage N0-1 pancreatic cancer. Participants were randomised to either adjuvant chemotherapy with either weekly 5-FU or gemcitabine three weeks prior and for 12 weeks post chemoradiotherapy sandwiched in between. Radiotherapy was delivered at a dose of 50.4Gy (at 1.8 Gy/fraction/day) concurrent with continuous infusional 5-FU at 250mg/m^2/day. Most patients (n= 381) had tumours confined to the pancreatic head. More patients with stage T3 and 4 disease received gemcitabine and more grade 4 haematologic toxicity was experienced in the gemcitabine arm (14% vs. 2%). Rates of treatment completion were comparable. Although no overall survival advantage of gemcitabine over 5-FU was seen if all pancreatic lesions were included, the subgroup of patients with pancreatic head tumours assigned to the gemcitabine group had a trend toward a more favourable survival (20.5 months vs. 16.9 months with a hazard ratio (HR) for death of 0.82; 95% CI, 0.65-1.03; p = 0.09). The 3-year rate of survival was also higher (31 vs. 21%) also favouring the gemcitabine group.

2.2 Adjuvant chemotherapy strategies

Older adjuvant cytotoxic regimes such as the triplet of doxorubicin, mitomycin and 5-fluorouracil (AMF) for six cycles to treat pancreatic and papillary cancers showed no overall survival advantage beyond two years, although there was a 1 and 2 year relapse-free survival advantage favouring chemotherapy over surgery alone.[7]

In addition to the survival advantage shown ESPAC-1, the Charité Onkologie (CONKO-001) study[8] published in 2007 demonstrated a survival benefit with adjuvant gemcitabine over surgery alone. Patients with R0 or R1 resections were assigned to observation alone or gemcitabine delivered at 1000mg/m^2/week (days 1, 8 and 15 of a 28 day cycle) for a total of six cycles. There was a trend toward an improved median overall survival (22.8 vs. 20.2 months p=0.06) as well as a statistically significant improvement in disease-free survival (13.4 vs. 6.9 months p <0.001) over surgery alone. Importantly the rate of 5-year survival was significantly better in those patients receiving adjuvant gemcitabine over observation alone (21% vs. 9%).

In the largest adjuvant pancreatic trial to date, ESPAC-3[9-10] involved 1088 patients with R0- or R1 resected pancreatic adenocarcinoma, randomising patients into either observation alone, 5-FU/LV, or gemcitabine. Notably the 5-FU was delivered as five bolus doses (425mg/m^2 with leucovorin 20mg/m^2 days 1-5 of a 28 day cycle) rather than as an infusion. 551 patients received 5-FU and 537 received gemcitabine with treatment for a total of six months. The observational arm was discontinued after the outcome of the CONKO-001 trial was made available. At a median follow up of 34.2 months after 753 deaths, there was no advantage seen between the intervention arms (23.0 vs. 23.6 months p=0.39). 12 and 24 month survival was 78.5% and 48.1% respectively in those who received 5-FU with 80.1%

and 49.1% respectively in the gemcitabine arm. The side effect profile however favoured gemcitabine in terms of grade 3-4 toxicity and hospitalisation. Grade 3 and 4 mucositis was seen in 10% of patients who received 5-FU (compared with no patients on gemcitabine). Grade 3-4 diarrhoea was also significantly higher in the 5-FU group. The gemcitabine treated group did however experience higher rates of grade 3 and 4 thrombocytopenia, although the absolute risk of this remained small (1.5 vs. 0%) (p=0.003). Quality-of-life was also comparable.

Thus, survival outcomes were not significantly improved by gemcitabine over 5-FU group in ESPAC-3. This outcome differs to that seen in the advanced setting.[13] One reason could be that the 5-FU intensity was greater in ESPAC-3 than that seen in the Burris *et al.* trial.

2.3 Recommendations

Adjuvant chemotherapy in resected pancreatic cancer is the standard of care, yet the role of chemoradiotherapy remains controversial. Gemcitabine for six cycles is preferable over 5-FU based treatment due to its more favourable toxicity profile. Although modest improvements in median survival have been shown, progression-free and 5-year survival rates are improved.

3. Medical therapy of locally advanced and metastatic disease: First-line strategies

3.1 Single-agent chemotherapy

5-fluorouracil (5-FU), capecitabine, and gemcitabine

5-fluorouracil (5-FU) has been used for half a century in advanced pancreatic cancer.[11] As a single agent, objective responses rates have typically been less than 10% with some historical data reporting higher response rates probably based on cruder estimations of disease burden such as physical examination and ultrasound. Typically responses were usually for less than six months.

Capecitabine is an oral fluoropyrimidine prodrug which is metabolised to 5-FU. A small phase II study[12] in patients with locally advanced or metastatic pancreatic cancer was performed in 42 patients at a dose of 1,250mg/m^2 given twice a day in 3-week cycles, with 2 weeks of treatment followed by a 1-week break. Disease response evaluation was based on either computerised tomography (CT) or physical examination. Of the 41 patients with evaluable disease the objective response rate (ORR) was 7.3% (3 patients), with 41% having stable disease. 38% had progressive disease within the first 7 weeks. Median survival was quoted at 182 days (95% CI, 85-274 days). 52% of patients developed hand-foot syndrome (HFS) (41% Grade 2-3) and 48 % had nausea (24% Grade 2-3). 12% had grades 2-3 mucositis.

The randomised trial leading to the acceptance of gemcitabine as standard therapy in advanced pancreatic cancer was published in 1997.[13] This study compared gemcitabine with bolus weekly 5-FU. Gemcitabine was favoured over 5-FU with a modest improvement in median survival (5.7 vs. 4.4 months, p=0.0025). More significantly, the rate of 1-yr survival was improved (18% vs. 2%), and importantly the rate of clinical symptom improvement (measured by at least four weeks of improvement in either pain, reduced analgesic use, improved weight loss or performance status) favoured the gemcitabine arm (24% vs. 5%).

3.2 Combination chemotherapy and epidermal growth factor receptor (EGFR) inhibition

Gemcitabine/erlotinib

Gemcitabine/other EGFR inhibitor combinations

Erlotinib, an oral tyrosine kinase inhibitor (TKI) of the epidermal growth factor receptor (EGFR), has to date been the only EGFR inhibitor combined with a cytotoxic to show, an albeit modest, survival advantage in a phase III study. [14] It was evaluated with gemcitabine in patients with locally advanced or metastatic disease. Patients received either gemcitabine at 1000mg/m^2 (weekly for 7 out of 8 weeks) then continued with weekly treatment (in 3 out of 4 weeks), or the equivalent strategy combined with erlotinib at 100mg or 150mg per day. The latter dose was provided to a cohort of Canadian patients. Median overall survival improved with the combination approach of erlotinib with gemcitabine, compared with gemcitabine alone [(6.24 months versus 5.91 months; HR 0.82 (95% CI, 0.69 to 0.99; P = 0.038)]. The superiority of 150mg erlotinib over 100mg was not proven. One could argue that the benefit on overall survival is not economically justified, however with a 1-year survival rate improvement from 17 to 23% (95% CI, 18% to 28%, 95% CI, 12% to 21%, P = 0.023), this has become an acceptable standard of care in many centres.

Gefitinib, another EGFR inhibitor TKI has less evidence, but was evaluated in combination with gemcitabine in a phase II study[15] which reported either disease stability or response in 18/53 patients. The median progression-free survival was 4.1 months and median overall survival was 7.3 months. The reported 1-year survival rate was 27%.

Phase II and III studies combining other EGFR inhibitors such as cetuximab[16] or lapatinib (a dual HER2/EGFR inhibitor)[17] in combination with gemcitabine have not provided an additional survival advantage. Similarly a trial adding cetuximab to a gemcitabine/ cisplatin doublet did not progress beyond a phase II trial, as time to progression was equivalent at 5 months, despite a higher disease control rate.[18] Dual EGFR inhibition with erlotinib and panitumumab has recently been examined in a randomised phase II study, with a modest 3.3 vs. 2.0 month PFS advantage, though mature survival data and statistical significance has not been published to date[19].

The role of erlotinib incorporated into the management of patients with locally advanced disease is being evaluated in the Groupe Cooperateur Multidisciplinaire en Oncologie (GERCOR) LAP07 phase III trial.[20] Patients are randomised initially to either induction gemcitabine or gemcitabine/erlotinib. In those patients who do not progress after four months, there is a secondary randomisation into a chemotherapy (with either gemcitabine or gemcitabine/erlotinib), or a chemoradiotherapy arm (with concurrent capecitabine) until tumour progression.

3.3 Combination chemotherapy: Gemcitabine-containing regimens

Gemcitabine/fluoropyrimidine doublets

Gemcitabine/platinum doublets

A number of gemcitabine-containing combinations with either fluoropyrimidines or platinum agents have been attempted. Individually these trials have not provided significant improvements in survival over gemcitabine alone. However subset-analyses of some of these trials, as well as a meta-analysis suggest that doublets may confer a meaningful survival improvement in the fittest patients with Karnofsky Performance Status (KPS) scores of 90% or above.[21]

Gemcitabine and 5-FU was examined in a phase III trial[22] which randomised 322 patients to a schedule of gemcitabine 1000mg/m^2 (three weeks out of four), with or without bolus 5FU 600mg/m^2/week), however did not produce a statistically significant improvement in overall survival compared with gemcitabine alone (6.7 vs. 5.4 months respectively p=0.09).

Gemcitabine and capecitabine was also examined in a phase III trial comparing a gemcitabine/capecitabine doublet with gemcitabine with previously untreated locally advanced or metastatic disease.[23] It suggested a significantly higher objective response rate (ORR) of 19.1% vs. 12.4%; (P = 0.034), as well as an improvement in progression-free survival (HR 0.78 95% CI, 0.66 to 0.93; P=0.004) favouring the doublet. However it only demonstrated a trend toward an improved overall survival (HR 0.86; 95% CI, 0.72 to 1.02; P=0.08). Another study of this combination also showed no significant difference in the primary end-point of overall survival [(8.4 months with the combination arm vs. 7.2 months with gemcitabine alone (p= 0.234)]. However a post-hoc subgroup analysis did reveal evidence for more favourable survival in the combination arm if performance status was better. Patients with KPS of 90-100% receiving combination therapy had a median overall survival of 10.1 vs. 7.4 months compared with gemcitabine alone (p= 0.014).[24]

Combination gemcitabine and cisplatin was assessed in 195 patients enrolled in a phase III trial comparing gemcitabine 1000mg/m^2 (days 1, 8 and 15 of a 28 day cycle) with gemcitabine 1000mg/m2 and cisplatin 50mg/m^2 (days 1 and 15). Tumour responses were similar in the combination (10.2%) vs. standard treatment arms (8.2%), with an improved progression-free survival and equivalent toxicity. However, despite a trend toward an improvement in overall survival (the primary endpoint of this study) within the combination arm (7.5 vs. 6.0 months), this did not reach statistical significance (p=0.15).[25]

Louvet *et al*[26] compared a combination gemcitabine/oxaliplatin doublet (GEMOX) with gemcitabine. Patients received either treatment with gemcitabine 1000mg/m^2 and oxaliplatin 100mg/m^2 every 2 weeks compared with weekly gemcitabine 1000mg/m^2. The combination was shown to improve response rates (26.8 vs. 17.3% respectively, P=0.04), as well as progression-free survival (5.8 vs. 3.7 months P=0.04). However differences in median overall survival were not statistically significant (9.0 vs. 7.1 months P= 0.13). The combination arm was associated with greater rates of grade 3-4 thrombocytopenia, vomiting and sensory neuropathy. Some patients received radiotherapy for local control at the oncologists' discretion after they had completed 3 months of systemic therapy. The overall survival data may have been influenced by a proportion of gemcitabine patients receiving platinum-containing second-line therapy, once they had progressed and were off study.

Gemcitabine in combination with irinotecan was assessed in a trial that randomised 360 patients to gemcitabine 1000mg/m^2 and irinotecan 100mg/m^2 on days 1 and 8 every 21 days or gemcitabine alone.[27] Rates of diarrhoea, nausea and vomiting were higher in the combination arm with no improvement in the overall survival.

3.4 Combination chemotherapy: Non-gemcitabine containing regimens

Irinotecan-docetaxel

FOLFIRINOX

An earlier non-gemcitabine containing regimen of irinotecan and docetaxel was examined in a phase II study randomising patients into two arms with or without cetuximab but response rates were 7 and 4.5% respectively. This did not meet a pre-determined goal to proceed to a phase III study.[28]

The recent French PRODIGE 4 (ACCORD 11) study[29] randomised 342 patients with metastatic pancreatic carcinoma, who had an Eastern Cooperative Oncology Group performance status score of 0 or 1, to either a regimen of gemcitabine (1000mg/m^2 weekly for 7 of 8 weeks followed by weekly treatment for 3 out of four weeks) or FOLFIRINOX. FOLFIRINOX patients received oxaliplatin (85mg/m^2), irinotecan (180mg/m^2), leucovorin (400mg/m^2), with bolus (400mg/m^2) then infusional (2400mg/m^2 over 46 hours) 5-FU. Treatment was delivered every two weeks. It is important to note that more patients in the FOLFIRINOX arm (42.5%) received granulocyte colony stimulating factor (G-CSF) support than those in the gemcitabine arm (5.3%).

Using overall survival as its primary end point, and with an intended treatment period of six months, FOLFIRINOX treated patients had an impressive median 11.1 month overall survival, compared with only 6.8 months in those treated with gemcitabine alone (HR for death, 0.57; 95% CI, 0.45 - 0.73; $p<0.001$). Progression-free survival was also superior (6.4 vs. 3.4 months (HR, 0.47; $P<0.0001$). Objective response rates were significantly higher in the FOLFIRINOX group (31.6%) compared with gemcitabine (9.4%) ($p<0.001$). This advantage was at the expense of higher rates of grade 3 or 4 neutropenia (febrile neutropenia of 5.4% vs. 0.6% $P=0.0001$), thrombocytopenia (9.1% vs. 2.4% $p=0.008$), neuropathy, diarrhoea and grade 2 alopecia. There was one toxicity-related death in each arm of the trial. Despite the increased toxicity, quality of life scores were more preserved at six months in the FOLFIRINOX-treated patients. This regimen is therefore being considered a suitable option for some patients, particularly those with a good performance status. A survey of US Oncologists recently revealed that 18% would now adopt FOLFIRINOX over a gemcitabine-erlotinib doublet in the first-line setting for patients with a performance status of ECOG 1.[30]

3.5 Recommendations

The standard of care in the first-line setting of advanced pancreatic cancer remains gemcitabine or gemcitabine with erlotinib for most patients. The alternative of 5-FU remains if gemcitabine is poorly tolerated. Those who are particularly fit with a performance status of ECOG 0-1, might be considered for a gemcitabine-platinum or a gemcitabine-capecitabine doublet (based on subset- and recent meta-analyses), or the non-gemcitabine regimen of FOLFIRINOX. Recent phase III evidence for the latter challenges the traditional paradigm of a gemcitabine-containing backbone, but it must be balanced with the higher risks of toxicity when recommending treatment. Enrolment in clinical trials should always be considered if possible.

4. Medical therapy of locally advanced and metastatic disease: Second-line strategies in gemcitabine-refractory disease

4.1 Oxaliplatin-based doublets

The strategy of continuing gemcitabine with the addition of oxaliplatin (GEMOX) was evaluated in patients who have progressed on gemcitabine alone in a phase II trial of 33 patients with locally advanced and metastatic disease.[31] A partial response was seen in 7 of the 31 patients with evaluable disease and stable disease for 2 months or more was seen in 11 patients. The median survival was 6 months.

Second-line combination oxaliplatin/5-FU was examined in the Charité Onkologie trial (CONKO-003).[32] This began as a phase III trial with the intention to compare a 5-FU-oxaliplatin doublet (the OFF regimen) with best supportive care (BSC).[33] The OFF regimen differs from FOLFOX being a 42-day cycle where infusional 5-FU (2000mg/m^2 over 24 hours) with bolus LV (200mg/m^2) is given days 1,8,15, and 22. Oxaliplatin (85mg/m^2) is given on days 8 and 22. The protocol was revised due to poor acceptance of the best supportive care arm and later altered to include a 5-FU/LV arm as the control. Despite this methodological alteration, the study when presented as an abstract, did show an improvement in overall survival from 13 to 26 weeks favouring the doublet arm.[33]

There is phase II evidence showing activity with a doublet of oxaliplatin and capecitabine in the gemcitabine-refractory setting.[34] In a study of 41 patients, capecitabine was given at 1000mg/m^2 BD days 1-14 with oxaliplatin 130mg/m^2 every 3 weeks (doses of 850mg/m^2 and 110mg/m^2 respectively were used in patients greater than 65). Reported median overall survival was 23 weeks (95% CI, 17.0-31.0) with a progression-free survival of 9.9 weeks (95% CI, 9.6-14.5 weeks). Six month and 1 year survival rates were 44% and 21% respectively (95% CI 31-62% and 11-38%). Another recent phase II study has also confirmed activity in a mixed cohort of patients with pancreatic and biliary tract carcinomas.[35]

4.2 Capecitabine/erlotinib

A phase II study of capecitabine (1000mg/m^2 BD days 1-14 of 21 day cycles) combined with erlotinib 150mg daily enrolled 32 patients.[36] The objective radiological response (ORR) was only 10% and median survival duration was 6.5months. 17% had CA 19-9 reductions of more than 50% of baseline. Diarrhoea, fatigue, rash and hand-foot syndrome were common toxicities. This has been suggested as an active first or second-line option, especially if gemcitabine is not tolerated.

4.3 Irinotecan – based therapy

Single agent irinotecan (150mg/m^2) given every 2 weeks has demonstrated activity in the second-line setting.[37] 33 patients were evaluated in a phase II study where 48% had either stable disease or a partial response. The median time to progression was 4 months. With combination 5-FU and irinotecan regimens, disease control rates of 44.3-50% with overall survivals of 6 months or more have been reported.[38] Some patients received this in the third-line setting. However, patients were highly selected and much of the data is retrospective.

Recently a nanoparticle liposomal encapsulated form of irinotecan (PEP02) was evaluated as a single agent in a phase II trial at 120mg/m^2 given every 2 weeks in 37 patients who had progressed on gemcitabine.[39] A 74% 3-month overall survival endpoint was reached with initial reports of a 52% disease control rate. However 31% and 25% of patients had grade 3 or more fatigue and neutropenia respectively. Further prospective randomised evidence is awaited.

4.4 Taxanes/nanoparticle – bound paclitaxel

There is phase II evidence of 18 patients utilising weekly paclitaxel monotherapy with good tolerability.[40] Five patients had stable disease with one patient who achieved a complete response lasting beyond one year. The reported median overall survival was 17.5 weeks. Treatment was well tolerated with only one patient developing grade 3 myelotoxicity. A further report described evidence for activity using single agent docetaxel, combination docetaxel-gemcitabine or capecitabine regimes, however this was a small heterogeneous group of patients and assessment was retrospective.[41]

SPARC (Secreted protein acidic and rich in cysteine) is frequently expressed by stromal fibroblasts adjacent to pancreatic adenocarcinoma cells, and immunohistochemical expression within the peritumoral stroma is an independent predictor for poorer survival, whereas expression by cancer cells is not. An analysis of 299 pancreaticoduodenectomy specimens showed that patients who expressed SPARC had a median survival of 15 months whereas patients who did not, had double the median survival of 30 months ($p < 0.001$).[42] Nanoparticle albumin-bound (nab) paclitaxel (Abraxane®; Abraxis BioScience) is believed to allow better paclitaxel delivery by allowing albumin to bind to SPARC. It also has the advantages of avoiding the Cremophor® - related hypersensitivity reactions associated with standard paclitaxel, as well as delivery with a shorter infusion time.

In a phase I/II study, patients with metastatic pancreatic adenocarcinoma were given first-line nab-paclitaxel (100-150mg/m2) in combination with gemcitabine 1000mg/m2 (days 1,8 and 15 of a 28 day cycle).[43] Of the 63 patients in the study, 35 had tissue available for immunohistochemical analysis. 29% of patients were SPARC positive. If SPARC positive, this predicted a metabolic response on positron emission tomography (PET) in 75% of those patients as well as a progression-free survival advantage of 6.2 vs. 4.8 months. A further phase II study of single agent nab-paclitaxel in patients who had progressed on gemcitabine however was less impressive with 63% of patients progressing by RECIST criteria at their first response assessment.[44] These patients were not preselected based on SPARC status.

The question of whether incorporating nanoparticle bound-paclitaxel into first-line chemotherapy with gemcitabine leads to a clinically meaningful improvement in survival is yet to be answered by a prospective randomised clinical trial currently awaiting completion.[45] Although tissue analysis for SPARC is included in this trial, the interventional arm will not be enriched with SPARC positive patients.

4.5 Recommendations

To date there is no established standard of care in the second-line setting or beyond. Treatment must therefore be tailored to each patient but may include oxaliplatin, fluoropyrimidine or taxane-based regimens, as outlined above. There is very limited evidence for irinotecan-based treatment. A 5-FU/oxaliplatin or capecitabine-erlotinib doublet is an option. Consideration for enrolment in a clinical trial should be given if available.

5. Future targets in pancreatic cancer

Because attempts at improving survival in pancreatic cancer with cytotoxic and biologic therapy have been modest at the most thus far, newer strategies of targeting the core signaling pathways implicated in pancreatic cancer are needed.

Previously, genetic mutations affecting genes such as TP53, KRAS, CDKN2A and SMAD4 were known to be associated, but a more recent genome-wide analysis has identified a broader range of aberrant pathways implicated in pancreatic cancer growth.[46] In most of the 24 cancers examined in this series, the majority of the genetic mutations were felt to be disrupting one or more of 12 core signaling pathways.

In pancreatic cancer, aberrations can occur in signal transduction and other pathways that promote cell survival and allow proliferation. These include KRAS,[47] PI3K/Akt/mTOR,[49-50] EGFR,[52] insulin-like growth factor (IGF-1) (which is co-expressed with Src),[52] hepatocyte growth factor (HGF) and vascular endothelial growth factor (VEGF).[53] There are embryonic developmental signaling pathways that also lead to progression such as the Hedgehog, Notch, and Wnt pathways.[54-57] Matrix metalloproteinases (MMPs) also play a part in promoting neovascularisation and tumour invasion, and abnormalities in core pathways involved in DNA repair as well as apoptosis control such as p53, SMAD/TGF-β and p14 AFR/p16 are also seen.[58-59]

Finally there is also documented activity or upregulation of other factors such as cyclo-oxygenase,[60] focal adhesion kinase (FAK) (which in turn interacts with the IGF-1 receptor),[61] telomerase,[62] as well as cholecystokinin, gastrin and gastrin receptors.[63]

5.1 Current evidence and future strategies targeting specific pathways in pancreatic cancer

- K-ras
- Epidermal growth factor receptor (EGFR)
- Angiogenesis/matrix metalloproteinases (MMPs)/integrins
- PI3k/Akt/mTOR
- Nf-kβ
- Cyclo-oxygenase
- TGF-β, SMAD4, MET, and IGF-1
- Src
- Hedgehog/wnt pathways/Notch
- Gastrin/cholecystokinin receptors

5.1.1 The ras pathway

K-ras is part of the Ras group of genes, which code for GTP-binding proteins in the cellular membrane. Ras is important in cellular differentiation and proliferation, as well as adhesion and the regulation of apoptosis. When activated by the associated EGFR, Ras leads to further downstream activation of Raf, MAP2K, MAPK and PI3K-Akt cascades. K-ras mutations lead to cell-cycle progression, and promote tumour cell survival. Mutated K-ras, seen in over 90% of pancreatic cancer is mostly identified in codon 12 but may also be seen in codons 13 and 61.[47]

There has been an attempt in an adjuvant phase II study to vaccinate against k-ras, in patients who harbour codon 12 k-ras mutations.[64] In 24 patients, this was felt to be safe, however less than half of patients had a detected immune response and the protective value of this strategy is unknown.

Another approach has been to inhibit the KRAS protein itself. This has been attempted through targeting its attachment to the cell membrane by inhibiting farnesyltransferase with tipifarnib - a farnysyltransferase inhibitor (FTI).[66] Inhibiting Ras-driven signal transduction and interfering with Ras-membrane binding with other small molecule drugs such a salirasib, or antisense/RNA inhibitors are early in clinical development.[65] Unfortunately to date the only strategy reaching a phase III study, combining tipifarnib with gemcitabine in advanced pancreatic carcinoma, did not provide any significant difference in either the clinical benefit rate, median progression-free, or overall survival.[66] This is likely due to alternate pathways that still allow the prenylation of Ras.

Downstream Ras pathway inhibition of mitogen-activated protein kinase (MAPK) with a MEK inhibitor has not shown any phase II activity.[67] This was despite preclinical evidence showing synergistic activity by dual inhibition with the EGFR TKI inhibitor gefitinib and the MAPK inhibitor CI-1040 (PD184532).[68]

5.1.2 The epidermal growth factor receptor (EGFR) pathway

Activation of this pathway leads to downstream signaling events through MAPK, PI3K-Akt and the STAT family of proteins. STAT proteins also have roles in cell proliferation, survival, motility, invasion and adhesion. Over-expression of this pathway and its ligands (EGF and TGF-α) are common in pancreatic cancer.[69-70] The clinical evidence for targeting the EGFR is outlined above. As previously mentioned, the addition of erlotinib or cetuximab to gemcitabine has resulted in only modest and no additional overall survival benefit respectively.

5.1.3 Angiogenesis, matrix metalloproteinases (MMPs) and integrins

VEGF overexpression is common in pancreatic adenocarcinoma and is associated with a poorer prognosis.[71] Despite this being an attractive target, multiple anti-angiogenic strategies added to a backbone of gemcitabine have been disappointing. Two phase III trials in advanced pancreatic adenocarcinoma, have shown no overall survival benefit with the addition of the VEGF monoclonal antibody bevacizumab[72] to either single-agent gemcitabine, or a doublet of gemcitabine with erlotinib.[73] The latter study did however demonstrate a difference in progression-free survival (HR, 0.73; 95% CI, 0.61 to 0.86; P = 0.0002).

Sorafenib is an oral multitargeted kinase inhibitor which inhibits the VEGF-receptor tyrosine kinase as well as Raf-1, the platelet-derived growth factor receptor (PDGFR), c-kit and FLT-

3. It has not shown any significant additive activity in a phase II study. [74] Similarly axitinib (a selective oral inhibitor of multiple VEGF receptors), has also failed to show improved efficacy when combined with gemcitabine in the phase III setting despite promise in an earlier phase II trial.[75-76] A phase III study randomised 546 patients with metastatic pancreatic cancer to gemcitabine with aflibercept (the VEGF 'trap') vs. gemcitabine with placebo (clinicaltrials.gov identifier NCT00574275). This was also terminated early due to no significant improvement in the primary or secondary end points of overall and progression-free survival.

Matrix metalloproteinases (MMPs) are enzymes that break down the extracellular matrix and are required for tumour spread and neovascularisation. However, randomised trials utilising the MMP inhibitor marimastat in metastatic disease did not show any added survival benefit over gemcitabine alone.[77-79] Whether there might be a role in the adjuvant setting remains unknown.

Volociximab is a monoclonal antibody that inhibits fibronectin binding to α5β1-integrin, which promotes apoptosis in tumour endothelial cells. A small, phase II study combining this agent with gemcitabine in 20 patients showed activity with stable disease in half of patients and a partial response in one patient. The median time to progression (TTP) was 4.3 months with 37% of patients alive at 12 months. However there is no prospective randomised evidence to date.[80] Cilengitide is another agent that interferes with integrin binding leading to proliferative endothelial cell apoptosis, but it was not shown to be of added benefit when combined with gemcitabine.[81] There are other integrin inhibitors in preclinical and early clinical stages of evaluation.

5.1.4 The PI3k/Akt/mTOR pathway

The phosphoinositide 3′-kinase (PI3k)/Akt/mammalian target of rapamycin (mTOR) pathway which is regulated upstream by KRAS is important in pancreatic tumorigenesis and angiogenesis. Activation in pancreatic cancer is common, and is associated with loss of the tumour suppressor PTEN, and with poorer outcomes as well as gemcitabine resistance.[82] Despite this, the mTOR inhibitors everolimus and temsirolimus have shown no objective responses in phase II studies, and when the former was combined with erlotinib, also no objective responses were seen.[83-84] It is felt that they are unlikely to have a role - at least as a single agent strategy - in this disease. The PI3K and Akt inhibitors (BKM-120 and MK-2206) are in phase I development. RX-0201 (an Akt-1 mRNA antisense oligonucleotide) is being evaluated in a phase II trial in combination with gemcitabine.[82]

5.1.5 NFkβ

Nuclear factor kappa light-chain enhancer of activated β cells (NFkβ) is also activated by the PI3k/Akt/mTOR pathway. Curcumin (diferuloyl methane) - a component of the common Indian spice turmeric - has been shown to inhibit NFkβ. A phase II study using 8g of curcumin as a single agent daily for two months found that this agent was tolerable in 25 patients, two of which received prolonged (up to 12 month) periods of stable disease. One patient achieved a partial response.[85] A further phase II study of 17 patients with curcumin in combination with gemcitabine showed that 5 patients either had stable or partial responses but another 5 patients could not tolerate treatment due to abdominal discomfort, and had to discontinue therapy.[86] A phase III trial of gemcitabine with or without a combination of curcumin and celecoxib (a cyclo-oxygenase-2 (COX-2) inhibitor) is currently in progress.[87]

5.1.6 Cyclo-oxygenase

The cyclo-oxygenase (COX) pathway is also important. Inhibition with celecoxib has been proven to suppress tumour proliferation as well as VEGF expression in pancreatic cancer.[88] However phase II trial responses in combination with gemcitabine have been mixed. The most favourable phase II study was performed in 42 patients (most with metastatic rather than locally advanced disease) who received gemcitabine 1000mg/m^2 (on days 1 and 8 only of a 3-week cycle) in combination with celecoxib 400mg BD. The clinical benefit rate in 30 patients was reported as 71% [95% CI, 58-84%]), and the median overall survival was 9.1 months (95% CI, 7.5-10.6 months).[89] However another phase II study showed that despite a clinical benefit rate of 52% in 25 patients, the 12 month survival rate was 15%, which did not reach predetermined efficacy in order to proceed to a phase III trial.[90]

5.1.7 Transforming growth factor-β (TGF-β), SMAD4, MET, and IGF-1

TGF-β binds to cell receptors that lead to downstream activation of SMAD4 which in turn moves into the cell nucleus to activate gene transcription. TGF-β is also involved with activating other pathways including Ras, PI3K and MAPK. Although tumour suppressive in epithelial cells, it is also involved in mediating invasion and metastasis. In pancreatic cancer, mutations in SMAD4 are seen in 50% and up to 4% of TGFβ receptors.[91] Mutations of the former can lead to reduced TGF-β tumour suppression as well as increased tumour cell invasiveness. Exploitation of this pathway with inhibitors such as antisense oligonucleotides specific to the TGF receptor are in early phase clinical development in several solid malignancies including pancreatic cancer.[92]

Overexpression of the c-MET proto-oncogene which codes for MET (mesenchymal-epithelial transition factor) is common in a number of solid malignancies such as colon, gastric, lung, breast, ovarian, bladder and pancreatic cancer.[93] The resultant protein - hepatocyte transcription factor receptor (HGFR) is stimulated by HGF which is produced by fibroblasts in the stromal microenvironent. This in turn, leads to further tumour growth, angiogenesis, invasion, and metastasis formation. Similarly, the insulin-like growth factor (IGF-1) and focal adhesion kinase (FAK) pathways which are implicated in tumour growth and survival are overexpressed in pancreatic cancer. Inhibitors such as the selective cMET inhibitor tivatanib (ARQ 197) and anti IGF-1 receptor antibody cixutumumab are also early in clinical development.

5.1.8 Src

Src is a proto-oncogene which codes for a non-receptor tyrosine kinase (RTK). Src proteins are a family of kinases involved in cell adhesion, and fibroblast division. Expression has been documented in a variety of cancers including pancreatic cancer, where overexpression is seen in 70%.[94] Overexpressed Src can lead to upregulation of the IGF-1 receptor.[52] Phase I trials of the BCR/Abl, c-kit and Src family inhibitor dasatinib have been performed in patients in a variety of solid tumours but at present another dual Src and Abl tyrosine kinase inhibitor SKI-606 (bosutinib) is undergoing phase I/II evaluation with gemcitabine as adjuvant therapy in the postoperative setting.[95]

5.1.9 Hedgehog/Wnt pathways/Notch

The hedgehog signaling pathway plays an important part in embryonic development but when aberrant, may be implicated in tumorigenesis. [96] Two transmembrane proteins work in tandem. Ptch (patched), which is tumour suppressing, inhibits the Smo (smoothened) protein which when activated by a Ptch mutation, allows hedgehog proteins to bind. This leads to downstream activation of GLI-1 which promotes nuclear transcription. One of the hedgehog proteins (Sonic Hedgehog - SHH) is expressed in 70% of pancreatic adenocarcinoma. Preclinical evidence points to the drug cyclopamine inhibiting Smo, but further trial evidence for hedgehog pathway inhibitors in pancreatic cancer patients is awaited.

The Wnt pathways are also important in normal embryonic development and mutations are implicated in tumorigenesis. If the Wnt-β-catenin cascade pathway is aberrant (65% of pancreatic cancer), abnormal overactivation of β-catenin occurs which promotes abnormal nuclear transcription.[97] There is preclinical evidence that blocking this pathway can lead to pancreatic cell death, which may be a future potential target for treatment. It is thought that chemokine receptor 4 (CXCR4) is key in tumour angiogenesis and metastasis. Specific blockade of this chemokine receptor or its ligand SDF-1 may be a further potential future clinical strategy. It is thought that inhibiting both these pathways may have anti cancer stem cell effects.[97]

Notch genes code for proteins also responsible for tumour differentiation, proliferation and apoptosis and the pathway requires the enzyme gamma-secretase to be activated. Notch 3 is also expressed in most pancreatic cancers with preclinical evidence of a potential role using siRNA and secretase inhibitors in therapy.[98]

5.1.10 Gastrin and cholecystokinin receptors

Targeting gastrin And the cholecystokinin receptor CCK-BR, with the intravenous agent JB95008 (gastrozole) has been attempted in advanced pretreated pancreatic cancer but was found to be no better than 5-FU in terms of survival.[99]

Another novel oral gastrin inhibitor named Z-360 has been was examined in a phase Ib/IIa study and found to be active when given in combination with gemcitabine, with a future randomised controlled trial planned.[100-101]

6. Biomarkers in pancreatic cancer

In contrast to other solid tumour malignancies, there have been relatively modest or poor responses achieved with molecularly targeted agents to date in unselected patients with pancreatic cancer. There is an urgent need for a personalised approach to better define biomarkers in order to predict patients that are more likely to benefit from a particular cytotoxic or molecular targeted therapy.

The biomarker with the most preclinical and clinical evidence is human equilibrative nucleoside transporter 1 (hENT1). Gemcitabine requires transmembrane nucleoside transport proteins to enter cells and to have a therapeutic effect. Both hENT1 and 2 allow this with hENT1 being more selective. A lack of hENT1 expression has been shown to interfere with gemcitabine influx, and is associated with reduced efficacy and decreased survival in patients.[102-105] However it is not yet clear whether immunohistochemical hENT1 expression or gene expression will be the most predictive measure, or whether there is a concordance between hENT1 expression in primary and metastatic disease.

Once gemcitabine is transported into the cell, it is phosphorylated by deoxycytidine kinase (dCK) to difluorodeoxycytidine. It is gemcitabine triphosphate's (dFdCTP) incorporation into DNA that leads to strand termination. DFdCTP is metabolised by cytidine deaminase (CDA). There is evidence of correlation between dCK and CDA levels, and also detected single nucleotide polymorphisms (SNPs) in genes that code for these and other proteins involved in gemcitabine transport and metabolism, and overall survival.[106] However, to date, attempts at increasing the effective intracellular concentration of gemcitabine and its metabolite dFdCTP have not translated into improved patient survival in the phase III trial setting. Fixed-dose rate (FDR) gemcitabine (1,500mg/m^2/150mins) only modestly improved overall survival (6.2 vs. 4.9 months, HR 0.83 stratified log-rank $p = 0.04$) compared with standard gemcitabine, and did not meet predetermined efficacy. It was also associated with greater haematological toxicity.[107]

A modified form of gemcitabine, CP-4126 (gemcitabine-5'-elaidic acid ester, Clavis Pharma) bypasses nucleoside transporters. It is undergoing phase II evaluation in patients with advanced pancreatic cancer, after a phase I study showed a good safety profile.[108-109]

Other promising predictive and prognostic biomarkers may include variations in cellular histone modification patterns.[110] Immunohistochemical analyses of histone H3 lysine 4 and 9, dimethylation and histone H3 lysine 18 acetylation were performed on tissue banks. Tissue was derived from patients with resected pancreatic tumours (including those in the RTOG 9704 study which compared adjuvant 5-FU and gemcitabine). Low levels of some histone modifications predicted a poorer disease-free survival if patients were treated with adjuvant 5-FU compared with gemcitabine.

DPC4 (SMAD4) gene expression has recently found to be prognostic and associated with local failure following adjuvant chemoradiotherapy, or with metastatic spread in locally advanced disease.[111-112] However prospective validation is still required, especially if therapeutic targeting of this pathway is a future therapeutic option. These, and other markers such as mismatch repair polymorphisms, are also yet to be prospectively validated.

7. Conclusion

Despite research into the medical management of pancreatic cancer, survival remains poor. Numerous agents and combinations have been attempted in early phase clinical trials, but to date, very modest improvements have been made in overall survival. Single agent gemcitabine still remains the standard of care for most patients in both the adjuvant and advanced settings with adjuvant chemoradiotherapy being more controversial. In the advanced settings, gemcitabine or gemcitabine with erlotinib are appropriate for most, but fit patients may benefit from gemcitabine-containing cytotoxic doublets. FOLFIRINOX is now considered an option in the fittest of patients, but its toxicity is significant. Although no standard of care exists in the second-line setting, fluoropyrimidines, oxaliplatin, erlotinib and taxanes including nab-paclitaxel show activity, often in combination regimens.

Increased knowledge of the molecular pathogenesis of pancreatic cancer has allowed new targets and therapeutic strategies to emerge. However, true progress in the personalised management of this disease will only be likely with equally important research into the identification, and validation of appropriate predictive and prognostic biomarkers.

8. References

[1] Jemal A, Siegel R, Ward E, et al. Cancer Statistics, 2010. *CA Cancer J Clin* 2010;60: 277-300

[2] Kasler MH, Ellenberg SS. Pancreatic cancer. Adjuvant combined radiation and chemotherapy following curative resection. *Arch Surg* 1985; 120(8):899-903.

[3] Douglass HO. Further evidence of effective adjuvant combined radiation and chemotherapy following curative resection of pancreatic cancer. Gastrointestinal Tumor Study Group. *Cancer* 59:2006-2010.

[4] Klinkenbijl JH, Jeekel J, Sahmoud T, et al. Adjuvant radiotherapy and 5-flurouracil after curative resection of cancer of the pancreas and periampullary region. Phase III trial of the EORTC gastrointestinal tract cancer cooperative group. *Ann Surg* 1999; 230(6):776

[5] Neoptolemos JP, Stocken DD, Friess H, et al. A randomized trial of chemoradiotherapy and chemotherapy after resection of pancreatic cancer. *N Engl J Med* 2004;350:1200-1210

[6] Regine WF, Winter KW, Abrams R, et al. RTOG 9704: a phase III study of adjuvant pre and post chemoradiation 5-FU vs. gemcitabine for resected pancreatic adenocarcinoma. *J Clin Oncol* 2009; 27 (18 Suppl)(abst 4007).

[7] Bakkevold KE, Arnesjo B. Dahl O, Kambestad B. Adjuvant combination chemotherapy (AMF) following radical resection of carcinoma of the pancreas and papilla of Vater - results of a controlled prospective, randomized multicenter study. *Eur J Cancer* 1993; 29A (5):698.

[8] Oettle H, Post S, Neuhaus P, et al. Adjuvant chemotherapy with gemcitabine vs. observation in patients undergoing curative intent resection of pancreatic cancer: a randomized controlled trial. *JAMA* 2007;297(3):267

[9] Neoptolemos JP, Buchler MW, Stocken DD, et al. ESPAC-3: a multicenter, international, open-label randomized, controlled phase III trial of adjuvant 5-fluorouracil/folinic acid versus gemcitabine in patients with resected pancreatic ductal adenocarcinoma. *J Clin Onco*l 2009;27(18 Suppl): (abst LBA4505).

[10] Neoptolemos JP, Stocken DD, Bassi C, et al.: Adjuvant chemotherapy with fluorouracil plus folinic acid vs. gemcitabine following pancreatic cancer resection: a randomized controlled trial. *JAMA* 2010, 304:1073-81

[11] Royal RE, Wolff RA, Crane CH: Cancer of the Pancreas, in De Vita VT Jr, Lawrence TS, Rosenberg SA (eds): Cancer: Principles and Practice of Oncology (ed 9). Philadelphia, PA, Lippincott Williams and Wilkins, 2011 pp 961-989

[12] Cartwright T, Cohn A, Varkey J, et al: Phase II study of oral capecitabine in patients with advanced or metastatic pancreatic cancer. *J Clin Onco*l 20:160-164, 2002

[13] Burris HA III, Moore MJ, Andersen J, et al. Improvements in survival and clinical benefit with gemcitabine as first-line therapy for patients with advanced pancreas cancer: a randomized trial. *J Clin Oncol* 1997;15:2403-2413.

[14] Moore MJ, Goldstein D, Hamm J, et al. Erlotinib plus gemcitabine compared with gemcitabine alone in patients with advanced pancreatic cancer: A phase III trial of the National Cancer Institute of Canada Clinical Trials Group. *J Clin Oncol* 2007; 25(15):1960
[15] Fountzilas G, Bobos M, Kalogera-Fountzila A. Gemcitabine combined with gefitinib in patients with inoperable or metastatic pancreatic cancer: a phase II Study of the Hellenic Cooperative Oncology Group with biomarker evaluation. *Cancer Invest.* 2008 Oct;26(8):784-93
[16] Philip PA, et al. Phase III study of gemcitabine plus cetuximab versus gemcitabine in patients with locally advanced or metastatic pancreatic adenocarcinoma: SWOG S0205 study [Abstract] *J. Clin Oncol.* 2007;25:a4509
[17] Safran H, Miner T, Bahary N. Lapatinib and gemcitabine for metastatic pancreatic cancer: A phase II study. *J Clin Oncol* 27, 2009 (suppl; abstr e15653)
[18] Cascinu S, Berardi S, Siena S. The impact of cetuximab on the gemcitabine/cisplatin combination in first-lie treatment of EGFR-positive advanced pancreatic cancer (APC): A randomized phase II trial of GISCAD. *J Clin Oncol.* 2007 ASCO Annual Meeting Proceedings Part . Vol 25, No 18S (June 20 Suppl), 2007:4544
[19] Kim GP, et al. Randomized phase II trial of panitumumab (P), erlotinib (E), and gemcitabine (G) versus erlotinib-gemcitabine in patients with untreated, metastatic pancreatic adenocarcinoma. *J Clin Oncol* 2011;29(Suppl 4): Abstract 238
[20] ClinicalTrials.gov identifier NCT00634725.
[21] Heinemann V, Boeck S, Hinke A, et al. Meta-analysis of randomised trials: evaluation of benefit from gemcitabine-based combination chemotherapy applied to advanced pancreatic cancer. *BMC Cancer* 2008;8:82
[22] Berlin J, Catalano P, Thomas J, et al. A phase III study of gemcitabine in combination with 5-FU versus gemcitabine alone in patients with advanced pancreatic carcinoma: Eastern Cooperative Oncology Group Trial E2297. *J Clin Oncol* 2002; 20:3270-3275
[23] Cunningham D, Chau I, Stocken DD, et al. Phase III randomized comparison of gemcitabine versus gemcitabine plus capecitabine in patients with advanced pancreatic cancer. *J Clin Oncol* 2009; 27: 5513-8
[24] Hermann R, Bodoky G, Rubstaller T, et al. Gemcitabine plus capecitabine versus gemcitabine alone in advanced pancreatic cancer. A randomized phase III trial. *J Clin Oncol* 2007; 25:2212-2217
[25] Heinemann V, Quietzsch D, Gieseler F, et al. Randomized phase III trial of gemcitabine plus cisplatin compared with gemcitabine alone in advanced pancreatic carcinoma. *J Clin Oncol.* 2006 Aug 20;24(24):3946-52
[26] Louvet C, Labianca R, Hammel P, et al: Gemcitabine in combination with oxaliplatin compared with gemcitabine alone in locally advanced or metastatic pancreatic cancer. Results of a GERCOR and GISCAD phase III clinical trial. *J Clin Oncol* 2005; 23:3509-3516
[27] Rocha Lima C, et al. A randomised phase 3 study comparing efficacy and safety of gemcitabine and irinotecan to gemcitabine alone in patients with locally advanced or metastatic pancreatic cancer who have not received prior systemic therapy. *Proc Am Soc Clin Oncol.* 2003;22:251 (abstract 1005)
[28] Conroy T, Desseigne F, Ychou M, et al. FOLFIRINOX versus gemcitabine for metastatic pancreatic cancer *N Engl J Med* 2011; 364:1817-1825

[29] Bendell JC, et al. Immediate impact of the FOLFIRINOX phase III data reported at the 2010 ASCO Annual Meeting on prescribing plans of American oncology physicians for patients with metastatic pancreas cancer (MPC). *J Clin Oncol* 2011; 29 (Suppl 4) Abstract 286

[30] Burtness BA, et al. Phase II ECOG trial of irinotecan/docetaxel with or without cetuximab in metastatic pancreatic cancer: updated survival and CA19-19 results [Abstract] *J. Clin. Oncol.* 2008;26:a4642.

[31] Gemcitabine and oxaliplatin (GEMOX) in gemcitabine refractory advanced pancreatic adenocarcinoma: a phase II study. Demois A, Peeters M, Polus M, et al. *B J Cancer* (2006): 94, 481-485.

[32] Oettle H, Pelzer U, Stieler J, et al. Oxaliplatin/folinic acid/5-fluorouracil (OFF) plus best supportive care versus best supportive care alone in second-line therapy of gemcitabine-refractory advanced pancreatic cancer (CONKO 003). *J Clin Oncol* 2005; 23(16 Suppl.) Abstract 4031

[33] Pelzer U, Kubica K, Stieler, et al. A randomised trial in patients with gemcitabine-refractory pancreatic cancer. Final results of the CONKO-003 study. *J Clin Oncol* 2008; 26(15 Suppl): Abstract 4508.

[34] Xiong HQ, Varadhachary GR, Blais JC, Hess KR, Abbruzzese JL, Wolff RA. Phase II trial of oxaliplatin plus capecitabine (XELOX) as second-line therapy for patients with advanced pancreatic cancer. *Cancer* 2008: 113:2046-52.

[35] Mane J, et al. Second-line chemotherapy with capecitabine (CAP) and oxaliplatin (OX) in patients with pancreatic or biliary tree adenocarcinoma (ADC). 2011 Gastrointestinal Cancers Symposium. *J Clin Oncol* 2011; 29 (suppl. 4): Abstract 308

[36] Kulke MH, Blaszkowsky LS, Ryan DP. et al. Capecitabine plus erlotinib in Gemcitabine-Refractory Advanced Pancreatic Cancer. *J Clin Oncol* 2007 25:4787-4792

[37] Yi SY, Park YS, Kim HS, et al. Irinotecan monotherapy as second-line treatment in advanced pancreatic cancer. *Cancer Chemother Pharmacol* 2009; 63:1141-5

[38] Neuzillet C, Hentic O, Rousseau B, et al. FOLFIRI regimen as second-/third-line chemotherapy in patients with advanced pancreatic adenocarcinoma refractory to gemcitabine and platinum salts. A retrospective series of 70 patients. 2011 Gastrointestinal Cancers Symposium. *J Clin Oncol* 2011; 29 (Suppl. 4): Abstract 272.

[39] Ko AH, Tempero MA, Shan Y, et al. A multinational phase II study of liposomal irinotecan (PEP02) for patients with gemcitabine-refractory metastatic pancreatic cancer. 2011 Gastointestinal Cancers Symposium. *J Clin Oncol* 2011; 29(suppl.4): Abstract 237.

[40] Oettle H, Arnold D, Esser M, et al. Paclitaxel as weekly second-line therapy in patients with advanced pancreatic cancer: a retrospective study. *Anticancer Drugs* 2000; 11:635-638.

[41] Said MW, Syrigos K, Penney R, et al. Docetaxel second-line therapy in patients with advanced pancreatic cancer: a retrospective study. *Anticancer Res* 2010; 30:2905-9

[42] Infante JR, Matsubayashi H, Sato N, Tonascia J, Klein AP, Riall TA, et al. Peritumoral fibroblast SPARC expression and patient outcome with resectable pancreatic adenocarcinoma. *J Clin Oncol* 2007; 25:319-25

[43] Von Hoff DD, Ramanathan R, Borad M, Laheru D, Smith L, Wood T, et al. SPARC correlation with response to gemcitabine plus nab-paclitaxel in patients with advanced metastatic pancreatic cancer: A phase I/II study. *J Clin Oncol* 27:15s, 2009 (suppl; abstr 4525)

[44] Hosein PJ, Lopes GD Jr., Gomez CM, et al. A phase II trial of nab-paclitaxel (NP) in patients with advanced pancreatic cancer who have progressed on gemcitabine based therapy. *J Clin Oncol* 28:15s, 2010 (suppl; abstr 4120)
[45] CA046: ClinicalTrials.gov identifier NCT00844649
[46] Jones S, et al. Core signaling pathways in human pancreatic cancers revealed by global genomic analyses. *Science.* 2008; 321:1801-180
[47] Almoguera C, et al. Most human carcinomas of the exocrine pancreas contain mutant c-K-ras genes. *Cell.* 1988;53:549-554
[48] Ruggeri BA, Huang L, Wood M, Cheng JQ, Testa JR. Amplification and overexpression of AKT2 oncogene in a subset of human pancreatic ductal adenocarcinomas. *Mol Carcinog.* 1998;21:81-86
[49] Schlieman MG, Fahy BN, Ramsamooj R, Beckett L, Bold RJ. Incidence, mechanism and prognostic value of activated Akt in pancreas cancer. *Br. J. Cancer.* 2003;89:2110-2115.
[50] Asano T, et al. The PI3-kinase/Akt signaling pathway is activated due to aberrant Pten expression and targets transcription factors NF-k□ and c-Myc in pancreatic cancer cells. *Oncogene.* 2004;23:8571-8580.
[51] Bloomston M, Bhardwaj A, Ellison EC, Frankel WL. Epidermal growth factor receptor expression in pancreatic carcinoma using tissue microarray technique. *Dig. Surg.* 2006;23:74-79.
[52] Hakam A, Fang Q, Karl R, Coppola D. Coexpression of IGF-1R and c-Src proteins in human pancreatic ductal adenocarcinoma. *Dig. Dis. Sci.* 2003;48:1972-8
[53] Furukawa T, Duguid WP, Kobari M, Matsuno S, Tsao MS. Hepatocyte growth factor and Met receptor expression in human pancreatic carcinogenesis. *Am J Pathol.* 1995;147:889-895.
[54] Thayer SP, et al. Hedgehog is an early and late mediator of pancreatic cancer tumorigenesis. *Nature.* 2003;425:851-856
[55] Dang T, Vo K, Washington K, Berlin J. The role of Notch3 signaling pathway in pancreatic cancer [Abstract] *J Clin. Oncol.* 2007;25:a21049
[56] Doucas H, et al. Expression of nuclear Notch3 in pancreatic adenocarcinomas is associated with adverse clinical features, and correlates with the expression of STAT3 and phosphorylated Akt. *J. Surg. Oncol.* 2008;97:63-68.
[57] Zeng G, et al. Aberrant Wnt/beta-catenin signaling in pancreatic adenocarcinoma. *Neoplasia.* 2006;8:279-289.
[58] Goggins M, et al. Genetic alterations of the transforming growth factor beta receptor genes in pancreatic and biliary adenocarcinomas. *Cancer Res.* 1998;58:5329-5332.
[59] Stathis A, Moore MJ. Advanced pancreatic carcinoma: current treatment and future challenges. *J. Nat. Rev. Clin. Oncol.* 7, 163-172 (2010); doi:10.1038/nrclinonc.2009.236
[60] Tucker ON, et al. Cyclooxygenase-2 expression is upregulated in human pancreatic cancer. *Cancer Res.* 1999;59:987-990
[61] FAK and IGF-IR interact to provide survival signals in human pancreatic adenocarcinoma cells. *Carcinogenesis.* 2008;29:1096-1107
[62] Hiyama E, et al. Telomerase activity is detected in pancreatic cancer but not in benign tumors. *Cancer Res.* 1997;57:326-331
[63] Caplin M, et al. Expression and processing of gastrin in pancreatic adenocarcinoma. *Br. J. Surg.* 2000;87:1035-1040.
[64] Abou-Alfa GK, Chapman PB, Feilchenfeldt J, et al. Targeting mutated K-ras in pancreatic adenocarcinoma using an adjuvant vaccine. *Am J Clin Oncol.* 2011 Ju;34(3):321-5

[65] Rudek MA, Khan Y, Goldsweig H et al. Integrated development of S-Trans, Trans-Farnesylthiosalicyclic acid (FTS, Salisarib) in pancreatic cancer. *J Clin Oncol* 26:2008 (May 20 suppl; abstr 4626)

[66] Van Cutsem E, et al. Phase III trial of gemcitabine plus tipifarnib compared with gemcitabine plus placebo in advanced pancreatic cancer. *J Clin. Oncol.* 2004;22:1430-1438.

[67] Rinehart J, et al. Multicenter phase II study of the oral MEK inhibitor, CI-1040, in patients with advanced non-small-cell lung, breast, colon, and pancreatic cancer. *J. Clin. Oncol.* 2004;22:4456-4462.

[68] Jimeno A, et al. Dual mitogen-activated protein kinase and epidermal growth factor receptor inhibition in biliary and pancreatic cancer. *Mol. Cancer Ther.* 2007;6:1079-1088.

[69] Korc M, et al. Overexpression of the epidermal growth factor receptor in human pancreatic cancer is associated with concomitant increases in the levels of epidermal growth factor and transforming growth factor alpha. *J. Clin. Invest.* 1992;90:1352-1360.

[70] Bloomston M, Bhardwaj A, Ellison EC, Frankel WL. Epidermal growth factor receptor expression in pancreatic carcinoma using tissue microarray technique. *Dig. Surg.* 2006;23:74-79

[71] Seo Y, Baba H, Fukuda T, Takashima M, Sugimaxhi K. High expression of vascular endothelial growth factor is associated with liver metastases and a poor prognosis for patients with ductal adenocarcinoma. *Cancer.* 2000;88:2239-45

[72] Kindler HL, et al. A double-blind, placebo-controlled, randomized phase III trial of gemcitabine (G) plus bevacizumab (B) versus gemcitabine plus placebo (P) in patients (pts) with advanced pancreatic cancer (PC): a preliminary analysis of Cancer and Leukemia Group B (CALGB) *J. Clin. Oncol.* 2007;25:4508-4509

[73] Van Cutsem E, Vervenne WL, Bennouna J et al. Phase III trial of bevacizumab in combination with gemcitabine and erlotinib in patients with metastatic pancreatic cancer. *J. Clin. Oncol.* 2009 May 1;27(13):2231-7. Epub 2009 Mar23.

[74] Wallace JA, et al. Sorafenib (S) plus gemcitabine (G) for advanced pancreatic cancer (PC): A phase II trial of the University of Chicago Phase II Consortium [Abstract] *J. Clin. Oncol.* 2007;25:a4608.

[75] Spano JP, et al. Efficacy of gemcitabine plus axitinib compared with gemcitabine alone in patients with advanced pancreatic cancer: an open-label randomised phase II study. *Lancet.* 2008;371:2101-2108.

[76] Kindler HL, Ioka T, Richel DJ. Axitinib plus gemcitabine versus placebo plus gemcitabine in patients with advanced pancreatic adenocarcinoma: a double-blind randomized phase III study. *Lancet Oncol* 2011:12:256-262

[77] Bramhall SR, Rosemurgy A, Brown PD, Bowry C, Buckels JA. Marimastat as first-line therapy for patients with unresectable pancreatic cancer: a randomized trial. *J. Clin. Oncol.* 2001;19:3447-3455.

[78] Bramhall SR, et al. A double-blind placebo-controlled, randomised study comparing gemcitabine and marimastat with gemcitabine and placebo as first line therapy in patients with advanced pancreatic cancer. *Br. J. Cancer.* 2002;87:161-167.

[79] Moore MJ, et al. Comparison of gemcitabine versus the matrix metalloproteinase inhibitor BAY 12-9566 in patients with advanced or metastatic adenocarcinoma of the pancreas: a phase III trial of the National Cancer Institute of Canada Clinical Trials Group. *J. Clin. Oncol.* 2003;21:3296-3302.

[80] Evans T, et al. Final results from cohort 1 of a phase II study of volociximab, an anti-α5β1 integrin antibody, in combination with gemcitabine (GEM) in patients (pts) with metastatic pancreatic cancer (MPC) [Abstract] *J. Clin. Oncol.* 2007;25:a4549.
[81] Friess H, et al. A randomized multi-center phase II trial of the angiogenesis inhibitor Cilengitide (EMD 121974) and gemcitabine compared with gemcitabine alone in advanced unresectable pancreatic cancer. *BMC Cancer.* 2006;6:285.
[82] Kotowski A, Ma W. Emerging therapies in pancreas cancer. *J Gastrointest Oncol* 2011;2:93-103
[83] Wolpin BM et al. Phase II study of RAD001 in previously treated patients with metastatic pancreatic cancer. *J Clin Oncol* 26:2008 (May 20 suppl; abstr 4614)
[84] Javie MM et al. Inhibition of the mammalian target of rapamycin (mTOR) in advanced pancreatic cancer: results of two phase II studies. *BMC Cancer* 2010 Jul 14;10:368
[85] Dhillon N, et al. Phase II trial of curcumin in patients with advanced pancreatic cancer. *Clin. Cancer Res.* 2008;14:4491-4499
[86] Epelbaum R, Vizel B, Bar-Sela G. Phase II study of curcumin and gemcitabine in patients with advanced pancreatic cancer [Abstracts] *J Clin Oncol* 2008;26:a15619.
[87] http://clinicaltrials.gov/ct2/show/NCT00486460
[88] Wei D, et al. Celecoxib inhibits vascular endothelial growth factor expression in and reduces angiogenesis and metastasis of human pancreatic cancer via suppression of Sp1 transcription factor activity. *Cancer Res.* 2004;64:2030-2038.
[89] Ferrari V, Valcamonico F, Amoroso V, et al. Gemcitabine plus celecoxib (GECO) in advanced pancreatic cancer: a phase II trial. *Cancer Chemother. Pharmacol.* 2006; 57(2):185-190
[90] Dragovich T, et al. Gemcitabine plus celecoxib in patients with advanced or metastatic pancreatic adenocarcinoma: results of a phase II trial. *Am. J. Clin. Oncol.* 2008; 31:157-162.
[91] Goggins M, et al. Genetic alterations of the transforming growth factor beta receptor genes in pancreatic and biliary tract adenocarcinomas. *Cancer Res* 1998;58:5329-5332.
[92] Hilbig A, et al. Preliminary results of a phase I/II study in patients with pancreatic carcinoma, malignant melanoma or colorectal carcinoma using systemic IV administration of AP 12009 *J Clin Oncol* 2008; 26:a4621
[93] Wong HH, Lemoine NR. Pancreatic cancer: molecular pathogenesis and new therapeutic targets. *Nat Rev Gastroenterol Hepatol* 2009 July 6 (7);412-422
[94] Lutz MP, Esser IB, Flossmann-Kast BB, et al. Overexpression and activation of the tyrosine kinase Src in human pancreatic carcinoma. *Biochem Biophys Res Commun* 1998;243:503-508.
[95] ClinicalTrials.gov Identifier NCT01025570
[96] Thayer SP, et al. Hedgehog is an early and late mediator of pancreatic tumorigenesis. *Nature* 2003;425:851-856
[97] Hermann PC et al. Distinct populations of cancer stem cells determine tumour growth and metastatic activity in human pancreatic cancer. *Cancer Stem Cell* 2007 Sep 13;1(3):313-23
[98] Dang T, Vo K, et al. The role of Notch 3 signaling pathway in pancreatic cancer *J Clin Oncol* 2007;25:a21049
[99] Chau I, et al. Gastrazole (JB95008), a novel CCK2/gastrin receptor antagonist, in the treatment of advanced pancreatic cancer: results from two randomised controlled trials. *Br J Cancer.* 2006;94:1107-1115.

[100] Kawasaki D, et al. Effect of Z-360, a novel orally active CCK-2/gastrin receptor antagonist on tumor growth in human pancreatic adenocarcinoma cell lines in vivo and mode of action determinations in vitro. *Cancer Chemother. Pharmacol.* 2008;61:883-892.

[101] Meyer T, et al. A phase IB/IIA, multicentre, randomised, double-blind placebo controlled study to evaluate the safety and pharmacokinetics of Z-360 in subjects with unresectable advanced pancreatic cancer in combination with gemcitabine [Abstract] *J Clin Oncol.* 2008;26:a4636

[102] Mackey JR, Mani RS, Selner M, et al. Functional nucleoside transporters are required for gemcitabine influx and manifestation of toxicity in cancer cell lines. *Cancer Res* 1998. 58, 4349-4357

[103] Tanaka M, Javle M, Dong, X, et al. Gemcitabine metabolic and transporter gene polymorphisms are associated with drug toxicity and efficacy in patients with locally advanced pancreatic cancer. *Cancer* 2010, 116, 5325-5335.

[104] Spratlin J, Sangha R, Glubrecht, D, et al. The absence of human equilibrative nucleoside transporter 1 is associated with reduced survival in patients with gemcitabine-treated pancreas adenocarcinoma. *Clin Cancer Res* 2004; 10: 6956-6961.

[105] Farrell JJ, Elsaleh H, Garcia M , et al. Human equilibrative nucleoside transporter 1 levels predict response to gemcitabine in patients with pancreatic cancer. *Gastroenterology* 2009; 136:187-196.

[106] Spratlin J, Mackey, JR. Human equilibrative nucleoside transporter 1 (hENT1) in pancreatic adenocarcinoma: Towards individualised treatment decisions. *Cancers* 2010, 2, 2044-2054; doi:10.3390/cancers2042044

[107] Poplin E, Feng Y, Berlin J, et al. Phase III, randomised study of gemcitabine and oxaliplatin versus gemcitabine (fixed dose rate infusion) compared with gemcitabine (30-min infusion) in patients with pancreatic carcinoma E6201: a trail of the Eastern Cooperative Oncology Group. *J Clin Oncol* 2009 10;27(23):Epub 2009 Jul 6

[108] Hendlisz A, Voest EE, Schellens A, et al. Phase I study if oral CP-4126, a gemcitabine analogue, in patients with advanced solid tumours. *J Clin Oncol* 28, 2010 (suppl; abstr e13078)

[109] ClinicalTrials.gov identifier: NCT00913198

[110] Manuyakorn A, Paulsu R, Farrell J, et al. Cellular histone modification patterns predict prognosis and treatment response in resectable pancreatic adenocarcinoma: results from RTOG 9704. *J Clin Oncol* 28: 1358-1365

[111] Herman JM, Hsu CC, Fishman EK, et al. Correlation of DPC4 status with outcomes in pancreatic adenocarcinoma patients receiving adjuvant chemoradiation. *J Clin Oncol* 29: 2011(suppl 4; abstr 168)

[112] Crane CH, Yordy JS, Varadhachary GR, et al. Use of DPC-4 immunostaining of diagnostic cytology specimens to predict the pattern of tumour progression in locally advanced pancreatic cancer patients (LAPC). *J Clin Oncol* 29: 2011 (suppl 4; abstr 209)

5

Temporal Trends in Pancreatic Cancer

Tadeusz Popiela and Marek Sierzega
Jagiellonian University Medical College
Poland

1. Introduction

Pancreatic cancer is one of the most common malignancies of the digestive system and, depending on the geographic area, fourth or fifth leading cause of cancer deaths (Lillemoe *et al*, 2000; Simon & Printz, 2001). Between 1960 and 1980, the incidence rates had increased significantly in most industrialised countries, including Poland. Corresponding 5-year survival rates demonstrated only slight variations and remained stable at about 1-3%. Surprisingly, results obtained from some population databases suggest that only about 30% of patients registered as pancreatic cancer have been adequately verified by histopathology (Wood *et al*, 2006). Moreover, since many studies included only small groups of patients, previous reports did not properly reflect the actual changes, including long-term results of treatment (Gudjonsson, 1995). As incidence rates were relatively high and the efficacy of therapeutic methods was questionable, pancreatic cancer was subject to numerous clinical trials (Jafari & Abbruzzese, 2004). However, no clear conclusions could be drawn in terms of the best therapeutic approach due to marked differences between individual studies (Gudjonsson, 1995).

Many epidemiological studies published over the last 50 years provided detailed data for some general trends related to incidence and mortality rates for pancreatic cancer. Changes in other areas of interest, such as variation in surgical and systemic therapy or long-term outcomes are much less examined. Taking into account these facts, an analysis of temporal trends for some surgical aspects of pancreatic disorders may provide significant information supplementing the results of previous studies.

2. Methods

A literature search was performed using two bibliographic databases, i.e. PubMed and Ovid. Databases were searched using combinations of the following keywords: (pancreatic neoplasm or pancreatic cancer) and (trends or time related changes). Additionally all patients diagnosed with pancreatic duct cell cancer (*adenocarcinoma ductale*) treated between 1972 and 2003 at the 1st Department of General and GI Surgery of Jagiellonian University Medical College in Kraków were reviewed. Other pancreatic tumours verified as non-duct cell cancers and periampullary neoplasms were excluded. Clinical and demographic data, including age, gender and type of therapeutic interventions, were collected from medical records. Tumours were staged according to the TNM classification of *Union Internationale Contre Le Cancer* (UICC) of 1997. The type and extent of surgical treatment was categorised based on commonly accepted criteria (Pedrazzoli *et al*, 1999). To analyse temporal trends for pancreatic cancer, the study interval was divided into three periods, i.e. period 1 (1972-1983), period 2 (1984-1993) and period 3 (1994-2003).

3. General epidemiological trends

Worldwide epidemiological studies on pancreatic cancer have demonstrated slightly higher incidence rates in males irrespectively of the geographic area (Katanoda & Dongmei, 2008; Katanoda & Yako-Suketomo, 2010; Levi *et al*, 2003; Michaud, 2004; Sahmoun *et al*, 2003).

	Period 1 1972-1983 (n=145)	Period 2 1984-1993 (n=294)	Period 3 1994-2003 (n=508)	P
Gender female	70 (48%)	106 (36%)	222 (44%)	0.027†
male	75 (52%)	188 (64%)	286 (56%)	
Age, median (95%CI)	58 (57-62)	60 (58-62)	63 (62-65)	<0.001‡
Location head	89 (61%)	199 (68%)	341 (67%)	0.147†
body	50 (35%)	71 (24%)	140 (28%)	
tail	6 (4%)	24 (8%)	27 (5%)	
Stage I	0 (0%)	7 (2%)	5 (1%)	0.047†
II	3 (2%)	2 (1%)	16 (3%)	
III	8 (6%)	11 (4%)	32 (6%)	
IV	134 (92%)	274 (93%)	455 (90%)	
Therapy surgical	117 (81%)	228 (78%)	376 (74%)	0.192†
conservative	28 (19%)	66 (22%)	132 (26%)	
Type of surgical procedures				
resective	11 (9%)	46 (20%)	115 (31%)	<0.001†
non-resective	106 (91%)	182 (80%)	261 (69%)	
Type of pancreatic resections				
PD	8 (73%)	22 (48%)	46 (40%)	
PPD	0 (0%)	4 (8%)	14 (12%)	0.557†
distal pancreatectomy	2 (18%)	10 (22%)	22 (19%)	
total pancreatectomy	1 (9%)	10 (22%)	33 (29%)	
Type of non-resective surgery				
laparotomy	38 (36%)	62 (34%)	81 (31%)	
biliary bypass	55 (52%)	64 (35%)	19 (7%)	<0.001†
gastro-enteric bypass	4 (4%)	13 (7%)	67 (26%)	
biliary and enteric bypass	9 (8%)	43 (24%)	94 (36%)	
Chemotherapy				
no	138 (95%)	222 (76%)	231 (45%)	<0.01†
yes	7 (5%)	72 (24%)	277 (55%)	
Median survival, months (95%CI)				
overall	5.2 (4.7-5.6)	6.2 (5.2-7.2)	7.6 (6.7-8.5)	<0.001§
pancreatic resections	26.6 (10.4-42.8)	14.3 (11.2-17.4)	20.0 (13.7-26.3)	0.041§
unresectable tumours	5.0 (4.5-5.6)	5.5 (4.6-6.5)	5.9 (5.1-6.6)	<0.001§

Table 1. Demographic and clinical data of patients with pancreatic cancer (PD -pancreatoduodenectomy, PPPD - pylorus-preserving PD, † chi-square test; ‡ ANOVA analysis of variance, § log-rank test)

Most authors agree that this phenomenon is mainly related to the exposure to carcinogens, particularly smoking. The role of the latter factor has been confirmed by increasing incidence trends in populations with a high proportion of smoking individuals and lowering incidence in countries where smoking is decreasing, i.e. Sweden (Bobak, 2003; Flook & van Zanten, 2009; Luo *et al*, 2008; Mulder *et al*, 2002; Simon & Printz, 2001).

Between 1972 and 2003, a total of 1708 patients with chronic pancreatic and periampullary disorders were hospitalised, including 947 patients with histopathologically verified pancreatic duct cell cancer (Popiela et al, 2007). Fifty-eight per cent of 947 patients with pancreatic cancer were males (n=549) and 42% (n=398) females. Although the proportion of males increased temporarily to 64% in period 2, it subsequently decreased to values observed in period 1 (tab. 1). The median age was 62 years (95% confidence interval [CI] 61 - 62) and demonstrated a significant increasing trend over time. Similarly to other authors, we have recorded a significant increase in the proportion of females diagnosed with pancreatic cancer over the last twenty years. The significant increasing trend for the median age shown in our series was similar to other reports where growing numbers of pancreatic resections were carried out in elderly patients (Delcore *et al*, 1991; DiCarlo *et al*, 1998; Sohn *et al*, 1998).

4. Changes in pathological findings

Numerous changes have been observed worldwide in the diagnostics of pancreatic cancer during the last five decades. The number of cases diagnosed at laparotomy carried out due to jaundice or epigastric complaints decreased sharply as abdominal ultrasound was introduced into routine clinical practice (Soreide *et al*, 2010). Subsequently, ultrasound was gradually replaced by less operator-dependent imaging techniques, such as computed tomography (CT) and magnetic resonance imaging (MRI). A gradual increase in the use of endoscopic ultrasonography (EUS) and positron emission tomography (PET) has been observed over the recent years, but their application is usually limited to some specific clinical situations. The proportion of patients diagnosed solely with US and CT nowadays varies between 75% and 85%, while other imaging techniques (MRI, PET, EUS) are used less frequently (David *et al*, 2009; Ngamruengphong *et al*, 2010).

The majority of lesions treated in our centre was located in the head of the pancreas (n=629, 66%), whereas cancers of the body and tail were found in 28% (n=261) and 6% (n=57) of cases, respectively. There were no significant differences in the proportions of tumours located in the head, body and tail of the pancreas over time (Popiela *et al*, 2007). However, other authors suggested some variation over time. Based on 43,946 cases of pancreatic cancer recorded between 1973 and 2002 in the Surveillance, Epidemiology, and End Results (SEER), Lau et al. found a 46% increase in the incidence of body/tail cancers (Lau *et al*, 2010). Reports from other geographic areas mostly failed to demonstrate any significant change in the prevalence of distally-located cancers.

Technical improvements in imaging methods and their wider accessibility should theoretically allow for an earlier diagnosis of pancreatic cancer leading to reduced proportions of advanced tumours and increased resectability rates. Surprisingly, most cohort studies failed to demonstrate any marked increase in the proportion of cancers at a lower stage (Cress *et al*, 2006; Janes *et al*, 1996; Niederhuber *et al*, 1995; Riall *et al*, 2006; Sener *et al*, 1999). The percentage of patients with stage IV tumours in our series, similarly to other reports, showed only a slight lowering trend. Although this phenomenon was accompanied by increasing resectability rates, the proportion of stage groups in patients undergoing pancreatic resections remained stable. Similarly to our findings, other authors reported only slight variations in staging patients with pancreatic cancer. In a population of 2986 cases of pancreatic cancer from the Digestive Cancer Registry of Burgundy (France) over a 30-year period (1976–2005) the overall proportion of stage I, II and III tumours was 1.3%, 2.2% and 5.4%, respectively (David *et al*, 2009). The proportion of stage I–II cancers slightly increased from 2.8% in the 1976–1980 period to 8.8% in the 2001–2005 period, though these changes were highly significant (P<0.001). Nevertheless, metastatic and/or non-resected cases decreased only by about 10% from 95.2% to 85.5%. The increasing trend of resectability rates found in this study was also confirmed by authors from various geographic areas. In a group of 16,758 patients treated between 1980 and 2000 in Sweden, the proportion of resectable tumours observed by Linder et al. increased from 7.2% to 15.1% (Linder *et al*, 2006). A similar trend was reported for the US population in a recent study involving 24,016 patients (Riall *et al*, 2006).

5. Surgical trends

Improved diagnostic methods increased the percentage of patients diagnosed with metastatic disease before surgery. Simultaneous development of endoscopic methods allows to perform biliary or duodenal stenting, and along with better imaging tests, has contributed to the decreasing rates of open surgery in patients with disseminated disease (Lefebvre *et al*, 2009).

Two hundred and twenty-six of 947 analysed patients (24%) were disqualified from surgical intervention. The remaining 721 (76%) patients were subject to surgical therapy and this proportion decreased insignificantly from 81% to 74% in the last decade. Pancreatic resections were performed in 172 (24%) patients and the resectability rate increased significantly from 9% to 31% between period 1 and 3, respectively. No significant changes in the type of pancreatic resections could be demonstrated for the whole cohort. However, an increasing proportion of pylorus-preserving pancreaticoduodenectomy (Traverso procedure) from 0% to 23% in the last period was found for lesions located in the head of the pancreas. The percentage of patients undergoing only exploratory laparotomy was stable over time with a mean value of 33%. The proportion of patients with biliary bypass significantly decreased with a concomitant increase in the ratio of gastro-enteric and double bypass procedures.

A gradual increase in endoscopic procedures is commonly reported in most reports. Linder et al. reported a significant reduction in the proportion of patient subject to surgical biliary bypass from 45.9% between 1980 and 1986 to 18.1% between 1994 and 2000 (Linder *et al*, 2006). These changes were accompanied by a lowering percentage of gastro-enteric bypass from 33.8% to 22.8%. Lefebvre et al. reported a similar decreasing trend for palliative surgery from 55% in 1978–1982 to 32% in 1998–2002 due to the more common use of endoscopic stenting (Lefebvre *et al*, 2009). We have found analogical variations in biliary bypass from 52% to 7%, but as opposed to Linder et al. the percentage of gastro-enteric and simultaneous biliary and enteric bypasses increased from 4% to 26% and from 8% to 36%, respectively. This change in the therapeutic strategy was related mainly to our analysis of patients requiring open surgery for upper gastrointestinal ileus and results of randomized clinical trials supporting the idea of prophylactic gastro-enteric bypass (Lillemoe *et al*, 1999; Popiela *et al*, 2002b; Van Heek *et al*, 2003). The increasing proportion of pylorus-preserving pancreaticoduodenectomy observed in the last decade for patients undergoing pancreatic head resections reflects the current belief that the procedure does not impair oncological radicality and, as suggest some authors, reduces adverse metabolic consequences of pancreatic resections (Schafer *et al*, 2002).

The most important aspect of surgery-related trends in pancreatic cancer is associated with markedly decreasing postoperative mortality. We have observed similar changes in the early postoperative outcomes and long-term survival as those reported by other authors (Popiela *et al*, 2002b; Sierzega *et al*, 2006). In particular, a significant lowering trend of postoperative mortality rates was found from values exceeding 10% in the early eighties to an average of 4.1% in the last decade (fig. 1) (Popiela, 1979; Popiela *et al*, 2004).

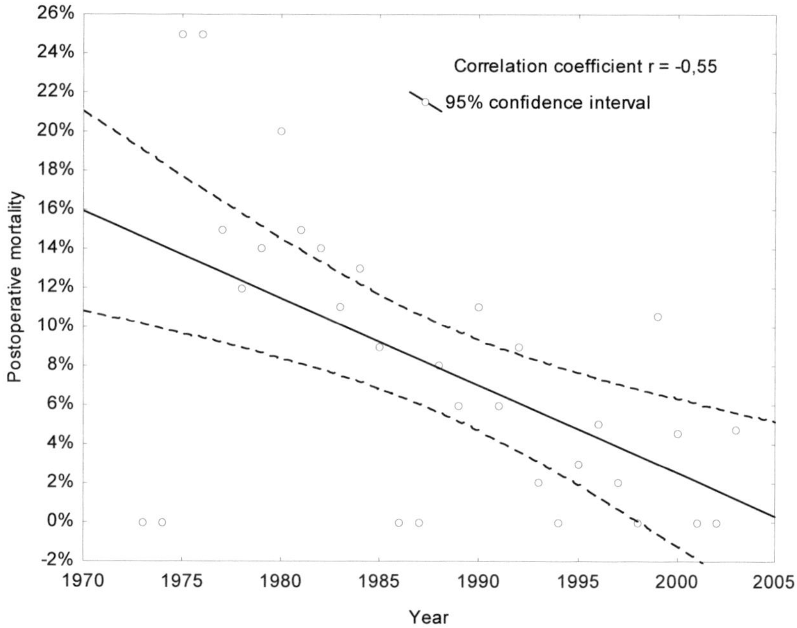

Fig. 1. Postoperative mortality rates for pancreatic resections in consecutive years

6. Trends in systemic therapy

Pancreatic surgery has reached a plateau in terms of long-term survival observed for patients with pancreatic cancer (Popiela *et al*, 2002a; Popiela *et al*, 2002c). Therefore, further improvements should only be expected from combined modality therapy. IN our series, various regimens of chemotherapy were used in 38% (n=356) of cases and the percentage of patients qualified of systemic therapy increased significantly from 5% in period 1 to 55% in period 3. Fluorouracil was the primary chemotherapeutic agent until 1997 and afterwards was replaced by multidrug regimens based on gemcitabine, cisplatin and irinotecan.

Although there is no uniform consensus on adjuvant therapy of pancreatic cancer, a recent meta-analysis of clinical trials have supported the benefits of chemotherapy found in our study (Stocken *et al*, 2005). The most recent analysis of data from the SEER registry in 1910 patients who underwent resections for pancreatic adenocarcinoma performed between 1991 and 2002 reflects the overall change in the proportion of patients qualified for systemic treatment after surgical intervention (Simons *et al*, 2010). The proportion of subjects receiving adjuvant chemoradiotherapy in US increased from 26% in 1991-1993 to 37% in 2000-2002. The role of palliative chemotherapy is also increasing as demonstrated in a recent meta-analysis of clinical trials, where chemotherapy significantly prolonged survival compared to symptomatic therapy (Yip *et al*, 2009). Another meta-analysis on gemcitabine combined with platinum agents provided additional proofs for combination therapy, as the concomitant use of both drugs significantly increased response rates and prolonged time to progression (Xie *et al*, 2006). Results of our studies showed that any gemcitabine based regimen of palliative chemotherapy produced better results than observed in control groups and the combination of gemcitabine and cisplatin was the most effective regimen (Popiela *et al*, 2001; Popiela *et al*, 2005). Increased rates of adjuvant and palliative chemotherapy have been reported by several authors (David *et al*, 2009; Lefebvre *et al*, 2009).

7. Changes in prognosis

The overall median survival in our series was 7.1 months (95%CI 6.6 to 7.6) and was significantly longer after pancreatic resections (median 14.8 months; 95%CI 11.5 to 16.9) than in the remaining cases (median 5.8 months; 95%CI 4.4 to 6.9). The overall 5-year survival rate was 4.5% and increased to 14.3% for resective cases. No patient with unresectable tumour survived 5 years from the time of diagnosis. Pairwise comparisons of survival functions demonstrated statistically significant differences between each stage according to UICC 1997 (fig. 2).

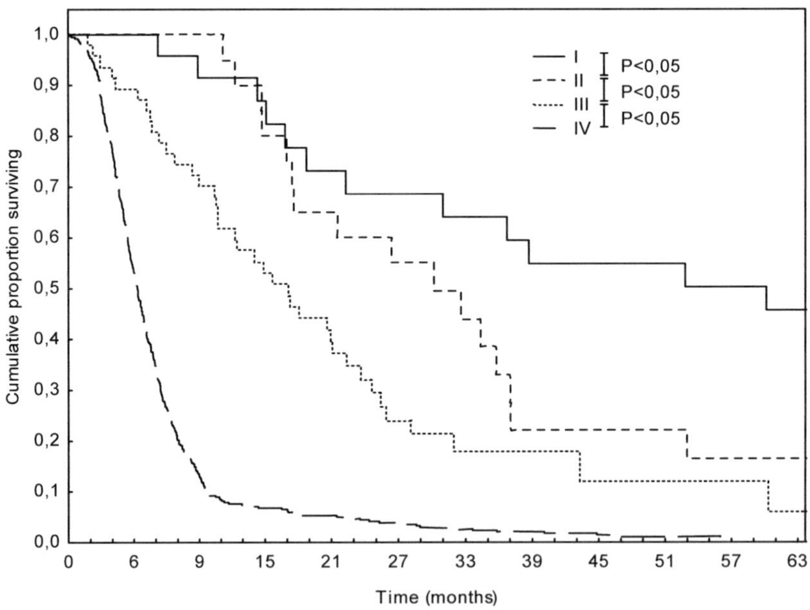

Fig. 2. Stage-specific survival for resectable pancreatic cancer

The 5-year survival rate for stage I was 50.3% with a median survival of 63.1 months (95%CI 7.6 to 118.6). Five-year survival rates of 16.5% and 5.9% for stage II and III, respectively, were significantly lower. Corresponding median survival times were 33.2 months (95%CI 21.0 to 45.5) and 20.1 months (95%CI 14.8 to 25.3). The median survival of patients with stage IV cancers was 6.2 months (95%CI 5.7-6.6) and no patient survived 5 years. The median and 5-year survival rates after curative resections (R0 according to UICC) were 27.9

months and 29.4%, respectively. The corresponding duration of median survival for microscopically (R1) and macroscopically (R2) non-radical resections of 11.4 and 11 months was significantly shorter. No patient survived 5 years after either R1 or R2 resection. A significant increasing trend for overall survival was found between period 1 and 3 (fig. 3, tab. 1). The correlation coefficient for the median survival of patients treated in consecutive years was 0.59 and this increasing trend was statistically significant (fig. 4). The median survival of patients undergoing pancreatic resections during the last decade (20 months, 95%CI 13.7 to 26.3) was significantly longer than for the period 1984-1993 (14.3 months, 95%CI 11.2 to 17.4). However, the differences between median survival during 1972-1983 and 1984-1993 or 1972-1983 and 1994-2003 were statistically insignificant (fig. 5). Nevertheless, the median survival of patients with unresectable tumours increased significantly between consecutive periods (fig. 6).

Long-term results in patients treated for pancreatic cancer demonstrate only slight variations over the last 30 years with 5-year survival rates of 1-3% (Gudjonsson, 1995; Lillemoe *et al*, 2000; Tsiotos *et al*, 1999). Nevertheless, the number of reports describing improving survival trends is growing (Riall *et al*, 2006; Wood *et al*, 2006). The 2.4-month increase in the overall median survival found in our patients was due to improvements observed in both resectable (from 14.3 months between 1984 and 1993 to 20 months between 1994 and 2003), and unresectable cases (from 5 months between 1972 and 1983 to 5.9 months in the last decade). The relatively high median survival (26.6 months) in resectable patients treated in period 1 was related to the small number of cases (11 patients). In a recent publication of 1423 patients undergoing pancreaticoduodenectomy for pancreatic cancer, the median survival increased significantly from 8 months in the eighties to 19 months in patients operated after 2000 with comparable proportions of stage groups (Winter *et al*, 2006). A similar trend was also reported by Riall et al. in a large study on unresectable

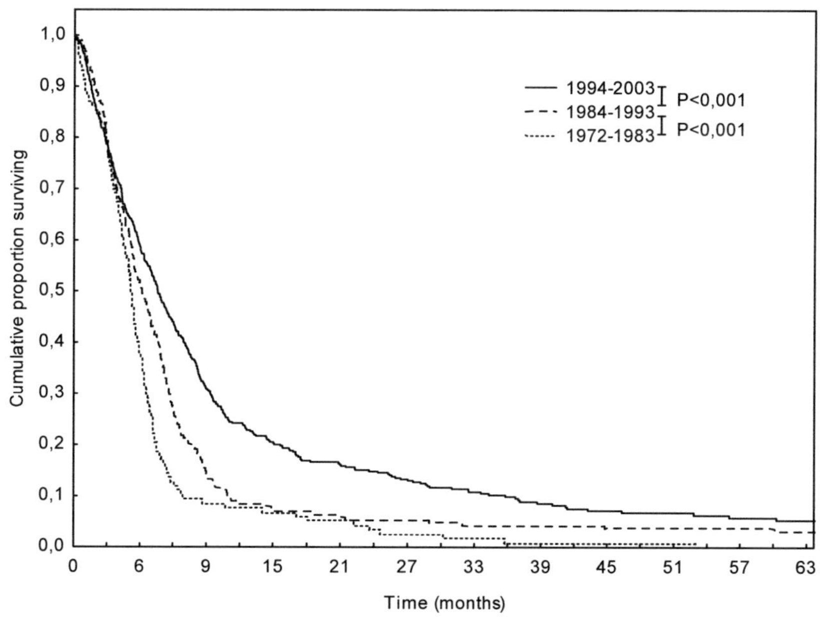

Fig. 3. Overall survival functions for individual time periods

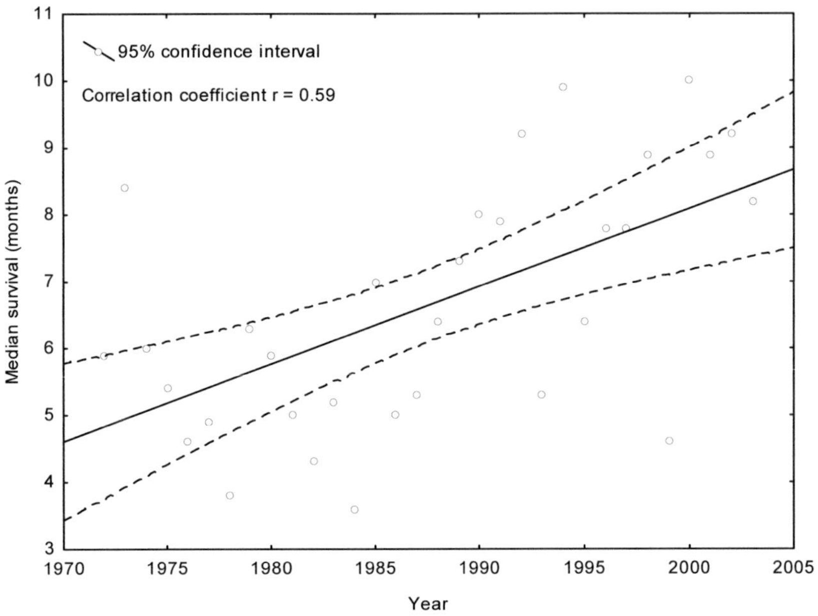

Fig. 4. Changes in median survival in consecutive years

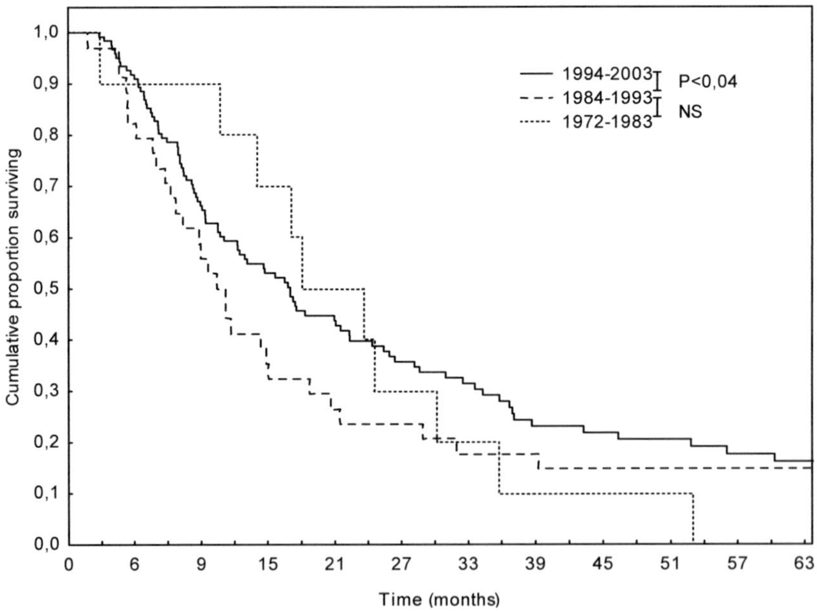

Fig. 5. Changes in survival in consecutive years for resectable tumours

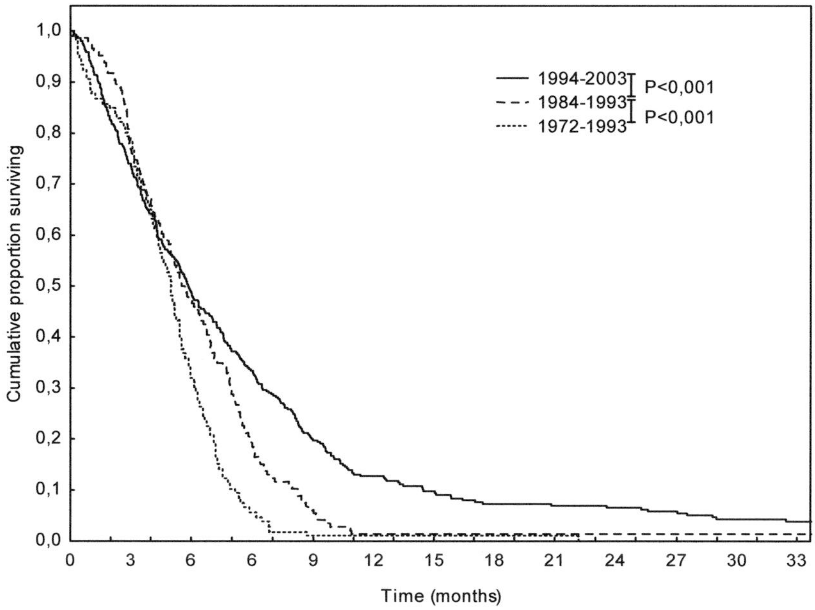

Fig. 6. Changes in median survival in consecutive years for unresectable tumours

pancreatic cancer (Riall *et al*, 2006). In 12043 cases of disseminated disease, the proportion of patients who survived 2 years increased from 1.4% between 1988 and 1991 to 2.3% between 1996 and 1999. A recent analysis of the SEER database showed a similar improving trend for overall survival in patients with pancreatic cancer (Lau *et al*, 2010). The overall 3-year survival rate increased from 4.3% to 6.2% from 1973 to 1987 to 1988 to 2002 for tumours of the pancreatic head and from 2.8% to 3.9% in pancreatic body/tail cancers. Similar observations were reported from the South Australian Cancer Registry covering the period from 1977 to 2006 with 4,166 pancreatic cancers (Luke *et al*, 2009) and 21,663 patients from the Cancer Registry of Norway for the period 1965–2007 (Soreide *et al*, 2010).

8. Conclusion

The analysis of 947 patients with pancreatic cancer treated between 1972 and 2003 demonstrated the existence of significant trends mainly for early postoperative and long-term outcomes. Postoperative mortality rates significantly decreased from values exceeding 10% in the early eighties to an average of 4.1% in the last decade. The overall median survival increased from 5.2 to 7.6 months and this change was reflected by improving outcomes in both resectable and unresectable disease. The observed changes are attributed mainly to the increasing role of combined therapy and emphasise the importance of such an approach.

Even with easily accessible imaging tests, the majority of patients with either cancer is still diagnosed at an advanced stage. Therefore, improved diagnostic procedures at the level of pre-hospital care are the key for actual improvement of patients' survival. Primary care physicians and specialists diagnosing patients with obstructive jaundice are of particular importance since endoscopic procedures commonly performed by gastroenterologists cannot be regarded as curative therapy and the need for surgical exploration should always be considered.

9. References

Bobak M (2003) Relative and absolute gender gap in all-cause mortality in Europe and the contribution of smoking. *Eur J Epidemiol* 18(1): 15-8

Cress RD, Yin D, Clarke L, Bold R, Holly EA (2006) Survival among patients with adenocarcinoma of the pancreas: a population-based study (United States). *Cancer Causes Control* 17(4): 403-9

David M, Lepage C, Jouve JL, Jooste V, Chauvenet M, Faivre J, Bouvier AM (2009) Management and prognosis of pancreatic cancer over a 30-year period. *Br J Cancer* 101(2): 215-8

Delcore R, Thomas JH, Hermreck AS (1991) Pancreaticoduodenectomy for malignant pancreatic and periampullary neoplasms in elderly patients. *Am J Surg* 162(6): 532-5; discussion 535-6

DiCarlo V, Balzano G, Zerbi A, Villa E (1998) Pancreatic cancer resection in elderly patients. *Br J Surg* 85(5): 607-10

Flook R, van Zanten SV (2009) Pancreatic cancer in Canada: incidence and mortality trends from 1992 to 2005. *Can J Gastroenterol* 23(8): 546-50

Gudjonsson B (1995) Carcinoma of the pancreas: critical analysis of costs, results of resections, and the need for standardized reporting. *J Am Coll Surg* 181(6): 483-503

Jafari M, Abbruzzese JL (2004) Pancreatic cancer: future outlook, promising trials, newer systemic agents, and strategies from the Gastrointestinal Intergroup Pancreatic Cancer Task Force. *Surg Oncol Clin N Am* 13(4): 751-60, xi

Janes RH, Jr., Niederhuber JE, Chmiel JS, Winchester DP, Ocwieja KC, Karnell JH, Clive RE, Menck HR (1996) National patterns of care for pancreatic cancer. Results of a survey by the Commission on Cancer. *Ann Surg* 223(3): 261-72

Katanoda K, Dongmei Q (2008) Comparison of time trends in pancreatic cancer incidence (1973-97) in East Asia, Europe and USA, from Cancer Incidence in Five Continents Vol. IV-VIII. *Jpn J Clin Oncol* 38(2): 165-6

Katanoda K, Yako-Suketomo H (2010) Comparison of time trends in pancreatic cancer mortality (1990-2006) between countries based on the WHO mortality database. *Jpn J Clin Oncol* 40(6): 601-2

Lau MK, Davila JA, Shaib YH (2010) Incidence and survival of pancreatic head and body and tail cancers: a population-based study in the United States. *Pancreas* 39(4): 458-62

Lefebvre AC, Maurel J, Boutreux S, Bouvier V, Reimund JM, Launoy G, Arsene D (2009) Pancreatic cancer: incidence, treatment and survival trends--1175 cases in Calvados (France) from 1978 to 2002. *Gastroenterol Clin Biol* 33(10-11): 1045-51

Levi F, Lucchini F, Negri E, La Vecchia C (2003) Pancreatic cancer mortality in Europe: the leveling of an epidemic. *Pancreas* 27(2): 139-42

Lillemoe KD, Cameron JL, Hardacre JM, Sohn TA, Sauter PK, Coleman J, Pitt HA, Yeo CJ (1999) Is prophylactic gastrojejunostomy indicated for unresectable periampullary cancer? A prospective randomized trial. *Ann Surg* 230(3): 322-8; discussion 328-30

Lillemoe KD, Yeo CJ, Cameron JL (2000) Pancreatic cancer: state-of-the-art care. *CA Cancer J Clin* 50(4): 241-68

Linder S, Bostrom L, Nilsson B (2006) Pancreatic cancer in sweden 1980-2000: a population-based study of hospitalized patients concerning time trends in curative surgery and other interventional therapies. *J Gastrointest Surg* 10(5): 672-8

Luke C, Price T, Karapetis C, Singhal N, Roder D (2009) Pancreatic cancer epidemiology and survival in an Australian population. *Asian Pac J Cancer Prev* 10(3): 369-74

Luo J, Adami HO, Reilly M, Ekbom A, Nordenvall C, Ye W (2008) Interpreting trends of pancreatic cancer incidence and mortality: a nation-wide study in Sweden (1960-2003). *Cancer Causes Control* 19(1): 89-96

Michaud DS (2004) Epidemiology of pancreatic cancer. *Minerva Chir* 59(2): 99-111

Mulder I, Hoogenveen RT, van Genugten ML, Lankisch PG, Lowenfels AB, de Hollander AE, Bueno-de-Mesquita HB (2002) Smoking cessation would substantially reduce the future incidence of pancreatic cancer in the European Union. *Eur J Gastroenterol Hepatol* 14(12): 1343-53

Ngamruengphong S, Li F, Zhou Y, Chak A, Cooper GS, Das A (2010) EUS and survival in patients with pancreatic cancer: a population-based study. *Gastrointest Endosc* 72(1): 78-83, 83 e1-2

Niederhuber JE, Brennan MF, Menck HR (1995) The National Cancer Data Base report on pancreatic cancer. *Cancer* 76(9): 1671-7

Pedrazzoli S, Beger HG, Obertop H, Andren-Sandberg A, Fernandez-Cruz L, Henne-Bruns D, Luttges J, Neoptolemos JP (1999) A surgical and pathological based classification of resective treatment of pancreatic cancer. Summary of an international workshop on surgical procedures in pancreatic cancer. *Dig Surg* 16(4): 337-45

Popiela T (1979) Early detection and surgical treatment of pancreatic cancer. *Pol Przeg Chir* 51: 1049-1054

Popiela T, Kedra B, Sierzega M (2001) Efficacy of gemcitabine in patients wit non-resectable pancreatic cancer: prospective clinical study. *Nowotwory* 51: 117-121

Popiela T, Kedra B, Sierzega M (2002a) Does extended lymphadenectomy improve survival of pancreatic cancer patients? *Acta Chir Belg* 102(2): 78-82

Popiela T, Kedra B, Sierzega M, Gurda A (2004) Risk factors of pancreatic fistula following pancreaticoduodenectomy for periampullary cancer. *Hepatogastroenterology* 51(59): 1484-8

Popiela T, Kedra B, Sierzega M, Kubisz A (2002b) Chirurgisch palliative Therapie beim Pankreaskarzinom: 25 Jahre Erfahrungen eines einzelnen Referenzzentrums. *Zentralbl Chir* 127(11): 965-70

Popiela T, Kedra B, Sierzega M, Kubisz A (2002c) Patienten mit nicht-fortgeschrittenen Pankreaskarzinomen profitieren von der ausgedehnten Lymphadenektomie. *Zentralbl Chir* 127(11): 960-4

Popiela T, Kulig J, Sierzega M, Legutko J (2005) A prospective randomized trial on two gemcitabine-based regimens of chemotherapy for unresectable pancreatic cancer. *Gastroenterology* 128(Supp 2): A-109

Popiela T, Kulig J, Sierzega M, Richter P, Legutko J (2007) Temporal trends of pancreatic cancer and cancer of the ampulla of Vater treated between 1972 and 2003. *Gastroenterol Pol* 14(4): 241-249

Riall TS, Nealon WH, Goodwin JS, Zhang D, Kuo YF, Townsend CM, Jr., Freeman JL (2006) Pancreatic cancer in the general population: Improvements in survival over the last decade. *J Gastrointest Surg* 10(9): 1212-23; discussion 1223-4

Sahmoun AE, D'Agostino RA, Jr., Bell RA, Schwenke DC (2003) International variation in pancreatic cancer mortality for the period 1955-1998. *Eur J Epidemiol* 18(8): 801-16

Schafer M, Mullhaupt B, Clavien PA (2002) Evidence-based pancreatic head resection for pancreatic cancer and chronic pancreatitis. *Ann Surg* 236(2): 137-48

Sener SF, Fremgen A, Menck HR, Winchester DP (1999) Pancreatic cancer: a report of treatment and survival trends for 100,313 patients diagnosed from 1985-1995, using the National Cancer Database. *J Am Coll Surg* 189(1): 1-7

Sierzega M, Popiela T, Kulig J, Nowak K (2006) The ratio of metastatic/resected lymph nodes is an independent prognostic factor in patients with node-positive pancreatic head cancer. *Pancreas* 33(3): 240-5

Simon B, Printz H (2001) Epidemiological trends in pancreatic neoplasias. *Dig Dis* 19(1): 6-14

Simons JP, Ng SC, McDade TP, Zhou Z, Earle CC, Tseng JF (2010) Progress for resectable pancreatic [corrected] cancer?: a population-based assessment of US practices. *Cancer* 116(7): 1681-90

Sohn TA, Yeo CJ, Cameron JL, Lillemoe KD, Talamini MA, Hruban RH, Sauter PK, Coleman J, Ord SE, Grochow LB, Abrams RA, Pitt HA (1998) Should pancreaticoduodenectomy be performed in octogenarians? *J Gastrointest Surg* 2(3): 207-16

Soreide K, Aagnes B, Moller B, Westgaard A, Bray F (2010) Epidemiology of pancreatic cancer in Norway: trends in incidence, basis of diagnosis and survival 1965-2007. *Scand J Gastroenterol* 45(1): 82-92

Stocken DD, Buchler MW, Dervenis C, Bassi C, Jeekel H, Klinkenbijl JH, Bakkevold KE, Takada T, Amano H, Neoptolemos JP (2005) Meta-analysis of randomised adjuvant therapy trials for pancreatic cancer. *Br J Cancer* 92(8): 1372-81

Tsiotos GG, Farnell MB, Sarr MG (1999) Are the results of pancreatectomy for pancreatic cancer improving? *World J Surg* 23(9): 913-9

Van Heek NT, De Castro SM, van Eijck CH, van Geenen RC, Hesselink EJ, Breslau PJ, Tran TC, Kazemier G, Visser MR, Busch OR, Obertop H, Gouma DJ (2003) The need for a prophylactic gastrojejunostomy for unresectable periampullary cancer: a prospective randomized multicenter trial with special focus on assessment of quality of life. *Ann Surg* 238(6): 894-902; discussion 902-5

Winter JM, Cameron JL, Campbell KA, Arnold MA, Chang DC, Coleman J, Hodgin MB, Sauter PK, Hruban RH, Riall TS, Schulick RD, Choti MA, Lillemoe KD, Yeo CJ (2006) 1423 pancreaticoduodenectomies for pancreatic cancer: A single-institution experience. *J Gastrointest Surg* 10(9): 1199-210; discussion 1210-1

Wood HE, Gupta S, Kang JY, Quinn MJ, Maxwell JD, Mudan S, Majeed A (2006) Pancreatic cancer in England and Wales 1975-2000: patterns and trends in incidence, survival and mortality. *Aliment Pharmacol Ther* 23(8): 1205-14

Xie DR, Liang HL, Wang Y, Guo SS, Yang Q (2006) Meta-analysis on inoperable pancreatic cancer: a comparison between gemcitabine-based combination therapy and gemcitabine alone. *World J Gastroenterol* 12(43): 6973-81

Yip D, Karapetis C, Strickland A, Steer CB, Goldstein D (2009) Chemotherapy and radiotherapy for inoperable advanced pancreatic cancer. *Cochrane Database Syst Rev*(4): CD002093

6

Current Perspectives and Future Trends of Systemic Therapy in Advanced Pancreatic Carcinoma

Purificacion Estevez-Garcia and Rocio Garcia-Carbonero
GI Oncology Unit, Medical Oncology Department,
Virgen del Rocio University Hospital,
Instituto de Biomedicina de Sevilla (IBIS), Seville,
Spain

1. Introduction

Pancreatic carcinoma is one of the most lethal solid tumors, with particularly high mortality-to-incidence rates. Indeed, about 278,684 people were diagnosed worldwide of pancreatic cancer in 2008, of whom 266,669 dyed from the disease in the same year (Ferlay et al, 2010). The greatest impact is observed in developed countries were pancreatic cancer has become the fourth leading cause of cancer-related death (Jemal et al, 2010).

Pancreatic ductal adenocarcinoma represents more than 90% of pancreatic malignancies. The majority arise in the head, neck or uncinate process (60-70%), being less commonly encountered in the body (5-10%) or tail (10-15%) of the gland (Solcia et al, 1997). Clinical presentation is often related to the location of the primary tumor within the gland, although many patients often undergo an initial period of nonspecific symptoms such as back pain or vague gastrointestinal distress. Jaundice may be a relatively early symptom for tumors located in the head or uncinate process of the pancreas. However, left-sided pancreatic tumors may remain asymptomatic for long periods of time. Other associated disorders include acute pancreatitis or diabetes mellitus, and when they develop in patients without risk factors or in conjunction with other associated symptoms such as pain, anorexia or weight loss, the possibility of an underlying malignancy should be considered. Thromboembolic complications are also very common and are associated with a poor prognosis, with an incidence ranging from 17% to 57% (Khorana & Fine, 2004). Anorexia, weight loss or gastric outlet obstruction generally occur late in the course of the disease. Nevertheless, even early symptoms in this tumor are usually indicative of advanced disease.

Clinical features of pancreatic adenocarcinoma translate its extremely high propensity for local invasion and distant spread, underscoring the great difficulty to obtain an early diagnosis. In fact, more than 70% of patients present with unresectable, locally advanced or metastatic disease at the time of diagnosis (Stathis & Moore, 2010), and 70-80% of resected tumors will eventually relapse following surgery. Once the tumor has progressed beyond surgical resectability, prognosis is rather poor, with median survival ranging from 6 to 9 months and 5-year overall survival rates of less than 5% (National Cancer Institute, 2010; Jemal et al, 2008).

In recent years there has been only minimal progress in the systemic treatment of metastatic pancreatic cancer. Current standard therapies have a limited impact on the natural history of this disease and improvements in systemic therapy are desperately needed in order to improve the prognosis of these patients. However, intense translational and clinical research has lead to a better and deeper understanding of the complex molecular biology of this tumor and shall help improve the development of new more effective drugs in this disease.

2. Conventional cytotoxic therapy

2.1 Monotherapy

Early randomized trials demonstrated that several 5-fluorouracil (5FU)-based combination chemotherapy regimens improved survival (hazard ratio [HR] = 0.64; 95%CI, 0.42 to 0.98) and quality of life of patients with advanced pancreatic cancer over best supportive care (BSC) alone (Sultana et al, 2007). Subsequent studies showed, however, that 5FU-based combination therapy did not result in better overall survival compared with 5FU alone (HR = 0.94; 95% CI, 0.82 to 1.08). 5FU monotherapy became, consequently, the standard of care for pancreatic cancer. Reported response rates widely ranged from 0% to 19% (Evans et al, 1997), partly due to the lack of standardized criteria to assess response in these early trials, with median survival times of 4.2 to 5.5 months (Burris et al, 1997).

During the 1990s several non-controlled trials suggested some promising activity of a new drug in pancreatic cancer, gemcitabine. The pivotal study by Burris et al was responsible for the change in practice from 5FU to gemcitabine based on a marginal survival advantage and an improvement in clinical benefit response favoring gemcitabine-treated patients. This trial enrolled 126 patients with chemotherapy-naïve advanced symptomatic pancreatic cancer who were randomly allocated to receive gemcitabine (1000 mg/m2/week x 7 followed by 1 week of rest, and then weekly x 3 every 4 weeks) or 5-FU (600 mg/m2/week) until disease progression, clinical deterioration or unacceptable toxicity (Burris et al, 1997). The primary efficacy outcome was clinical benefit response (CBR), a term introduced for the first time in this trial, which was a composite of measurements of pain (analgesic consumption and pain intensity), Karnofsky performance status and weight. No statistically significant difference was found between study arms in terms of objective response (gemcitabine 5.4% vs 5-FU 0%), but patients in the gemcitabine arm experienced improved CBR (24% vs 5%) and overall survival (5.65 months vs 4.41 months, p=0.0025), with 1-year survival rates also favoring gemcitabine-treated patients (18% vs 2%).

Further trials aimed to optimize gemcitabine administration schedule. Gemcitabine (difluorodeoxycytidine) is a nucleoside analogue capable of inhibiting ribonucleotide reductase to deplete nucleoside pools, and its phosphorylated metabolite is incorporated into DNA causing chain termination and inhibition of DNA synthesis, function and repair. Phosphorylation of gemcitabine to the monophosphate by deoxycytidine kinase is the rate-limiting step in the accumulation of the active diphosphate and triphosphate metabolites. Some early clinical studies observed the rate of gemcitabine triphosphate accumulation by mononuclear cells and leukemia cells was optimized using dose rates of 10 mg/m2/min.

Conversely, preclinical data had suggested a dose-response relationship independent of infusion duration. In light of these data, a randomized phase II trial conducted in 92 pancreatic cancer patients was designed to assess the efficacy of two dose-intense schedules of gemcitabine: a dose-intense schedule administering gemcitabine as a standard 30-minute infusion (2200 mg/2/week) versus gemcitabine administered at a fixed dose rate (FDR) of 10 mg/m2/min (1500 mg/m2/week 150-minute infusion) (Gelibter et al, 2005; Tempero et al, 2003). Patients in the FDR infusion arm experienced increased survival rates (18% vs 2% at 2 years, p=.007), consistent with the higher intracellular gemcitabine triphosphate concentrations observed in these patients, although at the expense of increased hematologic toxicity. However, a confirmatory phase III trial failed to confirm a survival advantage for the FDR regimen over the standard administration (Poplin et al, 2009).

2.2 Combination chemotherapy

Although the benefit of chemotherapy in patients with advanced pancreatic cancer is well established, the magnitude of the effect is rather small, with an absolute improvement of survival at 5 years of 3% to 6% (survival rates from 1975-77 to 1999-2005) (Oberstein & Saif, 2011). Over the past decade, multiple randomized trials have been performed to assess a number of gemcitabine-combination chemotherapy regimens in an effort to improve these modest results. These have included combinations with 5-FU (Berlin et al, 2002; Riess et al, 2005), capecitabine (Herrmann et al, 2007; Bernhard et al, 2008; Cunningham et al, 2009), cisplatin (Heinemann et al, 2006; Colucci et al, 2002, 2009), oxaliplatin (Louvet et al, 2005; Poplin et al, 2009), irinotecan (Rocha et al, 2004; Stathopoulos et al, 2006), exatecan (Abou Alfa et al, 2006) and pemetrexed (Oettle et al, 2005a). Individually, although many of these studies observed some improvement in terms of response rate and progression free survival favoring combination therapy, the great majority failed to demonstrate a survival benefit (Table 1).

The largest and most recent meta-analysis, however, confirm a modest although significant benefit in survival for gemcitabine combinations over gemcitabine alone (HR 0.91; 95%CI: 0.85 to 0.97; p=0.004) in patients with locally advanced or metastatic pancreatic cancer (Sultana et al, 2007; Heinemann et al, 2008b). The magnitude of this benefit was remarkably greater (HR 0.76; 95%CI: 0.67 to 0.87; p<0.0001) in patients with good performance status (representing 38% of all patients included in the meta-analysis). In subgroup analysis, platinum compounds (3 trials, 1077 patients; HR 0.85; 95%CI 0.74-0.96) and capecitabine (3 trials, 935 patients; HR 0.83; 95%CI 0.72-0.96) in combination with gemcitabine consistently showed improved survival over single-agent gemcitabine. Insufficient evidence was observed, nevertheless, to support combination of gemcitabine with 5FU or irinotecan.

The rationale for the combined use of gemcitabine and cisplatin is based on the preclinical evidence that gemcitabine not only increases cisplatin-induced DNA cross links, but also effectively inhibits their repair, and cisplatin, on the other hand, enhances the incorporation of gemcitabine triphosphate into DNA. In vitro studies show synergistic cytotoxicity and several non-controlled clinical studies suggested improved efficacy. Some early randomized studies observed increased response rates and progression free survival for patients treated with the cisplatin-gemcitabine combination as compared to those treated with gemcitabine alone (Colucci et al, 2002; Heinemann et al, 2006), with a non-significant trend towards a longer survival. However, more recent and larger trials have failed to confirm a significant

Reference	Treatment	Number of patients	Response Rate (%)	PFS (months)	OS (months)
Berlin *et al* (2002)	GEM vs GEM+5FU	327	5.6 vs 6.9	2.2 vs 3.4 (p=0.022)	5.4 vs 6.7 (p=0.09)
Herrmann *et al* (2007)	GEM vs GEM+ CAP	319	7.8 vs 10	3.9 vs 4.3 (p=0.103)	7.2 vs 8.4 (p=0.234)
Cunningham *et al* (2009)	GEM vs GEM+ CAP	533	12 vs 19 (p=0.034)	3.8 vs 5.3 (p=0.004)	6.2 vs 7.1 (p=0.08)
Colucci *et al* (2002)	GEM vs GEM+CIS	107	9.2 vs 26.4 (p=0.02)	1.8 vs 4.6 (p=0.048)	5 vs 7.5 (p=0.43)
Colucci et al (2010)	GEM vs GEM+CIS	400	10.1 vs 12.9 (p=0.37)	3.9 vs 3.8 (p=0.80)	8.3 vs 7.2 (p=0.38)
Heinemann *et al* (2006)	GEM vs GEM+CIS	195	8.2 vs 10.2	3.1 vs 5.3 (p=0.053)	6 vs 7.6 (p=0.15)
Louvet *et al* (2005)	GEM vs GEM+OX	313	17.3 vs 26.8 (p=0.04)	3.7 vs 5.8 (p=0.04)	7.1 vs 9 (p=0.13)
Poplin *et al* (2009)	GEM vs GEM FDR GEM+OX	832	6 vs 10 vs 9 (p=0.11)	2.6 vs 3.5 (p=0.04) vs 2.7 (p=0.1)	4.9 vs 6.2 (p=0.04) vs 5.7 (p=0.22)
Stathopoulos *et al* (2006)	GEM vs GEM+IRI	145	10 vs 15 (p=0.39)	2.8 vs 2.9 (p=0.79)	6.4 vs 6.5 (p=0.97)
Rocha Lima *et al* (2004)	GEM vs GEM+IRI	360	4.4 vs 16.1 (p<0.001)	3 vs 3.5 (p=0.352)	6.6 vs 6.3 (p=0.789)
Oettle *et al* (2005a)	GEM vs GEM+ PEM	565	7.1 vs 14.8 (p=0.004)	3.3 vs 3.9 (p=0.11)	6.3 vs 6.2 (p=0.847)
Abou Alfa *et al* (2006)	GEM vs GEM+EXA	349	4.6 vs 6.3	3.8 vs 3.7 (p=0.22)	6.2 vs 6.7 (p=0.52)

5FU, 5-fluoruracil; GEM, gemcitabine; CAPE, capecitabine; CIS, cisplatin; OX, oxaliplatin; IRI, irinotecan; EXE, exatecan; PEM, pemetrexed; RR, response rate; PFS, progression free survival; OS, overall survival.

Table 1. Selected phase III trials of gemcitabine-based chemotherapy in advanced pancreatic cancer

impact on overall survival, whereas combination therapy was associated with greater hematological toxicity (Colucci et al, 2010). Similar findings have been observed with the combination of gemcitabine with oxaliplatin (GEMOX). GEMOX was superior to gemcitabine in terms of response rate (26.8% v 17.3%; p=0.04), progression-free survival (5.8 v 3.7 months; p=0.04), and clinical benefit (38.2% v 26.9%; p=0.03), with a trend for an improved survival (9.0 v 7.1 months, p=0.13) (Louvet et al, 2005). Severe toxicities were however more commonly induced by the combination, particularly thrombocytopenia, emesis and neurotoxicity. More recently published trials, again, did not confirm these benefits for the GEMOX regimen (Poplin et al, 2009).

Combination of gemcitabine plus capecitabine is the other cytotoxic chemotherapy doublet that has shown some advantage over gemcitabine alone. Two recent phase III studies consistently demonstrated a gain in terms of progression free survival (PFS) for the combination, although the benefit in overall survival (OS) only achieved statistical significance in the meta-analysis of these trials (Cunningham et al, 2009; Herrmann et al, 2007). Cunningham et al randomized 533 patients to receive gemcitabine (1000 mg/m2 in 30-min infusion weekly x 3 every 4 weeks) plus capecitabine (830 mg/m2/12 hours day 1-21 every 28 days) versus gemcitabine alone. Combination therapy obtained higher response rates (19.1% vs 12.4%, p=0.034) and PFS (5.3 vs 3.8 months; HR 0.78, 95% CI 0.66-0.93, p=0.004) and a trend toward better OS of borderline significance (7.1 vs 6.2 months; HR 0.86, 95% CI 0.72-1.02, p=0.08). Herrmann and colleagues randomized 319 patients to receive either gemcitabine (1000 mg/m2 days 1 and 8 every 21 days) plus capecitabine (650 mg/m2/12 hours days 1-14 every 21 days) or gemcitabine alone (1000 mg/m2 weekly for 7 weeks and one week off, and then weekly x 3 every 4 weeks). No significant differences were observed among study arms in terms of response rate, clinical benefit or quality of life (Bernhard et al, 2008), and the primary endpoint of the study, OS, was not reached (8.4 vs 7.2 months, p=0.234). However, post hoc analysis did show a significant survival advantage for the gemcitabine-capecitabine combination in patients with good performance status (10.1 vs 7.4 months, p=0.004). In both studies toxicity in the combination arm was tolerable, with a low incidence of grade 3-4 adverse events, being neutropenia and diarrhea the most commonly encountered toxicities. In light of these results, treatment with gemcitabine plus capecitabine may be considered in fit patients with advanced pancreatic cancer.

Other multidrug combinations have also been investigated over the past years in several phase II-III trials, including PEFG (cisplatin, epirubicin, gemcitabine and 5-FU) (Reni et al, 2005), G-FLIP (irinotecan, gemcitabine, 5-FU, leucovorin and cisplatin) (Goel et al, 2007), and active schedules in other gastrointestinal cancers such as FOLFOX-6 (oxaliplatin, 5-FU and folinic acid) (Ghosn et al, 2007) or FOLFIRI.3 (irinotecan, 5-FU and folinic acid) (Taïeb et al, 2007). Increased tumor responses and progression free survival have been reported for some of these regimens (Reni et al, 2005), although at the expense of a worse toxicity profile with no impact on survival. However, the combination of Gemcitabine and *nab*-paclitaxel, an albumin-bound formulation of paclitaxel particles (Celgene, Summit, NJ), deserves special mention (Von Hoff et al, 2011). *nab*-Paclitaxel has shown antitumor activity in various advanced cancer types that overexpress the albumin-binding protein SPARC (secreted protein acidic and rich in cysteine), including breast, lung, and melanoma. Results of the phase I/II trial of this combination, with an overall response rate of 48%, a median survival of 12.2 months, and a 1-year survival rate of 48% at the MTD are among the highest ever reported for a phase II study in patients with advanced pancreatic cancer. Interestingly, SPARC expression in the stroma, but not in the tumor, was correlated with improved survival (median survival of 17.8 *v* 8.1 months for high- vs low- SPARC tumors, respectively; *P*= .0431), suggesting SPARC could be a potential new predictive biomarker of nab-paclitaxel activity. This promising results have prompted the conduction of a large international phase III study that is close to complete accrual. Also recently reported, results of the PRODIGE 4/ACCORD 11 trial comparing gemcitabine alone (1000 mg/m2 weekly x 7 every 8 weeks and then weekly x 3 every 4 weeks) to FOLFIRINOX (oxaliplatin 85 mg/m2, irinotecan 180 mg/m2, 5-FU 400 mg/m2 given as a bolus followed by 2400 mg/m2 given as a 46-hour continuous infusion; and leucovorin 400 mg/m2; every 2 weeks) demonstrated remarkable and significant improvements in response, progression free and overall survival rates favoring patients treated with FOLFIRINOX (31% vs. 9%, 6.4 months *vs.* 3.3 months, and 11.1 months *vs.* 6.8 months, respectively) (Conroy, 2011). These results are somewhat surprising, given the known modest activity of each of the individual drugs included in the regimen, and shall be confirmed. In addition, the higher toxicity profile of this combination limits its widespread use as standard of care in patients with metastatic disease, often frail. However, it may be an excellent option for carefully selected patients, particularly those with locally advanced borderline resectable disease. Anyhow, this is the first phase III randomized trial that has demonstrated a benefit in overall survival of unquestionable clinical relevance for patients with advanced pancreatic cancer, and it may change the classical paradigm of gemcitabine as the keystone in the management of advanced pancreatic cancer.

2.3 Gemcitabine-resistant disease

Once the disease progresses to gemcinatine-based therapy there is no accepted standard of care and most patients will not be suitable candidates for further therapy due to clinical deterioration. Second-line chemotherapy may be considered, however, in patients who maintain good performance status, although efficacy in this setting is questionable. Overall, it is estimated that approximately 30% of patients are in good condition (including good performance status and adequate organ function) for consideration of second-line treatment (Gounaris et al, 2010). A number of trials have been performed assessing the efficacy of different antineoplastic agents in this context. Most of the published evidence, however, consists of small phase II studies testing a variety of drugs in a heterogeneous population.

Oxaliplatin-fluoropyrimidine doublets are probably the chemotherapy regimens most widely evaluated in gemcitabine-resistant disease. Several small phase II studies showed some promising activity with different combinations of oxaliplatin and 5FU or capecitabine (FOLFOX, OFF, XELOX,..), with median survival (6-7 months) that did not substantially differed from that observed in chemotherapy-naïve patients (Tsavaris et al, 2005; Xiong et al, 2008). These results prompted the development of a phase III study (Charité Onkologie; CONKO 003) that aimed to evaluate the efficacy of the OFF regimen (oxaliplatin, fluorouracil and folinic acid) compared with best supportive care in gemcitabine-pretreated patients. Unfortunately, the control arm was closed after 46 of the planned 165 patients were enrolled due to clinician reluctance to enroll in a no-treatment arm (Oettle et al, 2005b). The results of this initial cohort, however, showed a substantial improvement in overall survival for treated patients (22 vs 10 weeks, p=0.0077). The trial design was then modified to include an alternative comparator arm consisting of 5FU plus folinic acid (FF regimen) and 165 patients were subsequently enrolled. Toxicity was acceptable with few grade 3-4 adverse events. Median progression-free survival and overall survival were significantly better in the OFF arm (13 vs 9 weeks, p=0.012, and 26 vs 13 weeks, p=0.014, respectively) (Pelzer et al, 2008).

Combining gemcitabine and oxaliplatin (GEMOX) has been another commonly evaluated therapeutic schedule. Two small non-controlled trials investigated the efficacy of oxaliplatin plus fixed-dose rate gemcitabine in patients who had progressed on single agent gemcitabine. Although reported response rates were relevant (21-24% of partial responses), toxicity was not negligible, with up to half of the patients developing at least one grade 3 adverse event (Demols et al, 2006, as cited in Gounaris et al, 2010; Fortune el al, 2009, as cited in Gounaris et al, 2010). These results, together with the findings of the phase III E6201 conducted in chemotherapy-naïve patients failing to demonstrate a survival advantage for the combination, do not warrant further evaluation of this regimen in the second-line setting (Poplin et al, 2009).

Irinotecan has been tested both as single agent and in combination with oxaliplatin or fluoropyrimidines showing some activity and an acceptable toxicity profile (Yi et al, 2009; Cantore et al, 2004). A direct comparison between oxaliplatin- and irinotecan-based regimens was made by Hwang and colleagues in a small randomized phase II trial (Hwang et al, 2009). Sixty patients were enrolled and randomly allocated to receive FOLFOX (oxaliplatin, folinic acid and infusional 5FU) or FOLFIRI.3 (the same folinic acid and 5FU schedule combined with irinotecan) after gemcitabine failure. No significant differences were observed among study arms neither in PFS (1.4 vs 1.9 months, $p>0.05$) nor in OS (4 months both regimens). In light of these results, both regimens may be reasonable options for second-line therapy in appropriately selected patients with advanced pancreatic cancer. Other irinotecan-based regimens including combinations with raltitrexed (Ulrich-Pur, 2003, as cited in Gounaris, 2010), docetaxel (Ko et al, 2008), docetaxel and mitomycin C (Reni et al, 2004) or ifosfamide (Cereda et al, 2011) have not achieved positive results in small phase II trials.

Rubitecan, an orally bioavailable camptothecin derivative, was the subject of the largest study conducted in gemcitabine-resistant pancreatic cancer, despite results of an initial single arm study were not particularly encouraging (median TTP and OS of 1.9 and 3 months, respectively). Subsequently, a large phase III study was launched the results of which have only been reported in abstract form (Jacobs et al, 2004). Four-hundred and nine patients were randomized to receive treatment with rubitecan or physician's best choice (chemotherapy 89%, supportive care only 11%). There were more responses in the rubitecan arm (11% vs. 1%) and the difference in median PFS, although clinically modest, reached statistical significance (1.9 vs. 1.6 months). There was no significant difference however in OS (3.5 vs 3.1 months, respectively).

Other tested drugs in this setting, such as taxanes or pemetrexed, have not shown particularly promising results in small studies (Gounaris et al, 2010; Boeck et al, 2007b; Mazzer et al, 2009). Multidrug combinations such as PEFG (cisplatin, epirubicin, 5-FU and gemcitabine) (Reni et al, 2008, as cited in Gounaris et al, 2010) or G-FLIP (gemcitabine, irinotecan, folinic acid, 5-FU and cisplatin) (Kozuch et al, 2001, as cited in Gounaris, 2010) appear to show improved efficacy with impressive median survival of 8.3 and 10.3 months, respectively. Selection bias may at least partially explain these outstanding results as reported toxicity was rather high, which in any case would limit their use in the general population.

3. Molecularly targeted therapies

Pancreatic adenocarcinoma is a malignant disease that results from the successive accumulation of gene mutations (Vogelstein & Kinzsler, 2004) evolving from premalignant lesions in the ductal epithelium to invasive cancer. These include activating mutations of KRAS2 oncogene (90% of pancreatic tumors), and inactivation of the tumor-suppresor genes CDKN2A (95%), TP53 (50-75%) or DPC4 (50%). More recent comprehensive genetic analysis have shown that molecular features in pancreatic cancer may be extremely complex and heterogeneous (Jones et al, 2008), although these genetic abnormalities may be classified in 12 core cancer signaling pathways involving not only pancreatic cancer cells but also other fundamental components of neoplasia such as cancer stem cells and tumor stroma (Hidalgo, 2010). As molecular pathways governing pancreatic cancer development are unraveled, novel targets emerge that may provide some promise to improve the dismal results obtained with conventional cytotoxic therapy.

3.1 EGFR-RAS-MEK-ERK pathway

EGFR (epidermal growth factor receptor), also known as HER-1 or ErbB-1, is activated by several ligands that include EGF (epidermal growth factor), TGF-α (transforming growth factor alpha), HB-EGF (heparin-binding EGF), amphiregulin, epiregulin, betacellulin and neuregulin. Activated EGFR forms homo- or heterodimeric complexes with other members of the ErbB family, triggering downstream signaling pathways such as Ras/MAP kinase, phosphatidylinositol 3'-kinase (PI3K)/Akt, Janus kinase (JAK)/Stat and phospholipase C/protein kinase C, that ultimately activate genes involved in cell proliferation, migration, adhesion, differentiation and apoptosis (Di Marco et al, 2010). Overexpression of EGFR and its ligands is very common in pancreatic cancer, and it is linked to increased tumor aggressiveness and poor prognosis. Preclinical studies have shown that blocking EGFR signaling inhibits growth and metastasis of pancreatic tumors in xenograft models and synergistic activity has been documented when combined with gemcitabine (Tempero et al, 2011).

Two strategies to antagonize EGFR signaling have been evaluated in the clinic to date: inhibition of the tyrosine kinase intracellular domain by small molecules and EGFR inhibition by monoclonal antibodies directed against the extracellular ligand binding domain. Erlotinib is an oral tyrosine kinase inhibitor [TKI] against EGFR, and the only targeted drug that has demonstrated some efficacy in pancreatic cancer thus far. The National Cancer Institute of Canada PA.3 trial was a phase III randomized study evaluating standard gemcitabine plus erlotinib (100 or 150 mg/day) versus gemcitabine plus placebo in 569 patients with chemo-naïve advanced pancreatic cancer (Table 2). Both PFS (PFS 3.75 vs 3.55 months, HR 0.77, p=0.004) and OS (6.24 vs 5.91 months, HR 0.82, p=0.038) were significantly improved in the experimental arm (Moore et al, 2007). Most common toxicity was, as expected, diarrhea and skin rash, which were of grade 1-2 in the majority of cases without negatively impacting patient´s quality of life. Interestingly, patients that developed grade 2 or higher skin rash had significantly longer survival compared to those who developed mild or no rash (10.5 vs 5.8 vs 5.3 months, respectively, HR 0.74, p=0.037). Levels of EGFR expression, however, were not correlated with survival. This was the pivotal study that granted erlotinib marketing authorization by regulatory authorities, although the small magnitude of benefit has precluded widespread acceptance by oncologists in Europe of the gemcitabine-erlotinib combination as the new standard of care for first line therapy of advanced pancreatic cancer.

One potential explanation for this modest effect of EGFR inhibition in pancreatic cancer is the fact that KRAS mutations occur in 70-90% of these tumors (Tempero et al, 2011). KRAS

Reference	Treatment	Number of patients	OS (months)	PFS (months)	RR (%)
Moore et al (2007)	GEM + PLA vs GEM+ERLOT	569	5.91 vs 6.24 (p=0.038)	3.55 vs 3,.75 (p=0.004)	8 vs 8.6
Philip et al (2007)	GEM vs GEM+CETUX	766	6 vs 6.5 (p=0.14)	3 vs 3.5 (p=0.058)	14 vs 12
Van Cutsem et al (2009)	GEM+ERLOT+PLA vs GEM+ERLOT+BEV	607	6 vs 7.1	3.6 vs 4.6 (p=0.0002)	8.6 vs 13.5
Kindler et al (2010)	GEM+PLA vs GEM+BEV	602	5.9 vs 5.8 (p=0.95)	2.9 vs 3.8 (p=0.07)	10 vs 13
Moore et al (2003)	GEM vs BAY 12-9566	277	6.59 vs 3.74 (p<0.01)	3.5 vs 1.68 (p<0.01)	-
Bramhall et al (2001)	GEM vs MARIMASTAT	414	5.5 vs 4.1	3.8 vs 1.9	25.8 vs 2.8
Bramhall et al (2002)	GEM vs GEM+MARIMASTAT	239	5.4 vs 5.4	3.1 vs 3	16 vs 11
Van Cutsem et al (2004)	GEM vs GEM+TIPIFARNIB	688	6 vs 6.3 (p=0.75)	3.6 vs 3.7 (p=0.72)	8 vs 6

GEM, gemcitabine; PLA, placebo; ERLOT, erlotinib; BEV, bevacizumab; RR, response rate; PFS, progression free survival; OS, overall survival

Table 2. Selected phase III trials of targeted agents in advanced pancreatic cancer

functions downstream of the EGFR signaling pathway, and mutations in the KRAS protein lead to constitutive activation independent of extracellular stimuli. This is a well established mechanism of resistance to EGFR blockade in colorectal cancer, and, indeed, EGFR-targeted therapy is only to be used in KRAS wild-type tumors. The potential predictive value of KRAS mutation status and EGFR gene copy number in pancreatic cancer was evaluated in 26% of the patients included in the PA.3 trial who had tumor samples available for analysis. KRAS mutations were detected in 79% of tested samples. EGFR copy number was not correlated with treatment effect. However, the HR of death between gemcitabine/erlotinib and gemcitabine/placebo was 1.07 for patients with KRAS-mutated tumors versus 0.66 for those with KRAS wild-type tumors. Although this difference did not reach statistical significance probably due to small numbers, this plausible trend shall be further evaluated to try to improve patient selection and therapeutic benefit.

Erlotinib has also been tested as second-line treatment of patients with advanced disease. Kulke et al evaluated the combination of erlotinib and capecitabine in 30 patients with gemcitabine-refractory pancreatic cancer. Objective radiologic responses were observed in 10% of patients and the median survival was 6.5 months. In addition, 17% of treated patients experienced decreases in tumor marker (CA 19-9) levels of more than 50% from baseline. However, common toxicities, particularly diarrhea and skin rash, were significant and required treatment dose reductions in 66% of patients (Kulke et al, 2007). More recently, this treatment regimen has been tested against erlotinib-gemcitabine in a phase III AIO trial. This trial included 279 chemotherapy naïve patients that were randomly allocated to receive capecitabine-erlotinib versus gemcitabine-erlotinib as the control arm. Crossover to gemcitabine or capecitabine alone was allowed at the time of progression. Neither time to treatment failure of second-line therapy (TTF2), which was the primary endpoint of the trial, nor OS were significantly different among study arms (TTF2 4.4 vs 4.2 months, HR 0.98, p=0.43; OS 6.9 vs 6.6 months, HR 0.96, p=0.78). Of note, overall survival was significantly correlated with KRAS mutation status (8.0 months vs 6.6 months for KRAS wild-type versus mutated tumors, respectively; HR 1.62; p=0.011). However, the study design, which included erlotinib in both treatment arms, does not allow to elucidate whether KRAS mutation status is predictive of efficacy of EGFR-targeted therapy or just a prognostic factor independent of therapy (Boeck et al, 2010). Anyhow, this regimen may represent an acceptable treatment option in patients who experience treatment failure with standard gemcitabine first-line therapy or for whom gemcitabine may not be an appropriate treatment option.

The other strategy to antagonize EGFR signaling consists of monoclonal antibodies directed against the extracellular domain of the receptor, such as cetuximab or panitumumab. They are currently approved for treatment of other advanced malignancies such as colorectal or head and neck cancer. Preclinical and early clinical trials suggested some efficacy too in pancreatic cancer. Disappointingly, a large phase III trial comparing the combination of cetuximab plus gemcitabine vs gemcitabine alone (Table 2), which enrolled 366 patients, did not demonstrate a benefit in survival for the combination regimen (Philip et al, 2007). Other approaches explored include dual EGFR inhibition (TKI inhibitors plus monoclonal antibodies). Preliminary results of a phase II randomized study suggest a small benefit in terms of PFS (3.3 months vs 2.0 months) for the addition of panitumumab to gemcitabine-erlotinib, although statistical significance was not reported and final data including overall survival are awaited for definitive conclusions (Kim et al, 2010).

Lapatinib, an oral TKI which reversibly inhibits both EGFR/HER1 and HER2/neu, has also been evaluated. Preclinical assays suggested activity alone and in combination with other drugs such as capecitabine. Moreover, a phase I trial combining lapatinib with either gemcitabine or GEMOX showed encouraging results with median survival of 10 months (Safran et al, 2008, as cited in Di Marco et al, 2010). More recently, preliminary results of a single arm phase II trial evaluating the combination of capecitabine and lapatinib as first-line treatment in advanced pancreatic cancer have been presented. Survival of 6 months was not reached in 7 of the 9 enrolled patients, and none of them obtained objective responses (McDermott et al, 2011). This data led to the premature termination of the study.

HER2 may be also targeted by monoclonal antibodies such as trastuzumab. HER2 is overexpressed in some pancreatic cancers, with results widely varying from 0 to 82% in different studies. One early trial evaluated gemcitabine plus trastuzumab in 34 metastatic pancreatic cancer patients with 2+/3+ Her2-positive tumors determined by immunohistochemistry. Only 4 patients (12%) presented Her2 neu 3+ expression. Partial responses were observed in 6% of patients (2/32) (Safran et al, 2004). Further studies would be needed to appropriately assess the role of this agent in pancreatic cancer.

Other therapeutic strategies have aimed to target some of the downstream effectors of EGFR. The high incidence of KRAS mutations in pancreatic cancer provided a strong rationale for the evaluation of KRAS inhibition. Tipifarnib was the first agent of this class to be tested. It is a farnesyl transferase inhibitor which demonstrated antiproliferative activity in a wide range of tumors in preclinical models. Farnesylation is an impotant post-traslational event required for Ras activation. A large phase III clinical trial, however, failed to demonstrate an improvement in survival of adding tipifarnib to gemcitabine over gemcitabine alone in patients with advanced pancreatic cancer (Table 2) (Van Cutsem et al, 2004). Some authors have postulated as a potential explanation for these negative results the fact that KRAS mutation could be an early event in the development of pancreatic cancer, becoming cancer cells less dependent on this pathway as the disease progresses. In addition, other mechanisms involved in the regulation of Ras activation (i.e. prenylation by other enzymes) may limit the therapeutic success of farnesyl transferase inhibition (Lobell R et al, 2001, as cited in Stathis & Moore, 2010).

Other agents targeting downstream effectors of the EGFR pathway currently under evaluation include MEK inhibitors. Phase I trials have established the recommended dose for further clinical development and have documented rash, diarrhea and central serous retinopathy as dose limiting toxicities, all of them reversible (Messersmith et al, 2011). Several phase I and II trial combining MEK inhibitors with standard chemotherapy and other targeted agents are ongoing, the results of which are awaited with great interest.

3.2 Antiangiogenic agents

Angiogenesis is a widely validated target for cancer therapy. Overexpression of vascular endothelial growth factor (VEGF) and its receptors (VEGFRs) has been described in pancreatic cancer and correlated with disease progression and poor prognosis. Bevacizumab is a recombinant humanized anti-VEGF monoclonal antibody and the most widely tested antiangiogenic agent. Promising data of several bevacizumab combination regimens in phase II clinical trials, with response rates of up to 24% and median survival of up to 11 months (Kindler et al, 2005; Walkins et al, 2010; Iyer et al, 2008, as cited in Di Marco et al, 2010), encouraged the development of two large phase III trials that unfortunately failed to yield positive results. The first one enrolled 602 patients that were randomized to receive gemcitabine plus bevacizumab or gemcitaine plus placebo. No significant differences were observed among study arms neither in PFS (PFS 3.8 vs 2.9 months) nor in OS (5.8 vs 5.9 months) (Kindler et al, 2010). The second one evaluated the addition of bevacizumab to the gemcitabine-erlotinib doublet (Table 2). Although PFS was better for the experimental arm (4.6 vs 3.6 months, HR 0.73, p=0.0002), the primary objective of the study was not met as the addition of bevacizumab did not improve overall survival (7.1 vs 6.0 months, HR 0.89, p=0.2) (Van Cutsem et al, 2009). A correlation between development of skin rash and improvement in survival was observed in this trial.

Other broadly tested agents that interfere with angiogenesis include small molecules targeting multiple kinases such as axitinib or sorafenib. Axitinib, an oral inhibitor of VEGFR-1, VEGFR-2 and VEGFR-3, was initially evaluated in a phase II randomized trial in combination with gemcitabine versus gemcitabine alone. This trial enrolled 103 patients and showed a small improvement in survival favoring the combination arm (6.9 vs 5.6 months), although this difference did not reach statistical significance (Spano et al, 2008). Nevertheless, a phase III trial was undertaken but was prematurely discontinued due to the lack of benefit observed in an interim analysis for the addition of axitinib to the standard gemcitabine therapy. Sorafenib has also been evaluated in combination with both gemcitabine and gemcitabine-erlotinib in different non-controlled trials with disappointing results (Wallace et al, 2007; Cohen et al, 2011). The lack of success of antiangiogenic strategies in pancreatic cancer could be potentially related to the fact that most tumors display intense fibrosis and are of hypovascular nature (Stathis & Moore, 2010).

3.3 Matrix metalloproteinases (MMP) inhibitors

MMPs are a family of zinc-dependent proteolytic enzymes implicated in the degradation of extracellular matrix proteins both in physiological and pathological conditions. Aberrant MMP expression contributes to neovascularization, dissemination and metastasis of a variety of solid malignancies (Stathis & Moore, 2010). Several compounds developed to inhibit MMPs have been completely unsuccessful in clinical trials over the last decade. Marimastat was the first agent to be tested (Table 2). Two large phase III trials enrolling over 900 patients showed marimastat, either alone or in combination with gemcitabine, was not able to improve survival or disease control of patients with advanced pancreatic cancer (Bramhall et al, 2001, 2002). Similar negative results were obtained with other agents of this class. Standard gemcitabine monotherapy was compared to BAY 12-9566, in a design that allowed for crossover after disease progression. Interim analyses demonstrated a deleterious effect on survival of the MMP inhibitor as compared to the control arm (OS 3.74 vs 6.59 months, $p<0.01$), and led to early trial termination (Moore et al, 2003). In light of this data, this approach has been definitively abandoned.

3.4 Other pathways

Phosphatidylinositol-3-kinase (PI3K)/Akt/mTOR

The PI3K/Akt/mTOR pathway is determinant for processes related to cell proliferation and inhibition of apoptosis, and constitutive activation of this pathway has been documented in pancreatic cancer (Royal et al, 2008). NVP-BEZ235 is a novel dual PI3K/mTOR inhibitor that has demonstrated activity in both human pancreatic cancer cell lines and mice models, and some synergy has been observed when combined with gemcitabine and antiangiogenic EMAP II (endothelial monocyte activating polypeptide II) (Awasthi et al, 2011). Further research will define the role of these new drugs in pancreatic cancer.

Src kinase

Src tyrosine kinase is a non-receptor protein implicated in tumor progression. It is overexpressed in more than two thirds of pancreatic adenocarcinomas. Src inhibitors (dasatinib, saracatinib) have been developed demonstrating antitumor activity in cancer cell lines and mice models (Royal et al, 2008). A recent phase II trial tested saracatinib (AZD0530) in 19 gemcitabine-refractory patients. No responses were seen and the minimum of 18% 6-month survival required for continuation of the trial was not achieved. A pharmacodiagnostic pre-selection strategy is planned to be implemented to better define patients most likely to respond (Nallapareddy et al, 2010).

IGF-1R

IGF-1R mediated signaling plays an important role in cell growth regulation and survival. Several monoclonal antibodies targeting IGF-IR have undergone clinical investigation (AMG479, MK0646, R1507). Based on promising preclinical and early clinical data, a phase III trial has been initiated to evaluate the combination of AMG479 plus gemcitabine in first-line metastatic pancreatic cancer (Hidalgo, 2010).

TNF-α

TNF-α shows potent anticancer activity, but high systemic toxicity limits its use. AdEgr.TNF.11D (TNFerade) is a gene delivery strategy to increase local peritumoral TNF concentrations through intratumoral injections of an adenoviral vector expressing hTNF, in an attempt to improve local activity while minimizing systemic effects. Effectiveness in combination with gemcitabine has been demonstrated in human pancreatic xenografts (Murugesan et al, 2009). A phase III trial is currently evaluating the addition of TNFerade to 5-FU plus radiotherapy in unresectable pancreatic cancer (Stathis & Moore, 2010).

Multikinase inhibitor

Masitinib is a multikinase inhibitor that has greater activity and selectivity against KIT than imatinib. Masitinib also potently inhibits PDGFR (platelet-derived growth factor receptor) and the intracellular kinase Lyn, and to a lesser extent, FGFR3 (fibroblast growth factor receptor 3). Synergistic activity with gemcitabine was demonstrated in preclinical assays. A phase II trial combining gemcitabine and masitinib in 22 patients reported median PFS of 6.4 months and OS of 7.1 months, with a 23% 18-months survival rate. Toxicity was acceptable, being cytopenia, diarrhea and rash the most common severe events (Hammel et al, 2009). A subsequent phase III trial is ongoing comparing gemcitabine with or without masitinib.

Death receptors

AMG655 is a monoclonal antibody against human death receptor 5 (DR5) that activates caspases and, as a result, induces apoptosis in tumor cells. It showed preclinical activity and synergy with gemcitabine. Early clinical data from a phase I trial that included 13 patients reported promising results for the combination of AMG655 with gemcitabine, with a response rate of 31%, median PFS of 5.3 months and a 6-month survival rate of 76.8%. Toxicity was however not negligible, with severe adverse events observed in 69% of patients (Kindler et al, 2009). A phase II is ongoing to assess efficacy and further characterize the safety profile of this combination.

Other pathways

Other pathways highly implicated in pancreatic tumorigenesis are at earlier stages of investigation. Hedgehog, Notch and Wnt signaling are important developmental pathways related to pancreatic cancer stem cells, and new agents are being developed to target these pathways (GDC-0449, IPI-926,..). Other agents in development include monoclonal antibodies against cell-membrane proteins such as mesothelin (MORAb-009). Specific mechanisms of cell killing are still not well defined but preclinical research suggest a role in pancreatic cancer (Hidalgo, 2010).

4. Conclusions

Pancreatic cancer continues to be a major challenge for oncologists as it is a highly chemoresistant malignancy carrying an extremely poor prognosis. Despite the intense research carried out over the last decades no major improvements have been achieved in patient's outcomes. Most patients present with locally advanced or metastatic disease and will therefore require systemic therapy. Conventional chemotherapy modestly improves survival and quality of life of patients with advanced disease. Gemcitabine has been the reference treatment for over a decade and little progress has been made since its introduction in clinical practice in 1997. Gemcitabine-combination therapy with capecitabine, platinum agents or erlotinib may be considered in patients with good performance status, although the small magnitude of benefit they confer shall be balanced against the increased toxicity they induce, particularly considering that prognosis is in any case rather poor and symptomatic relief shall be a major objective of disease management. FOLFIRINOX may be a preferred option for carefully selected fit patients, particularly those with locally advanced borderline resectable disease.

Nevertheless, there is much room for improvement, and more efforts in basic, translational and clinical research will be necessary in the following years for progress to be made. Indeed, a better understanding of the biology of pancreatic cancer shall enable the discovery of new targets of potential diagnostic or therapeutic interest. Meanwhile, as the molecular pathways governing pancreatic cancer are unraveled, efforts shall be made to improve selection of patients most likely to benefit from specific therapies (SPARC, kras,..). Small randomized phase II trials of both non-selected and enriched patient populations will help to adequately identify potentially active new agents. Phase III trials should only be initiated in appropriate patients based on strong clinical and biological grounds. In this context, the need for further collaborative research is highly warranted.

5. References

Abou Alfa GK, Letourneau R, Harker G et al. Randomized phase III study of exatecan and gemcitabine compared with gemcitabine alone in untreated advanced pancreatic cancer. J Clin Oncol 2006; 24: 4441-47.

Bang YJ, Van Cutsem E, Feyereislova A, Chung HC, Shen L, Sawaki A et al. Trastuzumab in combination with chemotherapy versus chemotherapy alone for treatment of HER2 positive advanced gastric or gastro-oesophageal junction cancer (ToGA): a phase 3, open-label, randomized controlled trial. Lancet 2010;376(9742):687-97.

Banu E, Banu A, Fodor A, et al. Meta-analysis of randomized trials comparing gemcitabine-based doublets versus gemcitabine alone in patients with advanced and metastatic pancreatic cancer. Drugs Asing 2007; 24: 865-79.

Berlin JD et al. Phase III study of gemcitabine in combination with fluoruracil versus gemcitabine alone in patients with advanced pancreatic carcinoma: Eastern cooperative oncology group trial E2297. J Clin Oncol 2002; 20: 3270-75.

Bernhard J, Dietrich D, Scheithauer W et al. Clinical benefit and quality of life in patients with advanced pancreatic cancer receiving gemcitabine plus capecitabine versus gemcitabine alone: a randomized multicenter phase II clinical trial-SAKK 44/00-CECOG/PAN.1.3.001. J Clin Oncol 2008; 26: 3695-701.

Boeck S, Weigang-Köhler K, Fuchs M, Kettner E, Quietzsch D, Trojan J et al. Second-line chemotherapy with pemetrexed after gemcitabine failure in patients with advanced pancreatic cancer: a multicenter phase II trial. Ann Oncol 2007; 18:745-51.

Boeck SH, Vehling-Kaiser U, Waldschmidt D, Kettner E, Märten A, Winkelmann C et al. Gemcitabine plus erlotinib (GE) followed by capecitabine (C) versus capecitabine plus erlotinib (CE) followed by gemcitabine (G) in advanced pancreatic cancer (APC): A randomized, cross-over phase III trial of the Arbeitsgemeinschaft Internistische Onkologie (AIO). J Clin Oncol 2010; 28(18 Suppl):LBA4011.

Bramhall SR, Rosemurgy A, Brown PD, Browry C & Buckels JA. Marimastat as first line therapy for patients with unresectable pancreatic cancer: a randomized trial. J Clin Oncol 2001;19:3447-55.

Bramhall SR, Schulz J, Nemunaitis J, Brown PD, Baillet M & Buckels JA. A double-blind placebo-controlled, randomized study comparing gemcitabine and marimastat with gemcitabine and placebo as first line therapy in patients with advanced pancreatic cancer. Br J Cancer, 2002; 87:161-7.

Brus C & Saif, MW. Second-line therapy for advanced pancreatic adenocarcinoma: where are we and where are we going? Journal of pancreatic cancer (JOP)(online), 2010; 11(4):321-323.

Burris HA 3rd, Moore MJ, Andersen J, Green MR, Rothenberg ML, Modiano MR, et al. Improvements in survival and clinical benefit with gemcitabine as first-line therapy for patients with advanced pancreas cancer: a randomized trial. J Clin Oncol 1997; 15: 2403-13.

Cantore M, Rabbi C, Fiorentini G, Oliani C, Zamagni D, Iacono C et al. Combined irinotecan and oxaliplatin in patients with advanced pretreated pancreatic cancer. Oncology 2004; 67:93-7.

Cereda S, Reni M, Rognone A, Fugazza C, Ghidini M, Ceraulo D, Brioschi M, Nicoletti R, Villa E. Salvage therapy with mitomycin and ifosfamide in patients with gemcitabine-resistant metastatic pancreatic cancer: a phase II trial. Chemotherapy 2011; 57 (2):156-61.

Colucci G, et al. Gemcitabine alone or with cisplatin for the treatment of patients with locally advanced and/or metastatic pancreatic carcinoma: A prospective, randomized phase III study of the Gruppo Oncologico dell'Italia Meridionale. Cancer 2002; 94: 902-10.

Colucci G, et al. Randomized phase III trial of gemcitabine plus cisplatin compared with single-agent gemcitabine as first-line treatment of patients with advanced pancreatic cancer: The GIP-1 study. J Clin Oncol 2010; 28 (10): 1645-51.

Conroy T, Desseigne F, Ychou M, Bouché O, Guimbaud R, Bécouarn Y, Adenis A et al. FOLFIRINOX versus gemcitabine for metastatic pancreatic cancer. N Engl J Med 2011; 364: 1817-25.

Cullinan S, Moertel CG, Wieand HS, et al. A phase III trial on the therapy of advanced pancreatic carcinoma. Evaluations of the Mallison regimen and combined 5-fluoruracil, doxorubicin, and cisplatin. Cancer 15:2207-12, 2007.

Cunningham D, Chau I, Stocken DD et al. Phase III randomized comparison of gemcitabine versus gemcitabine plus capecitabine in patients with advanced pancreatic cancer. J Clin Oncol 2009; 27: 5513-8.

Di Marco MC, Di Cicilia R, Macchini M, Nobili E, Vecchiarelli S, Brandi G and Biasco G. Metastatic pancreatic cancer: Is gemcitabine still the best standard treatment? (Review). Oncology Reports 2010; 23:1183-92.

Ducreux M, Mitry E, Ould-Kaci M et al. Randomized phase II study evaluating oxaliplatin alone, oxaliplatin combined with infusional 5-FU, and infusional 5-FU alone in advanced pancreatic carcinoma patients. Ann Oncol 15: 467-473, 2004

Ducreux M, Rouguer P, Pignon JP, et al. A randomized trial comparing 5-FU with 5-FU plus cisplatin in advanced pancreatic carcinoma. Ann Oncol 13: 1185-91, 2002.

Evans DB, Abbruzzese JL, Willett CG. Cancer of the pancreas. In: De Vita VT, Hellman S, Rosenberg SA (editors). Cancer: Principles and Practice of Oncology. 6th ed. Vol 1. Philadelphia: Lippincott, Williams & Wilkins; 1997. p. 1126-61.]ISBN: 0-7817-7207-9.

Ferlay J, Shin HR, Bray F, Forman D, Mathers C & Parkin DM. GLOBOCAN 2008 v1.2, Cancer incidence and mortality worldwide: IARC CancerBase No. 10 [Internet]. Lyon, France: International Agency for Research on Cancer, 2010. Available from: http://globocan.iarc.fr, accessed on 02/07/2011.

Gelibter A, Malaguti P, Di Cosimo S, et al. Fixed dose-rate gemcitabine infusion as first-line treatment for advanced-stage carcinoma of the pancreas and biliary tree. Cancer (Suppl) 2005; 104:1237-45.

Ghosn M, Farhat F, Kattan J, Younes F, Moukadem W, Nasr F and Chahine G. FOLFOX-6 combination as the first-line treatment of locally advanced and/or metastatic pancreatic cancer. J Clin Oncol 2007; 30: 15-20.

Goel A, Grossbard ML, Malamud S et al. Pooled efficacy analysis from a phase I-II study of biweekly irinotecan in combination with gemcitabine, 5-fluoruracil, leucovorin and cisplatin in patients with metastatic pancreatic cancer. Anticancer Drugs2007; 18: 263-71.

Gounaris I, Zaki K, Corrie P. Options for the treatment of gemcitabine-resistant advanced pancreatic cancer. Journal of the Pancreas (online) 2010 Mar 5; 11(2): 113-123.

Hammel P, Mornex F, Deplanque G, Mitriy E, Levy P, Seitz J et al. Oral tyrosine kinase inhibitor masitinib in combination with gemcitabine in patients with advanced pancreatic cancer: A multicenter phase II study. J Clin Oncol 2009; 27(15 Suppl.): Abstract 4617.

Heinemann V, Boeck S, Hinke A, Labianca R & Louvet C. Meta-analysis of randomized trials: Evaluation of benefit from gemcitabine-based combination chemotherapy applied in advanced pancreatic cancer. BMC Cancer, 2008; 8: 82.

Heinemann V, Boeck S. Perioperative management of pancreatic cancer. Ann Oncol 19 (Suppl. 7), vii273-vii278 (2008).

Heinemann V, Quetzsch D, Giseler F et al. Randomized phase III trial of gemcitabine plus cisplatin compared to gemcitabine alone in advanced pancreatic cancer. J Clin Oncol 2006; 24: 2946-52.

Herrmann R et al. Gemcitabine plus capecitabine compared with gemcitabine alone in advanced pancreatic cancer: a randomized, multicenter, phase III trial of the Swiss Group for Clinical Cancer Research and the Central European Cooperative Oncology Group. J Clin Oncol 2007; 25: 2212-17.

Hidalgo M. Pancreatic cancer. N Engl J Med, 2010; 362:1605-17.

Hwang J, Yoo C, Kim T, Lee J, Park D, Seo D et al. A randomized phase II trial of FOLFOX or FOLFIRI.3 as second-line therapy in patient with advanced pancreatic cancer previously treated with gemcitabine-based chemotherapy. J Clin Oncol 2009; 27:s4618.

Jacobs AD, Burris HA, Rivkin S, et al. A randomized phase III study of rubitecan vs best choice in 409 patients with refractory pancreatic cancer report from a North-American multi-center study. J clin Oncol 2004; 22:s4013.

Jemal A, Siegel R, Xu J, Ward E. Cancer statistics, 2010. *CA Cancer J Clin* 2010; 60:277-300. [PMID 20610543]

Jones S, Zhang X, Parsons DW, et al. Core signaling pathways in human pancreatic cancers revealed by global genomic analyses. *Science* 2008; 321:1801-6.

Kelsen D, Hudis C, Niedzwiecki D, et al. A phase III comparison trial of streptozocin, mitomycin and 5-fluoruracil with cisplatin, cytosine arabinoside, and caffeine in patients with advanced pancreatic carcinoma. Cancer 68: 965-969, 1991.

Khorana, AA & Fine RL. Pancreatic cancer and thromboembolic disease. *Lancet Oncology* 2004; 5: 655-63.

Kim GP, Foster NR, Salim M, Flynn PJ, Moore DF Jr, Zon R et al. Randomized phase II trial of panitumumab (P), erlotinib (E), and gemcitabine (G) versus erlotinib-gemcitabine in patients with untreated, metastatic pancreatic adenocarcinoma. J Clin Oncol 2011; (4 Suppl):29: abstract 238.

Kindler HL, Friberg G, Singh DA et al. Phase II trial of bevacizumab plus gemcitabine in patients with advanced pancreatic cancer. J Clin Oncol 2005; 23:8033-40.

Kindler HL, Garbo L, Stephenson J, Wiezorek J, Sabin T, Hsu M et al. A phase Ib study to evaluate the safety and efficacy of AMG655 in combination with gemcitabine (G) in patients (pts) with metastatic pancreatic cancer (PC). J Clin Oncol 2009;27(15 Suppl): abstract 4501.

Kindler HL, Niedzwiecki D, Hollis D, Sutherland S, Schrag D, Hurwitz H et al. Gemcitabine plus bevacizumab compared with gemcitabine plus placebo in patients with advanced pancreatic cancer: phase III trial of the Cancer and Leukemia Group B (CALGB 80303). J Clin Oncol 2010; 28(22):3617-22.

Ko AH, Dito E, Schillinger B, Venook AP, Bergsland EK & Tempero MA. Excess toxicity associated with docetaxel and irinotecan in patients with metastatic, gemcitabine-refractory pancreatic cancer: results of a phase II study. Cancer Invest 2008; 26:47-52.

Louvet C et al. Gemcitabine in combination with oxaliplatin compared with gemcitabine alone in locally advanced or metastatic pancreatic cancer: Results of a GERCOR and GISCAD phase III trial. J Clin Oncol 2005; 23: 3509-16.

Maisey N, Chau I, Cunningham D et al. Multicenter randomized phase III trial comparing protracted venous infusion (PVI) fluoruracil (5-FU) with PVI 5-FU plus mitomycin in inoperable pancreatic cancer. J Clin Oncol 20: 3130-36, 2002.

Mazzer M, Zanon E, Foltran L, De Pauli F, Cardellino G, Iaiza E et al. Second-line pemetrexed-oxaliplatin combination for advanced pancreatic adenocarcinoma. J Clin Oncol 2009; 27: e15597.

McDermott RS, Calvert P, Parker M, Webb G, Moulton B, McCaffey J. A phase II study of lapatinib and capecitabine in first-line treatment of metastatic pancreatic cancer (ICORG 08-39). J Clin Oncol 2011; 29 (4 Suppl): Abstract 315.

Messersmith WA, Falchook GS, Fecher LA, Gordon MS, Vogelzang NJ, DeMarini DJ et al. Clinical activity of the oral MEK1/MEK2 inhibitor GSD1120212 in pancreatic and colorectal cancer. J Clin Oncol 2011; 29(4 Suppl): abstract 246.

Moore MJ, Goldstein D, Hamm J et al. Erlotinib plus gemcitabine compared with gemcitabine alone in patients with advanced pancreatic cancer: a phase III trial of the National Cancer Institute of Canada Clinical Trials Group. J Clin Oncol 2007;25:1960-66.

Moore MJ, Hamm J, Dancey J, Eisenberg PD, Dagenais M, Fiels A et al. Comparison of gemcitabine versus the matrix metalloproteinase inhibitor BAY 12-9566 in patients with advanced or metastatic adenocarcinoma of the pancreas: a phase III trial of the National Cancer Institute of Canada Clinical Trials Group. J Clin Oncol 2003;21(17):3296-302.

Murugesan SR, King CR, Osborn R et al. Combination of human tumor necrosis factor-alpha (hTNF-alpha) gene delivery with gemcitabine is effective in models of pancreatic cancer. Cancer Gene Therapy 2009; 16:841-7.

Nallapareddy J, Arcaroli B, Touban A, Tan NR, Foster C, Erlichman JJ et al. A phase II trial of saracatinib (AZD0530), an oral Src inhibitor, in previously treated metastatic pancreatic cancer. J Clin Oncol 2010; 28 (15 Suppl): abstract 165.

National Cancer Institute. Pancreatic cancer treatment (PDQ®). Health professional version. Bethesda, MD, USA (Accessed: June 12, 2010)

Oberstein PE & f Saif MW. First-line treatment for advanced pancreatic cancer. Highlights from the "2011 ASCO Gastrointestinal Cancers Symposium". San Francisco, CA, USA. Journal of the pancreas; vol 12, number 2, march 2011:96-100. [ISSN 1590-8577]

Oettle H et al. A phase III trial of pemetrexed plus gemcitabine versus gemcitabine in patients with unresectable or metastatic pancreatic cancer. Ann Oncol 2005; 16: 1639-45.

Oettle H, Pelzer U, Stieler J, Hilbig A, Roll L, Schwaneret I et al. Oxaliplatin/folinic acid/5-fluoruracil [24 h] (OFF) plus best supportive care versus best supportive care alone in second-line therapy of gemcitabine refractory advanced pancreatic cancer (CONKO 003). J Clin Oncol 2005; 23 (16 Suppl):4031.

Pelzer U, Kubica K, Stieler J, Schwaner I, Heil G, Görner M et al. A randomized trial in patients with gemcitabine-refractory pancreatic cancer. Final results of the CONKO 003 study. J Clin Oncol 2008; 26 (15 Suppl): 4508.

Philip PA, Beneditti J, Fenoglio-Preiser C et al. Phase III study of gemcitabine (G) plus cetuximab (C) versus gemcitabine in patients (pts) with locally advanced or metastatic pancreatic adenocarcinoma (PA): SWOG S0205 study. J Clin Oncol 2007; 25(18 Suppl):LBA4509.

Poplin E et al. Phase III, randomized study of gemcitabine and oxaliplatin versus gemcitabine (fixed-dose rate infusion) compared with gemcitabine (30-minute infusion) in patients with pancreatic carcinoma E6201: a trial of the Eastern Cooperative Oncology Group. J Clin Oncol 2009; 27: 3778-85.

Reni M, Cordio S, Milandri C, et al. Gemcitabine versus cisplatin, epirubicin, fluoruracil, and gemcitabine in advanced pancreatic cancer: a randomized controlled multicentre phase III study. Lancet Oncol 2005; 6: 369-76.

Reni M, Panucci MG, Passoni P, Bonetto E, Nicoletti R, Ronzoni M et al. Salvage chemotherapy with mitomycin, docetaxel and irinotecan (MDI regimen) in metastatic pancreatic adenocarcinoma: a phase I and II trial. Cancer Invest 2004; 22:688-96.

Riess H et al. A randomized, prospective, multicenter, phase III trial of gemcitabine, 5-fluoruracile (5-FU), folinic acid versus gemcitabine alone in patients with advanced pancreatic cancer [abstract] J Clin Oncol 2005; 23 (Suppl 16): a4009.

Rocha Lima CM et al. Irinotecan plus gemcitabine results in no survival advantage compared with gemcitabine monotherapy in patients with locally advanced or metastatic pancreatic cancer despite increased tumor response rate. J Clin Oncol 2004; 22: 3776-83.

Royal RE, Wolff RA & Crane CH. Pancreatic cancer. In: DeVita VT, Lawrence TS, Rosenberg SA (Editors). Cancer principles and practice of oncology 8th edition Lippincott - Williams and Wilkins: 1086-1124.

Safran H, Iannitti D, Ramanathan R, Schwartz JD, Steinhoff M, Nauman C et al. Herceptin and gemcitabine for metastatic pancreatic cancers that overexpress HER2/neu. Cancer Invest 2004; 22:706-12.

Solcia E, Capella C & Kloppel G. Tumors of the exocrine pancreas. In Tumors of the Pancreas (Ed. Rosai J & Sobin LH) 145 (Armed Forces Institute of Pathology, Washington 1997).

Spano JP et al. Efficacy of gemcitabine plus axitinib compared with gemcitabine alone in patients with advanced pancreatic cancer: an open-label randomized phase II study. Lancet 2008; 371:2101-08.

Stathis A & Moore MJ. Advanced pancreatic carcinoma: current treatment and future challenges. *Nature Reviews*, 2010; 7:163-172.

Stathopoulos GP et al. A multicenter phase III trial comparing irinotecan-gemcitabine (IG) with gemcitabine (G) monotherapy as first-line treatment in patients with locally advanced or metastatic pancreatic cancer. Br J Cancer 2006; 95: 587-592.

Sultana A, Tudur Smith C, Cunningham D, et al. Meta-analyses of chemotherapy for locally advanced and metastatic pancreatic cancer. J Clin Oncol 2007; 25:2607-2615.

Sultana A, Tudur Smith C, Cunningham D, et al. Systematic review, including, meta-analyses, on the management of locally advanced pancreatic cancer using radiation/combined modality therapy. Br J Cancer 2007; 96:1183-90.

Taïeb J, Lecomte T, Aparicio T et al. FOLFIRI.3, a new regimen combining 5-fluoruracil, folinic acid and irinotecan, for advanced pancreatic cancer: results of an Association des GastroEnterologues Oncologues (Gastroenterologist Oncologist Association) multicenter phase II study. Ann Oncol 2007; 18: 498-503.

Tempero M, Berlin J, Ducreux D, Haller D, Harper D, Khayat et al. Pancreatic cancer treatment and research: an international expert panel discussion. Ann Oncol 2011; 22(7):1500-6.

Tempero M, Plunkett W, Ruiz Van Haperen V, Hainsworth J, Hochster H, Lenzi R & Abbruzzese J. Randomized phase II comparison of dose-intense gemcitabine: thirty-minute infusion and fixed dose rate infusion in patients with pancreatic adenocarcinoma. J Clin Oncol 2003; 21:3402-08.

Tsavaris N, Kosmas C, Skopelitis H, et al. Secon-line treatment with oxaliplatin, leucovorin and 5-fluorouracil in gemcitabine-pretreated advanced pancreatic cancer: A phase II study. Invest New Drugs 2005; 23:369-75.

Van Cutsem E, van de Velde H, Karasek P, Oettle H, Vervenne WL, Szawlowski A et al. Phase III trial of gemcitabine plus tipifarnib compared with gemcitabine plus placebo in advanced pancreatic cancer. J Clin Oncol 2004; 22:1430-38.

Van Cutsem E, Vervenne WL, Bennouna J et al. Phase III trial of bevacizumab in combination with gemcitabine and erlotinib in patients with metastatic pancreatic cancer. J Clin Oncol 2009; 27:2231-37.

Vogelstein B & Kinszler KW. Cancer genes and the pathways they control. *Nat Med* 2004; 10:789-99.

Von Hoff DD, Ramanathan R, Borad M, Laheru D, Smith L, Wood T et al. SPARC correlation with response to gemcitabine (G) plus nab-paclitaxel (nab-P) in patients with advanced metastatic pancreatic cancer: a phase I/II study. J Clin Oncol 2009; 27 (15 Suppl): 4525.

Von Hoff DD, Ramanathan RK, Borad MJ, Laheru DA, Smith LS, Wood TE, Korn RL, Desai N, Trieu V, Iglesias JL, Zhang H, Soon-Shiong P, Shi T, Rajeshkumar NV, Maitra A, Hidalgo M. Gemcitabine Plus nab-Paclitaxel Is an Active Regimen in Patients With Advanced Pancreatic Cancer: A Phase I/II Trial. J Clin Oncol. 2011 Oct 3. [Epub ahead of print] PubMed PMID: 21969517

Walkins DJ, Starling N, Chau I, Thomas J, Webb J, Oates JR et al. The combination of chemotherapy doublet (gemcitabine plus capecitabine) with a biologic doublet (bevacizumab plus erlotinib) in patients with advanced pancreatic adenocarcinoma: the TARGET study. J Clin Oncol 2010; 28 (15 Suppl): 4036.

Xiong HQ, Varadhachary GR, Blais JC, Hess KR, Abbruzzese JL and Wolff RA. Phase II trial of oxaliplatin plus capecitabine (XELOX) as second-line therapy for patients with advanced pancreatic cancer. Cancer 2008; 113: 2046-52.

Yi SY, Park YS, Kim HS, Jun HJ, Kim KH, Chang MH et al. Irinotecan monotherapy as second-line treatment in advanced pancreatic cancer. Cancer Chemotherapy Pharmacology 2009; 63: 1141-5.

Zhang Y, Yang Q, Jiang Z, Ma W, Zhou S, Xie de R. Overall survival of patients with advanced pancreatic cancer improved with an increase in second-line chemotherapy after gemcitabine-based therapy. Journal of pancreatic cancer (JOP) 2011; 12(2):131-7.

7

Immunotherapy of the Pancreatic Cancer

Yang Bo
HepatoBiliary Department of Surgery
3rd Affiliated Hospital of Soochow University, Changzhou, Jiangsu, China

1. Introduction

Pancreatic cancer, which we refer to pancreatic ductal adenocarcinoma, is the forth most common cause of cancer-realated-death disease. In 2010, there were 43,140 new cases and 36,800 patients died of pancreatic cancer in USA(1). Although surgical resection may be the only available treatment for this horrible disease, there are beyond 80% patients when dignosised cannot be cured by surgical treatment(2). In the past 50 years, despite of the progress in surgery skill, hospital morbidity and mortality rates were decreased from 59% and 24% to 36% and 2%, respectively(3) , in the patients received the most optimal surgical operation, the median survival ranged from 15 to 19 months, and 5-year survival rate was still approximately 20%(4). Even if Gemcitabine became the new standard of chemotherapy in pancreatic cancer in 1997(5). The outcome of the pancreatic cancer is still dismal, overall five-year survival rate is blow 5%. With an increasing incidence of pancreatic cancer in the world and conventional treatments often have limited effects and substantial toxicity, a strong need exists for novel therapies. Biological approaches, including gene therapy and immunotherapy, which are targeting pancreatic cancer at a molecular or protein level, are rapidly evolving and seem to be promising strategies for this devastating and virtually unexceptionally lethal malignancy.

2. Immune target and Immune response in pancreatic cancer

Cancer is fundamentally a gene associated disease, it has become increasingly clear that some genomic instability and aberrant gene expression lead to biologic behaviour abnormality in tumor cells. In pancreatic cancer, Several genes have high mutation rate in different phase, so the tumor cell may express abnormal antigens that make them immunologically distinct and potential targets for the host immune system.

K-Ras: The mutation of K-ras oncogene (homologous to the ras gene of Kirsten murine sarcoma virus) occurs in 75-100% of pancreatic cancer(6). With the progression from minimally dysplasia epithelium(PanIN 1A, 1B) to more severe dysplasia(PanIN 2, 3) and invasive cancer(7), the mutation rate of K-ras oncogene is increaseing successively, denotes k-ras oncogene plays a very important role in tumor origination and progression(8).

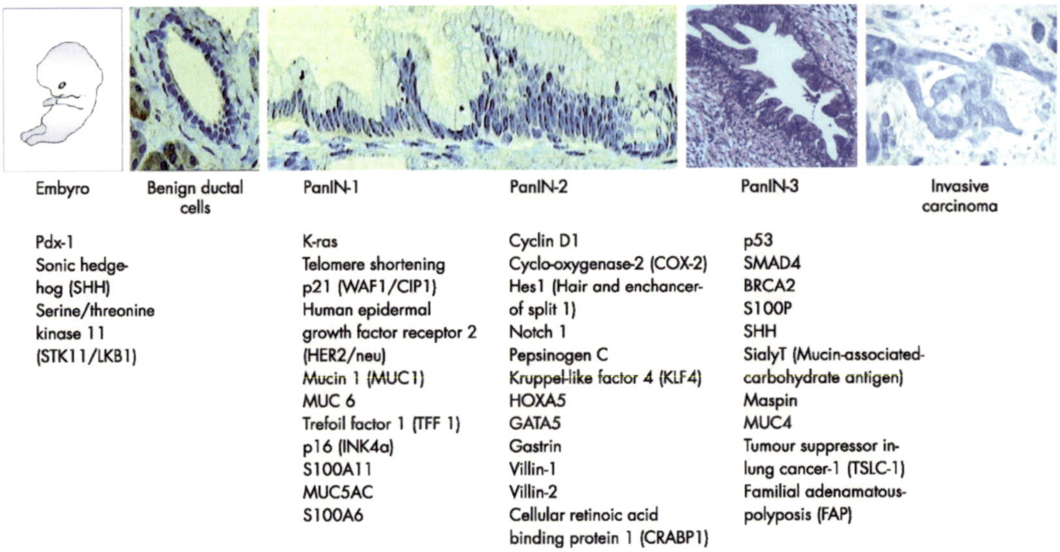

Picture 1. Associated genes in pancreatic cancer progression. from Paula Ghaneh, et al. Biology and management of pancreatic cancer. Gut 2007;56:1134-1152.

K-ras gene encodes a 21 kDa membrane-bound guanosine triphosphate(GTP) -binding protein. Before localization at cell membrane, K-ras protein must be farnesylated or geranylgeranylated on the same cysteine residue, it is involved in the transduction of signal from growth factor receptors and other signal inputs, as an upstream activator, it will activat several signaling pathways including Raf/MEK/ERK, P13K/Akt and RalEGF/Ral(9)to regulate gene expression and prevent apoptosis. The mutation of the K-ras oncogene, which occers mostly at codon 12 but also occasionally at codon 13 and 61, will lead to impaired GTPhosphatase(GTPase) activity, resulting in lock the protein locked in GTP-bound state and thus activating downstream signalling cascades(10). According to the META Analyse, point mutation occurred in codon 12 mainly divided into several types, the wild type GGT is replaced by GAT(47%), GTT(28%), CGT(15%), TGT(7%), AGT(2%) and GCT(1%). so in the protein, the 12th amino acid Guanine is replaced by Aspartic acid, Valine, Arginine, Cysteine, Alanine, Serine(11). The K-RAS function changes due to the abnormality in protein structure. The mutation also provide the epitope which might be the target in immunotherapy.

MUC1: Mucins are large glycoproteins with carbohydrate content and marked diversity both in the apoprotein and in the oligosaccharide moieties(12). MUC1 is a heavily glycosylated type I membrane protein with several extracellular tandem repeat domains, which is expressed by nearly all human glandular epithelial and its expression is limited to the apical membrane of the cells. In pancreatic cancer, MUC1 expression is upregulated with an expression pattern over the entire cell surface(13). The core peptide of MUC1 not only serves as a counter-receptor for myelin-associated glycoprotein in pancreatic cancer and is related to perineural invasion(14), but also block death receptor-mediated apoptosis by binding to caspase 8 and FADD(15). MUC1 molecular has sialic acid-containing oligosaccharides in a highly O-glycosylated tandem-repeat domain, the structure has wide range and a large molecular weight(16). Although the core protein of MUC1 is similar in both normal and tumor cells, there is a remarkable diversity in oligosaccharide moieties between normal and cancer cells(17).

Mesothelin: Mesothelin is a 40-kDa glycosyl phosphatidylinositol anchored cell surface protein and is a c-terminus menbrane-bound form of a 69-kDa precursor protein encoded by the Mesothelin gene(MSLN). Normally, mesothelin is only expressed on mesothelial cells which lining peritoneal, pleural and pericardial cavities(18). The biologic functions are not clearly understood. Some early studies have shown mesothelin playing role in tumor adhesion and dissemination(19). In pancreaticobiliary adenocarcinomas, the expression rate of mesotheline is 100%, whereas none in normal pancreas and chronic pancreatitis(20).

2.1 Immune escape and immunosuppression

In the past 50 years, with the advances in cellular, molecular biology of cancer and development of immunology, people comes to realizes the relationship between tumor and immune cells is just like a cat and mouse game. The human immune system assume the responsibility to get rid of the extrinsic and endogenic abnormal antigen, it can produce actived immunocyte or immune material such as antibody to react anomalous antigen and finally eliminate the target, but the fact is not under our desire. (Picture 2)

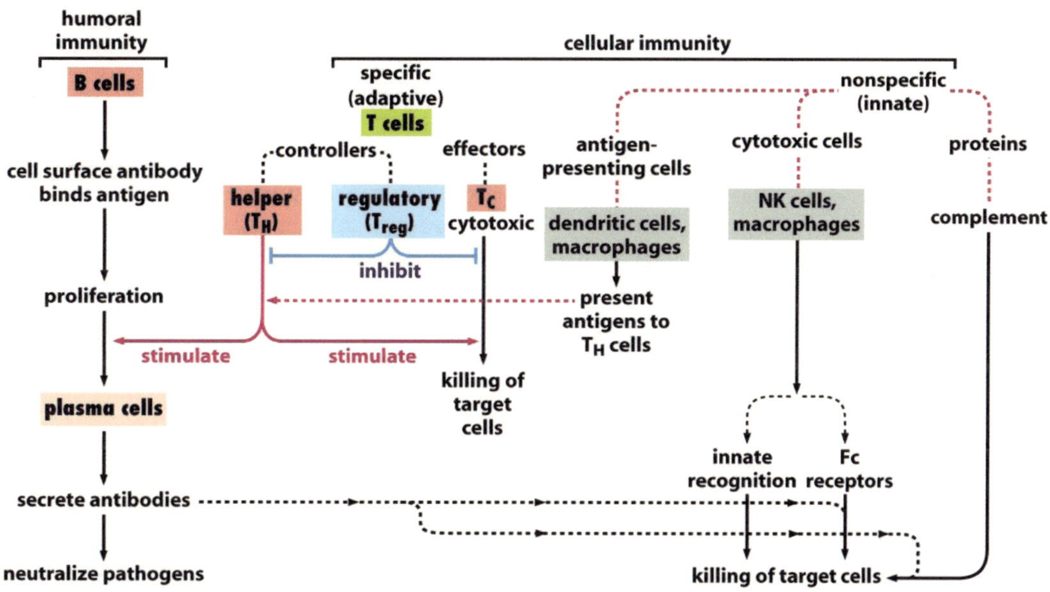

Picture 2. Immune system：From Robert A. Weinberg, The Biology of Cancer. 2007

At the genesis of the cancer, under ideal condition, the innate immune system responds to "danger signals", macrophages and fibroblasts are enlisted to construct the microenvironment surrounding the cancer cell, just like inflmmation, many cytokines and growth factors are produced to activate innate effector cells with antitumor activity, stimulate professional antigen-presenting cells (APCs, mainly dendritic cell) to capture tumor-derived antigens and migrate to draining lymph nodes to priming an adaptive response by activating T and B lymphocytes. Unfortunately, the growth factors can also stimulate cancer cells proliferation and progression. The cancer cells are so clever that can learn to avoid detection or to escape or overwhelm the immune response. Immunosuppressive tumor-associated macrophages (TAMs), myeloid-derived suppressor cells (MDSC), and regulatory T cells (Treg) reside in tumors, and their products along with tumor derived products (such as VEGF, TGFbeta and IL-10), create a microenvironment that resists immune activation and attack.

Many strategies are found to escape from immune surveillance[21]. 1) Physical exclusion of immune cells from tumor site. It has been proved in epithelial cancer that basal-membrane-like structures around the tumor can prevent lymphocytes from infiltrating and tumor-specific T cells expanding[22]. 2) Poor immunogenicity by reducing expression of major histocompatability complex(MHC) or co-stimulatory proteins[23] and disruption of natural killer(NK) and natural killer T (NKT) cell recognition[24]. The other ways are to change themselves by losing whole protein or TAA expression, which changes in immunodominant T-cell epitopes that alter T-cell recognition, antigen processing or binging to the MHC. 3) Secreting soluble immunosuppressive proteins such as interleukin (IL-10) to prevent inflammatory response from triggering, or vascular endothelial growth factor(VEGF) to interfere with dendritic cells(DC) activation and differentiation[25]. 4) Increasing expression of STAT3 protein to block the production of pro-inflammatory molecules[26].

If the specific reaction had been established, being attacked by activated NK cells, antibodies or cytotoxic T lymphocytes, cancer cells can escape elimination according to down-regulating targeted antigens, rendering tuomr-reative cell anergic[27], or inducing responding T cell apotosis specifically. The pro-apoptotic function of FasL on carcinoma cells has been demonstrated in both in virto and in vivo, FasL expressed cancer cells can induce apoptosis of lymphocytes in Fas-dependent manner[28], and in patient's biopsies, the present of FasL on cancer cells is in parallel with reduced number[29] and apoptosis [30]of tumor-infiltrating immune cells (TICs). In pancreatic ductal carcinoma, the expression of FasL is 82% in primary versus 100% in hepatic metastases and is associate with shorter survival[31]. At last, the eventual developed tumor reflects immunoediting with selection of poorly immunogenic and/or immune-resistant malignant cells[32].

Treg cells: CD4+25+Foxp3+ regulatory T cells (Tregs) have been discovered in the 1960s, which can suppres T-cell response and compromise the development of effective tumor immunity[33]. these cells are distinguished in high expressed CD4, CD25, CTLA-4, the glucocorticoid-induced TNF-related receptor (GITR) and the forkhead transcription Foxp3. they can arise in response to persistent antigen stimulation in the absence of inflammatory signals, especially in the presence of TGF-β[34]. The tumor-induced expansion of regulatory T cells by conversion of CD4+CD25+ lymphocytes is thymus and proliferation independent[35].

Tregs play a critical role in the induction of tolerance to tumor-associated antigens and suppression of antitumor immunity. Additional evidence showed that Tregs were increased locally within the tumor microenvironment by a mechanism that seems dependent on TGF-beta receptor expression and the presence of tumor derived TGF-beta. The murine pancreas cancer cell line Pan02 produces high levels of TGF-beta both in vitro and in vivo. In contrast, the esophageal murine cancer cell line, Eso2, does not. Immunohistochemical staining of Foxp3 in explanted tumors showed an identifiable population of Treg in the Pan02 (TGF-beta positive) tumors but not Eso2 (TGF-beta negative). Naive CD4+25-Foxp3- T cells, when adoptively had transferred into Rag-/- mice, were converted into Foxp3+ Treg in the presence of Pan02 but not Eso2 tumors. Induction of Treg in Pan02 mice was blocked by systemic injection of an anti-TGF-beta antibody. If Rag-/- mice were instead reconstituted with naive CD4+25- T cells expressing a mutated TGF-beta receptor, induction of Foxp3+ Treg in Pan02 bearing mice was blocked. Collectively, The observations supported the role of TGF-beta in the induction of Treg in pancreas adenocarcinoma(36).

Recent studies have shown that increased numbers of tumor-infiltrating Tregs were associated with poorer prognosis in pancreatic cancer(37)(38), so the presence of Tregs in pancreatic cancers highlighes the importance of targeting the suppressive function of these cells in future immunotherapy research.

In Yamamoto's study, a cytotoxicity assay, enzyme-linked immunosorbent spot (ELISPOT) assay and measuring cytokine secretion, were used to study the efficacy of Treg depletion by anti-CD25 antibody added to a dendritic cell/tumor cell (DC/TC) fusion hybrid vaccine in a murine pancreatic cancer model. All the mice treated with the combined therapy of fusion hybrid vaccine and Treg depletion rejected tumor growth in a challenging test, although the rejection rate was 20% both for mice that received the fusion hybrids alone or Treg depletion alone. In addition, combined therapy showed a significantly improved survival in comparison to other treatment or control groups. The NK cell activity for DC/TC fusion + Treg depletion was significantly higher than that for the other treatment groups. Cytotoxic T lymphocyte (CTL) activity for DC/TC could potentially be enhanced by the addition of Treg depletion therapy. The treatments including DC/TC fusion induced IFN-gamma secreting effector cells in ELISPOT assays. Furthermore, a cytometric beads array assay used to measure cytokine secretion showed that DC/TC fusion + Treg depletion stimulated the highest levels of IFN-gamma Th1/Th2 ratios and Th17. The results demonstrate that Treg depletion combined with DC/TC fusion hybrid vaccine enhanced the efficacy of immunotherapy in pancreatic cancer by activating CTLs and NK cells(39).

In both human pancreatic adenocarcinoma and a murine pancreatic tumor model (Pan02), tumor cells produce increased levels of ligands for the CCR5 chemokine receptor and, reciprocally, CD4(+) Foxp3(+) Tregs, compared with CD4(+) Foxp3(-) effector T cells, preferentially express CCR5. When CCR5/CCL5 signaling is disrupted, either by reducing CCL5 production by tumor cells or by systemic administration of a CCR5 inhibitor , Treg migration to tumors is reduced and tumors are smaller than in control mice. Thus, the study demonstrates the importance of Tregs in immune evasion by tumors, how blockade of Treg migration might inhibit tumor growth, and, specifically in pancreatic adenocarcinoma, the role of CCR5 in the homing of tumor-associated Tregs. Selective targeting of CCR5/CCL5 signaling may represent a novel immunomodulatory strategy for the treatment of cancer(40).

In murine mesothelin-expressing pancreatic tumor model (Panc02), vaccine with the immune-relevant mesothelin-derived peptides and in sequence with low-dose cyclophosphamide (CY) and an anti-CD25 IL-2Rα monoclonal antibody (PC61), which are known to deplete subpopulations of T regulatory cells (Tregs), showed that combined Treg-depleting therapies synergize to enhance vaccine efficacy(41).

Myeloid-derived suppressor cells: Myeloid-derived suppressor cells(MDSCs) are a heterogeneous population of cells that expand during cancer, inflammation and infection, and have a remarkable ability to suppress T-cell responses[42]. They contributes negative regulation of immune response and can be activated by factor produced by activated T cells and tumor stromal cells[43].

Myeloid derived suppressor cells (MDSC), which are observed with increased prevalence in the peripheral blood and tumor microenvironment of cancer patients, including pancreatic cancer. Accumulation of MDSC in the peripheral circulation has been related to extent of disease, and correlates with stage. MDSC have primarily been implicated in promoting tumor growth by suppressing antitumor immunity. There is also compelling evidence MDSC are also involved in angiogenesis and metastatic spread. Two main subsets of MDSC have been identified in cancer patients: a monocytic subset, characterized by expression of CD14, and a granulocytic subset characterized by expression of CD15. Both subsets of MDSC actively suppress host immunity through a variety of mechanisms including production of reactive oxygen species and arginase. Just as in humans, accumulation of monocytic and granulocytic MDSC has been noted in the bone marrow, spleen, peripheral circulation, and tumors of tumor bearing mice. Successful targeting of MDSC in mice is associated with improved immune responses, delayed tumor growth, improved survival, and increased efficacy of vaccine therapy. By further elucidating mechanisms of MDSC recruitment and maintenance in the tumor environment, strategies could be developed to reverse immune tolerance to tumor[44].

In a comprehensive analysis of circulating myeloid-derived suppressor cells (MDSCs) and T regulatory cells (Tregs) in pancreatic, esophageal and gastric cancer Patients Peripheral blood was collected from 131 cancer patients (46 pancreatic, 60 esophageal and 25 gastric) and 54 healthy controls. PBMC were harvested with subsequent flow cytometric analysis of MDSC (HLADR(-) Lin1(low/-) CD33(+) CD11b(+)) and Treg (CD4(+) CD25(+) CD127 (low/-) FoxP3(+)) percentages. MDSCs and Tregs were statistically significantly elevated in pancreatic, esophageal and gastric cancer compared with controls, and MDSC numbers correlated with Treg levels. Increasing MDSC percentage was associated with increased risk of death, and in a multivariate analysis, MDSC level was an independent prognostic factor for survival. A unit increase in MDSC percentage was associated with a 22% increased risk of death (hazard ratio 1. 22,95% confidence interval 1.06-1.41). The result showed MDSCs are an independent prognostic factor for survival[45].

In mice with spontaneous pancreatic tumours, mice with premalignant lesions as well as wild-type mice, Myeloid-derived suppressor cells (MDSC)were analysed. An increase in the frequency of MDSC early in tumour development was detected in lymph nodes, blood and pancreas of mice with premalignant lesions and increased further upon tumour progression. The MDSC from mice with pancreatic tumours have arginase activity and suppress T-cell responses, which represent the hallmark functions of these cells. The study suggests that immune suppressor mechanisms generated by tumours exist as early as premalignant lesions and increase with tumour progression and highlight the importance of blocking these suppressor mechanisms early in the disease in developing immunotherapy protocols[46].

Nagaraj reported use of the synthetic triterpenoid(CDDO-Me) can completely abrogated immune suppressive activity of MDSC in vitro, CDDO-Me reduced reactive oxygen species in MDSCs but did not affect their viability or the levels of nitric oxide and arginase.

Treatment of tumor-bearing mice with CDDO-Me did not affect the proportion of MDSCs in the spleens but eliminated their suppressive activity. This effect was independent of antitumor activity. CDDO-Me treatment decreased tumor growth in mice. Experiments with severe combined immunodeficient-beige mice indicated that this effect was largely mediated by the immune system. CDDO-Me substantially enhanced the antitumor effect of a cancer vaccines. treatment of pancreatic cancer patients with the synthetic triterpenoid (CDDO-Me) didn't affect the number of MDSCs in peripheral blood but significantly improved the immune response. The research demonstrated MDSCs is the key of the immunotherapy(47).

3. Nonspecific immunotherapy - Innate Immune system and cytokine

Nature kill cells are the central component of the innate immunity and play an important role in cancer immunosurveilance. It has been reported that NK cells can recognize and control tumor growth by direct cellular cytotoxicity and secrete immunostimulatory cytokines such as IFN-γ. The further researches have demonstrated NK cells can eliminate tumor cell by inhibiting cellular proliferation, angiogenesis, promoting apoptosis and stimulate the adaptive immune system. In mouse experimental models, NK cell-mediated elimination of tumor cells induced the subsequent development of tumor-specific T cell responses to the parental tumor cells as a bridge between innate and adaptive immune responses(48).

In 1984, K. Funa has found patients with pancreatic adenocarcinomas expressing deficiencies in the NK-IFN system at least three levels:(1)diminished basal NK activities, (2)decreased sensitivity of NK to IFN in virto, (3)decreased atypical IFN production by *staphylococcus aureus* cowan I (SACoI)(49).

In a recent clinical trial, a patient exhibited regression of several pancreatic cancer metastases following the administration of the immune modulator Ipilimumab (anti-CTLA-4 antibody). Tumor infiltrating lymphocytes (TIL-2742) and an autologous tumor line (TC-2742) were expanded from a regressing metastatic lesion excised from this patient. Natural killer (NK) cells predominated in the TIL (92% CD56(+)) with few T cells (12% CD3(+)). A majority (88%) of the NK cells were CD56(bright)CD16(-). TIL-2742 secreted IFN-γ and GM-CSF following co-culture with TC-2742 and major histocompatibility complex mismatched pancreatic tumor lines. After sorting TIL-2742, the purified CD56(+)CD16(-)CD3(-) subset showed reactivity similar to TIL-2742 while the CD56(-)CD16(-)CD3(+) cells exhibited no tumor recognition. In co-culture assays, TIL-2742 and the NK subset expressed high reactivity to several pancreatic cancer cell lines and could lyse the autologous tumor as well as pancreas cancer lines. Reactivity was partially abrogated by blockade of TRAIL. This represents the first report of CD56(+)CD16(-) NK cells with apparent specificity for pancreatic cancer cell lines and associated with tumor regression following the treatment with an immune modulating agent(50).

Clinical and experimental evidence demonstrate the extent of NK cell activity in peripheral blood is associated with cancer risk in adults(51). In recent years, novel studies have discovered the phenotypic status and functionality of NK cells in tumor site and also in peripheral blood of cancer patients. Research has shown that only a few infiltrating NK cells which are unlikely to greatly contribute to eliminate the tumoe cells(52). Due to NK's inefficient homing into malignant tissues, the situation may be overcome by cytokine-mediated activation in immunotherapeutical regimen(53). However, novel studies of tumor-associated NK cells demonstrated a striking phenotype, supporting the notion that tumor-induced alterations of activating NK cell receptor expression may hamper immune surveillance and promote tumor progression.

Bhat R reported the finding:besides its intrinsic oncolytic activity, parvovirus H-1PV is able to enhance NK cell-mediated killing of pancreatic adenocarcinoma cells. The experiment show that H-1PV infection of Panc-1 cells increases NK cell capacity to release IFN-γ, TNF-α and MIP-1α/β. Multiple activating receptors are involved in the NK cell-mediated killing of Panc-1 cells. Indeed, blocking of the natural cytotoxicity receptors-NKp30, 44 and 46 in combination, and NKG2D and DNAM1 alone inhibit the killing of Panc-1 cells. Interestingly, H-1PV infection of Panc-1 cells overcomes the part of inhibitory effects suggesting that parvovirus may induce additional NK cell ligands on Panc-1 cells. The enhanced sensitivity of H-1PV-infected pancreatic adenocarcinoma cells to NK cell-dependent killing could be traced back to the upregulation of the DNAM-1 ligand, CD155 and to the downregulation of MHC class I expression. The data suggests that NK cells display antitumor potential against PDAC and that H-1PV-based oncolytic immunotherapy could further boost NK cell-mediated immune responses and help to develop a combinatorial therapeutic approach against pancreatic cancer(54).

NK cells can eliminate tumor cells through their ability to mediate antibody-dependent cellular cytotoxicity(ADCC). Nk cell recognition of an antibody-coated target cell results in rapid NK cell activation and degranulation(55). NK-cell mediated ADCC play a part in mechanisms of tumor-targeted mAbs which targeting CD20, Her2/neu, epidermal growth factor receptor(EGFR)(56)(57). Because HLA class I is a ligand for inhibitory receptor family, killer cell immunoglobulin-like receptor of NK cells(58), loss of HLA class I expression can lead to escape of antigen-dependent cytotoxicity of CD8+ CTL and increase the possibility as a target of NK cell cytotoxicity. In pancreatic cancer, total HLA class I loss is 6% in primary versus 43% in metastastic tumors;0 in G1, 33% in G2 and 67% in G3(59).

In research of nonspecific immunotherapy, many cytokines were used to elevate the ability of the immune system. it is possible to activate tumor-specific antitumor immune responses by systemic injection of cytokine or introduction of cytokine gene into tumors through activating natural killer(NK) cells and tumor-specific CD4+ T cells and cytotoxic T lymphocytes(CTL). Different cytokines may stimulate antitumor immune responses by different mechanisms.

Granulocyte Marcophage Colony-Stimulating Factor(GM-CSF) and IL-2 are the most popular cytokines used in cancer immunotherapy. GM-CSF, which can stimulate bone marrows differentiating and maturing to neutrophils, monocytes and dendritic cells, is used to generate cancer immunotherapy called GAVX(60). In clinical trials using the GAVX, induction of systemic antitumor immune response and clinical activity was observed in pancreatic cancer, melanoma, and renal cell carcinoma. In a study of combination of chemotherapy and immunotherapy, two GM-CSF secreting pancreas cancer cell lines (CG8020/CG2505) as immunotherapy were administered alone or in sequence with Cy in patients with advanced pancreatic cancer. Results showed GM-CSF secreting pancreas cancer cell lines demonstrated minimal treatment-related toxicity in patients with advanced pancreatic cancer. Also, mesothelin specific T cell responses are detected/enhanced in some patients treated with CG8020/CG2505 immunotherapy. In addition, Cy modulated immunotherapy resulted in median survival in a Gemzar resistant population similar to chemotherapy alone[61].

Interlukin-2 (IL-2) is a growth factor that stimulates innate immunity cells. Different dose of IL-2 has been proved either enhance or decrease cellular and humoral immune functions. Rosenberg used it developing lymphokine-activated killer(LAK) therapy for cancer[62]. In a randomized study, preoperative subcutaneously IL-2 immunotherapy at 12 million IU for 3 consecutive days before surgery is able to abrogate the effects of the surgical trauma and recover a normal immunofunction in pancreatic cancer patients[63]. Recombinant interleukin-2 (rIL-2) was used in a study which aimed to evaluate the toxicity of pre- and postoperative rIL-2 treatment and the effects on innate immunity both in peripheral blood and in cancer tissue of patients with resectable pancreatic adenocarcinoma. Seventeen patients received high dose rIL-2 preoperative subcutaneous administration and two low dose postoperative cycles. NK cell and eosinophil count were evaluated in blood and in pancreatic surgical specimens. The result showed toxicity was moderate. In the early postoperative period, blood NK cells and eosinophils significantly increased compared to basal values ($p < 0.02$). Preoperative high dose rIL-2 administration is able to counteract surgery-induced deficiency of NK cells and eosinophils in peripheral blood in the early postoperative period, although it cannot overcome local mechanisms of immune tumor escape in cancer tissue. The amplification of innate immunity, induced by immunotherapy, may improve the control of metastatic cells spreading in the perioperative period[64].

As a bridge between innate and adaptive immune response[65], IL-12 is independently identified as natural killer-stimulating factor (NKSF) and cytotoxic lymphocyte maturation factor[66], which induces proliferation of NK and T1 cells and production of cytokines, especially IFN-γ , and also enhances the generation and activity of CTLs, through activation of STAT4[67].

The combination of IL-12 and IL-27 can modify the polarization of Th2 effectors by both reduction of IL-5, GM-CSF and IL-13 and induction of IFN-gamma production, which lasted after cytokine removal. Besides, the combined treatment functionally modulated the Th2 polarization of CEA-specific CD4(+) T cells and enhanced pre-existing Th1 type immunity[68].

In recent study, IL-12 was coformulated with the biodegradable polysaccharide chitosan which could enhance the antitumor activity of IL-12 while limiting its systemic toxicity. Antitumor efficacy of IL-12 alone and IL-12 coformulated with chitosan (chitosan/IL-12) was assessed in mice bearing established pancreatic (Panc02) tumors. Additional studies involving depletion of immune cell subsets, tumor rechallenge, and CTL activity were designed to elucidate mechanisms of regression and tumor-specific immunity. Coformulation with chitosan increased local IL-12 retention from 1 to 2 days to 5 to 6 days. Weekly i. t. injections of IL-12 alone eradicated ≤10% of established Panc02 tumors, while i. t. chitosan/IL-12 immunotherapy caused complete tumor regression in 80% to 100% of mice. Depletion of CD4(+) or Gr-1(+) cells had no impact on chitosan/IL-12-mediated tumor regression. However, CD8(+) or NK cell depletion completely abrogated antitumor activity. I. t. chitosan/IL-12 immunotherapy generated systemic tumor-specific immunity, as >80%

of mice cured with i. t. chitosan/IL-12 immunotherapy were at least partially protected from tumor rechallenge. Furthermore, CTLs from spleens of cured mice lysed MC32a and gp70 peptide-loaded targets. The reasearch has demonstrated Chitosan/IL-12 immunotherapy increased local retention of IL-12 in the tumor microenvironment, eradicated established, aggressive murine tumors, and generated systemic tumor-specific protective immunity(69).

4. Specific immunotherapy

Specific immunotherapy, which seems be more important in cancer treatment research, could be divide into 3 parts:monoclonal antibody, adoptive cellular therapy, and vaccine. Infusion of antibody or activated cells is called Passive Immunotherapy, on the other, vaccine can induce active immunotherapy. The simplest model of immune cell-mediated antigen-specific tumor rejection consists of three elements: appropriate antigen specific for the tumor, efficient antigen presentation and the generation of potent effector cells.

4.1 Active immunotherapy

Vaccine: The development of human therapeutic cancer vaccines has come a long way since the discovery of major histocompatability complex (MHC) restricted tumor antigens. As an new method to reconsituting immunity, cancer vaccionation can actively harness the intrinsic power of the immne system to recognize and destroy tumors. The ideal designed vaccine should actively generate antigen-specific immune response to abnomal protein expressed in tumor cells, including activating distinct components of the immune system:antigen presenting cells, B cells and T cells, producing the advantages of high specificity, minimal toxicity and permanently effective immunologic memory. Antigen could be delivered in the form of DNA or peptide, as well as tumor cells or antigen-pulsed DCs.

GM-CSF is an important growth factor for granulocytes and monocytes, and has a crucial role in the growth and differentiation of DCs. Kimura M has found in vivo growth of AsPC-1 cells, which retrovirally transduced with the GM-CSF gene, was inhabited and associated with increased survival of the nude mice(70).

A series of clinical trails have been reported by researchers in John Hopkins in recent 10 years. Jaffee et al conducted a phase I study using allogeneic GM-CSF-secreting whole-cell tumor vaccine for pancreatic cancer. As vaccines, Two pancreatic cancer lines(PANC 10.05 and 6.03), which had been genetically modified to express GM-CSF, were given to patients who had undergone pancreaticoduodenectomy eight weeks prior. Three of the eight patients who received $\geq 10\times10^7$ vaccine cells developed post-vaccination delayed-type hypersensitivity (DTH) responses associated with increased disease free survival time, and remained disease-free for longer than 25 months after diagnosis. Side effects were mainly limited to local skin reactions at the site of vaccination(71). Further phase II study of 60 patients with resected pancreatic adenocarcinoma, patients received five treatments of 2.5×10^8 vaccine cells, together with 5-Fu and radiotherapy. The reported median survival was 26 months, with a 1- and 2-year survival of 88% and 76% respectively(72). In latest report, a single institution phase II study of 60 patients with resected pancreatic adenocarcinoma was performed, each treatment consisted of a total of 5×10^8 GM-CSF-secreting cells distributed equally among 3 lymph node regions. Subsequently, had received

5-FU based chemoradiation, patient received 5 immunotherapy. The median disease-free survival was 17.3 months with median survival of 24.8 months. The administration of immunotherapy was well tolerated. Besides, the postimmunotherapy induction of mesothelin-specific CD8+ T cells in HLA-A1+ and HLA-A2+ patients correlates with disease-free survival. The research concluded that an immunotherapy approach intergated with chemoradiation is safe and helpful for resected pancreas cancer(73).

VEGF Vascular endothelial growth factor receptor 2 (VEGFR2) is an essential factor in tumor angiogenesis and in the growth of pancreatic cancer. Immunotherapy using epitope peptide for VEGFR2 (VEGFR2-169) is expected to improve the clinical outcome. A phase I clinical trial combining of VEGFR2-169 with gemcitabine was conducted for patients with metastatic and unresectable pancreatic cancer. Gemcitabine was administered at a dose of 1000 mg/m(2) on days 1, 8, and 15 in a 28-day cycle. The VEGFR2-169 peptide was subcutaneously injected weekly in a dose-escalation manner (doses of 0.5, 1, and 2 mg/body, six patients/one cohort). No severe adverse effect of grade 4 or higher was observed. Of the 18 patients who completed at least one course of the treatment, 15 (83%) developed immunological reactions at the injection sites. Specific cytotoxic T lymphocytes (CTL) reacting to the VEGFR2-169 peptide were induced in 11 (61%) of the 18 patients. The disease control rate was 67%, and the median overall survival time was 8. 7 months. This combination therapy for pancreatic cancer patients was tolerable at all doses. Peptide-specific CTL could be induced by the VEGFR2-169 peptide vaccine at a high rate, even in combination with gemcitabine. From an immunological point of view, the optimal dose for further clinical trials might be 2 mg/body or higher(74).

Ras peptide is the first agent tested in immunetherapy in pancreatic cancer. Gjertsen used an intradermal vaccine of APCs loaded ex vivo with synthetic ras peptide corresponding to the mutation found in patients. In this phase I/II trial , two of five patients with advanced pancreatic cancer showed induced immune response(75). In further phase I/II trial in 48 pancreatic cancer patients with different clinic stages, ras peptide in combination with GM-CSF could induce peptide-specific immunty in 58% patients. Compared to non-responders, survival time were prolonged in patients with advanced disease, the association between prolonged survival and an immune response against the vaccine suggests that a clinical benefit of ras peptide vaccination may be obtained for this group of patients(76).

In 24 Patients with resected pancreatic cancer, with K-ras mutations at codon 12, were vaccinated once monthly for 3 months with a 21-mer peptide vaccine containing the corresponding K-ras mutation of the patient's tumor. Immune responses were evaluated by delayed-type hypersensitivity (DTH) tests and the enzyme-linked immunosorbent spot assays. Results showed there were no grade 3-5 vaccine-specific toxicities. The only National Cancer Institute grade 1 and 2 toxicity was erythema at the injection site (94%). Nine patients (25%) were evaluable for immunologic responses. One patient (11%) had a detectable immune response specific to the patient's K-ras mutation, as assessed by DTH. Three patients (13%) displayed a DTH response that was not specific. Median recurrence free survival time was 8. 6 months (95% confidence interval, 2.96-19.2) and median overall survival time was 20. 3 months (95% confidence interval, 11.6-45.3). It suggested K-ras vaccination for patients with resectable pancreatic adenocarcinoma proved to be safe and tolerable with however no elicitable immunogenicity and unproven efficacy(77).

In another phase II study, a specific mutant ras peptide vaccine was tested as an adjuvant immunotherapy in pancreatic and colorectal cancer patients. Five pancreatic and seven colorectal cancer patients were vaccinated subcutaneously with 13-mer mutant ras peptide, corresponding to their tumor's ras mutation. Vaccinations were given every 4 weeks, up to a total of six vaccines. The result showed no serious acute or delayed systemic side effects were seen. Five out of eleven patients showed a positive immune response. Furthermore, the five pancreatic cancer patients have shown a mean disease-free survival (DFS) of 35. 2^+ months and a mean overall survival (OS) of 44.4^+ months. The study suggested it is feasible to use mutant ras vaccine in the adjuvant setting. This vaccine is safe, can induce specific immune responses, and it appears to have a positive outcome in overall survival(78). In a follow-up study, Twenty-three patients who were vaccinated after surgical resection for pancreatic adenocarcinoma (22 pancreaticoduodenectomies, one distal resection). The vaccine was composed of long synthetic mutant ras peptides designed mainly to elicit T-helper responses. Seventeen of 20 evaluable patients (85%) responded immunologically to the vaccine. Median survival for all patients was 27.5 months and 28 months for immune responders. The 5-year survival was 22% and 29%, respectively. Strikingly, 10-year survival was 20% (four patients out of 20 evaluable) versus zero (0/87) in a cohort of nonvaccinated patient treated in the same period. Three patients mounted a memory response up to 9 years after vaccination. The observation indicates that K-ras vaccination may consolidate the effect of surgery and represent an adjuvant treatment option for the future(79).

MUC1 In order to create MUC1-specific immune response, a vaccine composed of MUC1 peptide and SBAS2 adjuvant was tested in a phase I study, There was an increase in the percentage of CD8+ T cells and MUC1-specific antibody(80).

The other approach to induce MUC1-specific immune response is antigen-pulsed DCs. A Phase I/II clinical trial of a MUC1 peptide-loaded DC vaccine was carried out in 12 pancreatic and biliary cancer patients following resection of their primary tumors. The vaccine was well tolerated and no toxicity was observed. Prior to vaccination, patients entered onto this trial had a significantly higher percentage of FoxP3+CD4+T cells compared to age matched healthy controls. The percentage of these cells also increased transiently following each injection, returning to baseline or below before the next injection. Vaccinated patients have been followed for over four years and four of the twelve patients are alive, all without evidence of recurrence(81).

Another phase I/II trial used human autologous DCs transfected with MUC1 cDNA as vaccine, 4 of 10 patients showed a two- to ten-fold increase in the frequency of mucin-specific IFN-γ-secreting CD8+ T cells, suggesting an immune response(82). But in a phase III trial of 255 patients using vaccine consisted of recombinant vaccinia and fowlpox viruses coexpressing CEA/MUC1/TRICOM, researchers failed to improve overall survival compared to palliative chemotherapy or best supportive care(83).

In Kondo H's clinical trial, Peripheral blood mononuclear cells (PBMCs) of twenty patients with unresectable or recurrent pancreatic cancer were separated into adherent cells for induction of MUC1-DCs and floating cells for MUC1-CTLs. MUC1-DCs were generated by culture with granulocyte monocyte colony stimulating factor (GM-CSF) and interleukin-4 (IL-4) and then exposed to MUC1 peptide and TNF-alpha. MUC1-CTLs were induced by co-culture with YPK-1 and then with interleukin-2 (IL-2). MUC1-DCs were injected intradermally and MUC1-CTLs were given intravenously. The result showed one patient with multiple lung metastases experienced a complete response. Five patients had stable disease. The mean survival time was 9.8 months. No grade II-IV toxicity was observed. The research suggested adoptive immunotherapy with MUC1-DC and MUC1-CTL may be feasible and effective for pancreatic cancer(84).

Mesothelin It is first reported by Thomas that specific CD8+ T-cell response which targeting mesothelin epitopes in pancreatic cancer can be induced via cross-presentation by an approach that recruits APCs to the vaccination site(85). Combinated with anti-glucocorticoid-induced TNF receptor antibody (anti-GITR), the mesotheline DNA vaccine can induce immune pretection in mice with sungeneic mesothelin-expressing pancreatic cancer. 50% of animals treated with mesothelin were tumor-free 25 days after tumor injection compared to 0 in untreated mice(86).

DNA vaccines employing single-chain trimers (SCT) have been shown to bypass antigen processing and presentation and result in significant enhancement of DNA vaccine potency. In a study, a DNA vaccine employing an SCT targeting human mesothelin and characterized the ensuing antigen-specific CD8+ T cell-mediated immune responses and anti-tumor effects against human mesothelin-expressing tumors in HLA-A2 transgenic mice. The results showed that vaccination with DNA employing an SCT of HLA-A2 linked to human mesothelin epitope aa540-549 (pcDNA3-Hmeso540-beta2m-A2) generated strong human mesothelin peptide (aa540-549)-specific CD8+ T cell immune responses in HLA-A2 transgenic mice. Vaccination with pcDNA3-Hmeso540-beta2m-A2 prevented the growth of HLA-A2 positive human mesothelin-expressing tumor cell lines in HLA-A2 transgenic mice in contrast to vaccination with DNA encoding SCT linked to OVA CTL epitope. Thus, the employment of SCT of HLA-A2 linked to the human mesothelin epitope aa540-549 represents a potential opportunity for the clinical translation of DNA vaccines against human mesothelin-expressing tumors, including pancreatic cancer(87).

4.2 Passive immunotherapy

Passive immunotherapy could be accomplished by infusion monoantibody and tumor specific T-cell which was actived in vitro. With advances in structural and functional genomics, recent work has focused on targeted molecular therapy using monoclonal antibodies. Many monoantibodies were used to target molecules on the tumor cell surface and normal tissue stroma, which are related to pancreatic cancer oncogenesis, tumor growth or resistance to chemotherapy, as well as molecules involved in regulating inflammation and host immunoresponses. Although progress made by monoantibody in pancreatic cancer treatment, especially in preclinical studies, its clinical application requires further investigation. Besides the function bind to target antigen to block the corresponding signal transduction pathways, antibody-dependent cellular cytotoxicity (ADCC) can also be observed in some pancreatic cancer cell lines.

4.2.1 Antibody

Monoclonal antibodies against human tumor targets were initially in rodents, which will induce immunologic responses from patient against mouse antibodies. With the drvelopment of recombinant DNA technology, this problem was solved and chimeric antibodies, antibody fragments or intact fully human antibodies were produced and tested clinically. Base on moral principles, antibodies were used as adjunctive treement with chemotherapy agents, small molecule signal transduction inhibitors, or radiation in clinical trails, to study if can help patients lengthen the survival. The targets are generally classified into three major categories:cell surface proteins;antigen associated with the tumor stroma;antigen on tumor-associated vasculature and angiogenic ligands(88).

4.2.1.1 Anti-EGFR antibodies

Cetuximab is a chimeric mouse-human antibody against an epitope located in extra-celluar part of EGFR. In preclinical studies, cetuximab could decrease cell proliferation and phosphorylation of EGFR, and blocked the binding of the adaptor protein Grb2 to EGFR upon activation by EGF(89). Another preclinical study, the combination of cetuximab together with gemcitabine and radiation effectively prolonged the tumor xenograft volume doubling time (30.1±3.3days), compared with gemcitabine monotherapy (11.6±3.1days), radiation monotherapy (16.7±3.1days), cetuximab with gemcitabine (20.1±3.1days)and cetuximab with radiation (22.5±3.3days)(90).

In many clinical trails, synergistic effects were observed using combination of cetuximab therapy and chemotherapy agents. In a multicenter phase II trial, Patients with measurable locally advanced or metastatic pancreatic cancer who had never received chemotherapy for their advanced disease and had immunohistochemical evidence of EGFR expression were treated with cetuximab at an initial dose of 400 mg/m(2), followed by 250 mg/m(2) weekly for 7 weeks. Gemcitabine was administered at 1,000 mg/m(2) for 7 weeks, followed by 1 week of rest. In subsequent cycles, cetuximab was administered weekly, and gemcitabine was administered weekly for 3 weeks every 4 weeks. In sixty-one patients who were screened for EGFR expression, 58 patients (95%) had at least 1+ staining, and 41 were enrolled onto the trial, result showed Five patients (12.2%) achieved a partial response, and 26 (63.4%) had stable disease. The median time to disease progression was 3.8 months, and the median overall survival duration was 7.1 months. One-year progression-free survival and overall survival rates were 12% and 31.7%, respectively. The most frequently reported grade 3 or 4 adverse events were neutropenia (39.0%), asthenia (22.0%), abdominal pain (22.0%), and thrombocytopenia (17.1%). Cetuximab in combination with gemcitabine showed promising activity against advanced pancreatic cancer(91).

Another multicenter pahse II study which is combination treatment with cetuximab and gemcitabine/oxaliplatin. Patients which had histological or cytological diagnosis of metastatic pancreatic adenocarcinoma received cetuximab 400 mg m(-2) at first infusion followed by weekly 250 mg m(-2) combined with gemcitabine 1000 mg m(-2) as a 100 min infusion on day 1 and oxaliplatin 100 mg m(-2) as a 2-h infusion on day 2 every 2 weeks. The intention-to-treat analysis of 61 evaluable patients showed an overall response rate of 33%, including 1 (2%) complete and 19 (31%) partial remissions. There were 31% patients with stable and 36% with progressive disease or discontinuation of the therapy before re-staging. The presence of a grade 2 or higher skin rash was associated with a higher likelihood of achieving objective response. Median time to progression was 118 days, with a median overall survival of 213 days. A clinical benefit response was noted in 24 of the evaluable 61 patients (39%). Although the addition of cetuximab to the combination of gemcitabine and oxaliplatin is well tolerated, the reasearch failed to increase response or survival in patients with metastatic pancreatic cancer[92].

But the effect of the cetuximab is limited by the affinity of expressed EGFR in pancreatic cancer, other factors including mutation of K-ras, PTEN expression or host complement level. these may be the reasons of failure in some trails. In a phase II trail, within the cetuximab group and noncetuximab group, no significant differences were found in objective response rate (17.5% Vs12.2%), median progression-free survival (3.4 months Vs 4.2 months), median overall survival (7.5 months Vs 7.8 months)[93], The result can't prove a synergistic effect in combination of cetuximab and gemcitabine/cisplatin treatment in pancreatic cancer.

Another phase III trail of Patients with unresectable locally advanced or metastatic pancreatic adenocarcinoma were randomly assigned to receive gemcitabine alone or gemcitabine plus cetuximab. A total of 745 eligible patients were accrued. No significant difference was seen between the two arms of the study with respect to the median survival time (6. 3 months for the gemcitabine plus cetuximab arm v5.9 months for the gemcitabine alone arm; hazard ratio = 1.06; 95% CI, 0.91 to 1.23; P = .23, one-sided). Objective responses and progression-free survival were similar in both arms of the study. Although time to treatment failure was longer in patients on gemcitabine plus cetuximab (P=.006), the difference in length of treatment was only 2 weeks longer in the combination arm. Among patients who were studied for tumoral EGFR expression, 90% were positive, with no treatment benefit detected in this patient subset. The author think in patients with advanced pancreas cancer, the anti-EGFR monoclonal antibody cetuximab did not improve the outcome compared with patients treated with gemcitabine alone. Alternate targets other than EGFR should be evaluated for new drug development[94].

Matuzumab(EMD 72000) is a humanized IgG1 mAb against EGFR. Laboratory studies have shown promising inhibitory effects on tumor growth and angiogenesis, include L3. 6pl in an orthotopic rat model[95]. In an phase I clinical trail, matuzumab was given at a dose of 400-800 mg once weekly for 8 weeks, followed by gemcitabine 1000mg/m2 weekly for two cycles. The partial response or stable disease in 12 evaluated advanced pancreatic cancer patients was 66.7%[96].

4.2.1.2 Anti-ErbB2/HER2 antibodies

Trastuzumab(Herceptin) is a humanized mAb, which has shown significant growth inhibition of a pancreatic cancer cell line and xenografts established with the same line. In a study focusing on HER2 overexpressing pancreatic cancer, trastuzumab was combined with fluoropyrimidine S-1 to treat cancer cells in vivo and in vitro, pancreatic cell growth inhibition is observed not only by inhibition of the HER2 signal transduction pathway, but also by antibody-dependent cellular cytotoxicity(ADCC) induced by trastuzumab[97]. In another research, although in four pancreatic cell lines, trastuzumab didn't express inhibitor effect and synergistic effect with gemcitabine, ADCC were observed in three cells which expressed HER2 in mice. In Capan-1 xenografted mice, trastuzumab inhibited tumor growth significantly and prolonged survival[98].

Larbouret reported combination treatment of matuzumab and trastuzumab could enhance the inhibitory effect on HER2 phosphorylation, lead to significantly decrease xenograft tumor sizes or induce more complete remissions when compared to antibody alone, then prolonged survival in BxPC-3 and MIA PaCa-2 pancreatic cancer cells xenograft mice(99). The further study which took placed in nude mice, bearing human pancreatic carcinoma xenografts, combined anti-EGFR (cetuximab) and anti-HER2 (trastuzumab) or gemcitabine were given as trement and tumor growth was observed. Result showed in first-line therapy, mice survival was significantly longer in the 2mAbs group compared with gemcitabine (P<0.0001 for BxPC-3, P=0.0679 for MiaPaCa-2 and P=0.0019 for Capan-1) and with controls (P<0.0001). In second-line therapy, tumor regressions were observed after replacing gemcitabine by 2mAbs treatment, resulting in significantly longer animal survival compared with mice receiving continuous gemcitabine injections (P=0.008 for BxPC-3, P=0.05 for MiaPaCa-2 and P<0.001 for Capan-1). Therapeutic benefit of 2mAbs was observed despite K-Ras mutation. Interestingly, concerning the mechanism of action, coinjection of F(ab')(2) fragments from 2mAbs induced significant tumor growth inhibition, compared with controls (P=0.001), indicating that the 2mAbs had an Fc fragment-independent direct action on tumor cells. This preclinical study demonstrated a significant improvement of survival and tumor regression in mice treated with anti-EGFR/anti-HER2 2mAbs in first- and second-line treatments, compared with gemcitabine, independently of the K-Ras status(100).

4.2.1.3 Anti-MUC1 antibodies

PAM4 is a murine antibody to MUC1 obtained from mice immunized with purified mucin from a human pancreatic cancer xenograft sample. In a preclinical study, 90Yttrium-labelled PAM4 monoclonal antibody was combined with gemcitabine in mice bearing Capan-1, the result showed increased inhibition of tumor growth and prolonged survival of the mice(101). The recent clinical trail took place in 21 patients with advanced pancreatic cancer. 111In-hPAM4 showed normal biodistribution with radiation dose estimates to red marrow and solid organs acceptable for radioimmunotherapy and with tumor targeting in 12 patients. One patient withdrew before (90)Y-hPAM4; otherwise, 20 patients received (90)Y doses of 15 (n=7), 20 (n=9), and 25 mCi/m(2) (n=4). Treatment was well tolerated; the only significant drug-related toxicities were (NCI CTC v.3) grade 3 to 4 neutropenia and thrombocytopenia increasing with (90)Y dose. There were no bleeding events or serious infections, and most cytopenias recovered to grade 1 within 12 weeks. Three patients at 25 mCi/m(2) encountered dose-limiting toxicity with grade 4 cytopenias more than 7 days, establishing 20 mCi/m(2) as the maximal tolerated (90)Y dose. Two patients developed HAHA of uncertain clinical significance. Most patients progressed rapidly and with CA19-9 levels increasing within 1 month of therapy, but 7 remained progression-free by CT for 1.5 to 5.6 months, including 3 achieving transient partial responses (32%-52% tumor diameter shrinkage). The study concluded (90)Y-Clivatuzumab tetraxetan was well tolerated with manageable hematologic toxicity at the maximal tolerated (90)Y dose, and is a potential new therapeutic for advanced pancreatic cancer(102).

In a Phase I trial for patients with stage III and IV pancreatic cancer, another antibody C595, which is targeting the protein core of MUC1, was conjugated with the α-particle-emitting

213bismuch. In vitro study showed specific cytotoxic to MUC1-expressing pancreatic cancer cells in a concentration-dependent manner compared to controls[(103)].

4.2.1.4 Anti-mesothelin antibodies

SS1P is a recombinant immunotoxin that consists of an anti-mesothelin scFv(ss1) fused to PE38, a 38Kda portion of Pseudomonas exotoxin. Sing-chain Fv(scFv)v was isolated from a phage display library obtained from the spleen of mice immunized with mesothelin-expression plasmid. After binding to mesothelin and subsequent internalisation into cells, it inhibits protein synthesis and results in apoptosis.

In preclinical study, SS1P plus radition in treating mesothelin-expressing tumor xenografts, combination treatment significantly prolonged the doubling time of tumors[(104)];meanwhile, synergic result was observed when treat with gemcitabin, the tumors were induced regression completely[(105)].

In the further phase I clinical study, SS1P was administered by intravenous infusion in 34 patients with mesothelin-expressing tumor, including 2 pancreatic cancer patients, the results showed that it was well-tolerated with self-limiting pleuritis as dose-limiting toxicity, 12% tumor size decresed from 20-50% and lasted for more than 4 weeks, 56% patients showed stable disease and 29% of the patients had progressive disease[(106)].

Another monoclonal antibody against mesothelin, MORAb-009, is a chimeric of a mouse and human mAb derived from a phage-display library and re-engineered[(107)]. In a phase I clinical trial, treatment of MORAb-009 in patients with advanced mesothelin-expressing cancers has been determined if safety, dose-limiting toxicity (DLT), and maximum tolerated dose (MTD). A total of 24 subjects were treated including 13 mesothelioma, 7 pancreatic cancer, and 4 ovarian cancer patients. The median number of MORAb-009 infusions was 4 (range 1-24 infusions). At the 400 mg/m(2) dose level, 2 subjects experienced DLT (grade 4 transaminitis and a grade 3 serum sickness). Thus, although there were other contributing causes of these adverse events, 200 mg/m(2) was considered the MTD. Other adverse events at least possibly related to MORAb-009 included 7 drug hypersensitivity events (all grade 1 or 2) and a thromboembolic event (grade 4). Eleven subjects had stable disease. There was a dose-dependent increase in serum MORAb-009 concentration. The result suggested that MORAb-009 is well tolerated and the MTD when administered weekly is conservatively set at 200 mg/m(2). Phase II studies of MORAb-009 in different mesothelin-expressing cancers are ongoing[(108)].

4.2.2 Adoptive cell transfer

In cellular antitumor immunity, T-cells must first be activated by bone marrow—derived APCs that present tumor antigens and provide essential co-stimulatory signals, migrate and gain access to the tumor microenvironment, and overcome obstacles to effective triggering posed by the tumor. Dendritic cells, which are the strongest antigen presenting cells in the body. Their generation for anti-tumor immunity has been the focus of a vast array of scientific and clinical studies. DC's specialized capacity to cross-present exogenous Ags onto major histocompatability (MHC) class I molecules for the generation of T-Ag-specific cytotoxic T lymphocytes (CTLs) has made it possible to produce actived T cell in vitro and in vivo. Adoptive immunotherapy involves harvesting the patient's peripheral blood T-lymphocytes, stimulating and expanding the autologous tumor-reactive T-cells, finally transferring them back into the patient.

4.2.2.1 K-ras-specific CTLs

In vitro, Immature DCs had pulsed with synthesized mutant K-ras peptide (YKLVVVGAV). When the DCs were matured, Kras antigen epitope can express on the DC's surface effectively and Cytotoxic T lymphocytes (CTLs) can be induced when autogeneic and homologous T cells co-cultured with the mutant K-ras peptide-pulsed DCs. The reasearch demonstrated the induced CTLs can kill the pancreatic cancer cell line Patu8988 which expresss the same K-ras mutation type effectively in virto and in vivo. Without damage the normal tissue cells, the killing rate of activated K-ras specific CTLs to the tumor cell when the ratios of CTL: Patu8988 cells were 10:1, 20:1, and 50:1 were (21.2+/-1.9)%, (32.4 +/- 2.1)%, and (45.7+/-5.3)% respectively, all while the killing efficiency significantly superior to those of the non-specific activated T lymphocyte (all $P < 0.05$). Eight days after CTL injection into the nude mice the tumor size of the intratumor injection group was (68 +/- 13) mm^3, significantly smaller than those of the control group and IL-2 activated non-specific CTL intra-tumor injection group [(87+/-14) mm^3 and (79 +/- 19) mm^3, both $P < 0.05$]. The survival rates of the nude mice of the K-ras specific CTL intra-tumor injection group, CTL caudal vein injection group, and IL-2 activated non-specific CTL intra-tumor injection group were all significantly higher than that of the control group (all $P < 0.05$), and the survival rate of the K-ras specific CTL intra-tumor injection group was significantly higher than that of the IL-2 activated non-specific CTL intra-tumor injection group ($P < 0.05$). Immunohistochemical staining confirmed that K-ras specific CTL had the ability to move toward tumor. The result showed antigen-specific-CTLs induced in virto and transferred into the patient can used be a effective treatment for pancreatic cancer(109).

4.2.2.2 MUC1-specific CTLs

In MUC1 expressing Tumor-bearing mice , there were low affinity MUC1-specific CTLs that have no effect on the spontaneously occurring pancreatic tumors in vivo. However, adoptive transfer of these CTLs was able to completely eradicate MUC1-expressing injectable tumors in MUC1 transgenic mice, and these mice developed long-term immunity. These CTLs were MHC class I restricted and recognized peptide epitopes in the immunodominant tandem repeat region of MUC1. The MET mice appropriately mimic the human condition and are an excellent model with which to elucidate the native immune responses that develop during tumor progression and to develop effective antitumor vaccine strategies(110).

In a study of 11 patients with lung metastases from different cancer, CTLs were generated in virto using cultured DCs, synthetic peptide, peripheral blood lymphocytes, IL-2 and anti-CD3 antibody. The patients received either Muc-1, CEA, gpl00, Her-2 or SART-3-PDAK cells generated in vitro, All transfers of peptide-pulsed dendritic cell-activated killer(PDAK) cells, which showed peptide/HLA-specific lysis, were well-tolerated in all patients, and adverse effects (elevation of transaminase, fever, and headache) were observed primarily at grade 1, but in no case greater than grade 2. One partial response (PR) of lung metastasis occurred in a pancreatic cancer patient who received 3x10(7) Muc-1-PDAK cells/kg. The cytolytic units of PDAK cells in this patient appeared to be substantially higher compared to those in PD patients. The results suggest that adoptive immunotherapy using PDAK cells for cancer patients with antigen-positive lung metastasis is safe and feasible[111].

However, in another clinical study, data demonstrate that MUC1 peptide-based immunization elicits mature MUC1-specific CTLs in the peripheral lymphoid organs. The mature CTLs secrete IFN-gamma and are cytolytic against MUC1-expressing tumor cells in vitro. Unfortunately, active CTLs that infiltrate the pancreas tumor microenvironment become cytolytically anergic and are tolerized to MUC1 antigen, allowing the tumor to grow. The CTL tolerance could be reversed at least in vitro with the use of anti-CD40 co-stimulation. The pancreas tumor cells secrete immunosuppressive cytokines, including IL-10 and TGF-beta that are partly responsible for the down-regulation of CTL activity. In addition, they down-regulate their MHC class I molecules to avoid immune recognition. CD4+CD25+T regulatory cells, which secrete IL-10, were also found in the tumor environment. Together these data indicate the use of several immune evasion mechanisms by tumor cells to evade CTL killing. Thus altering the tumor microenvironment to make it more conducive to CTL killing may be key in developing a successful anti-cancer immunotherapy[112].

4.2.2.3 Telomerase-specific CTLs

In a syngeneic pancreatic tumor mouse model, T-cells were produced in vitro by coculturing human lymphocytes with telomerase peptide-pulsed dendritic cells(DCs) or in vivo by injection of peptide, animals treated with telomerase-specific T cells showed significantly delayed disease progression[113].

4.2.2.4 Mesothelin-specific CTLs

With the identification of novel mesothelin CTL epitopes, T-cell lines generated from one of these epitopes were shown to lyse pancreatic tumor cells. Several agonist epitopes were defined and were shown to (a) have higher affinity and avidity for HLA-A2, (b) activate mesothelin-specific T cells from normal individuals or cancer patients to a greater degree than the native epitope in terms of induction of higher levels of IFN-gamma and the chemokine lymphotactin, and (c) lyse several mesothelin-expressing tumor types in a MHC-restricted manner more effectively than T cells generated using the native peptide. External beam radiation of tumor cells at nontoxic levels was shown to enhance the expression of mesothelin and other accessory molecules, resulting in a modest but statistically significant increase in tumor cell lysis by mesothelin-specific T cells. The result supports and extends observations that mesothelin is a potential target for immunotherapy of pancreatic cancers, as well as mesotheliomas. Combination of immunotherapy and chemoradiotherapy may be a better choice for the patients[114].

4.3 Future perspective

Although it is used as adjuvant treatment in preclinical or clinical trail, immunotherapy may be the next great hope for pancreatic cancer treatment. While monoclonal antibodies, cytokines, vaccines and CTL have individually shown some promise, it's hard to say which is better in nonspecific and specific immunotherapy. It seems to be the best strategy to obtained more efficient results in combination with a variety of antigens, or vaccine and antibody combinations. A nonspecific and specific immunotherapy combination offers another potent strategy. With the combination, the ultimate achievable goal may be a durable anti-tumor immune response that can destory and prevent it from recurrence over the course of a patient's life.

According to the existed profiles, The key of the immunotherapy on pancreatic cancer is to break through cancer microenvironment's defence. Suppressing the function of immuno-suppression cells, such as immunosuppressive tumor-associated macrophages (TAMs), myeloid-derived suppressor cells (MDSCs), and regulatory T cells (Tregs) reside in tumors is as important as inducing the specific immune agent, such as antibody or CTL.

Combating with each other, tumor and immune system are like two warriors on the other side of balance. What we can do is to break the balance and help the immune system win the war. Traditional methods, surgical operation, chemoradiation, can decrease the number of the tumor cells to the minimum while do harmful to immune system in the same time. So as the followed treatment, the passive immunotherapy may be the best choice to supply enough actived immune agents in a short period to kill the metastatic cancer cells. When patient recovered, Cytokines and vaccine will help to establish long - term specific immune response to keep watch on and get rid of residuary cancer cells. Owing to pancreatic cancer cells expressing different abnormal antigens, the combination of 2 or more epitopes vaccines will obstain better effect to prevent from recurrence. and metastasis.

5. References

[1] American Cancer Society Facts & Figures 2010. Atlanta, American Chemical Society ; 2010
[2] Li D, Xie K, Wolff R, et al. Pancreatic Cancer. Lancet 2004;363(9414):1049-57
[3] Crist DW , Sitzmann JV, Cameron JL. Improved hospital morbidity, mortality, and survival after the Whipple procedure. Ann Surg. 1987;206(3):358-365.
[4] Yeo CJ, Abrams RA, Grochow LB, et al. Pancreaticoduodenectomy for pancreatic adenocarcinoma:postoperative adjuvant chemoradiation improves survival. A prospective, single-institution experience. Ann surg 1997;225(5):621-633
[5] Burris HA 3rd , Moore MJ, Andersen J, et al. Improvements in survival and clinical benefit with gemcitabine as first-line therapy for patients with advanced pancrease cancer:a randomized trial. J Clin Oncol. 1997;15(6):2403-2413.
[6] Almoguera C, Shibata D, Forrester K, et al. Most human carcinomas of the exocrine pancreas contain mutant c-K-ras genes. Cell 1988;53(4):549-554.
[7] Hruban RH, Goggins M, Parsons J, et al. Progression model for pancreatic cancer. Clin Cancer Res 2000;6(8):2969-72.
[8] Digiuseppe JA, Hruban RH, Offerhaus GJ, et al. Detection of K-ras mutations in mucinous pancreatic duct hyperplasia from a patient with a family history of pancreatic carcinoma. Am J pathol. 1994;144(5):889-895.

[9] Peyssonnaux C, Provot S, Felder-Schmittbuhl MP, et al. Induction of postmitotic neuroretina cell proliferation by distinct Ras downstream signaling pathways. Mol Cell Biol 2000;20(19):7068-7079.
[10] Malumbres M, Barbacid M. RAS oncogenes:the first 30 years. Nat Rev Cancer 2003;3(6):459-465.
[11] Hruban RH, van Mansfeld AD, Offerhaus GJ, et al. K-ras oncogene activation in adenocarcinoma of the human pancreas. A study of 82 carcinomas using a combination of mutant-enriched polymerase chain reaction analysis and allele-specific oligonucleotide hybridization. Am J Pathol. 1993;143(2):545-54.
[12] Hollingsworth MA, Swanson BJ. Mucins in cancer :protection and control of the cell surface. Nat Rev Cancer. 2004;4(1):45-60.
[13] Levi E, Klimstra DS, Andea A, et al. MUC1 and MUC2 in pancreatic neoplasia. J Clin Pathol 2004;57(5):456-462.
[14] Swanson BJ, McDermott KM, Singh PK, et al. MUC1 is a counter-receptor for myelin-associated glycoprotein(Siglec-4a) and their interaction contributes to adhesion in pancreatic cancer perineural invasion. Cancer Res 2007;67(21):10222-10229.
[15] Aqata N, Ahamad R, Kawano T, et al. MUC1 oncoprotein blocks death receptor-mediated apoptosis by inhibiting recruitment of caspase-8. Cancer Res 2008; 68(15):6136-6144.
[16] Burdick MD, Harris A, Reid CJ, et al. Oligosaccharides expressed on MUC1 produced by pancreatic and colon tumor cell line. J Biol Chem. 1997;272(39):24198-24202.
[17] Julian J, Carson DD. Formation of MUC1 metabolic complex is conserved in tumor-derived and normal epithelial cells. Biochem Biophys Res Commun. 2002;293(4):1183-1190.
[18] Hassan R, Bera T, Pastan I. mesothelin:a new target for immunotherapy. Clin Cancer Res 2004;10(12 Pt 1):3937-3942.
[19] Rump A, Morikawa Y, Tanaka M, et al. Binding of ovarian cancer antigen CA125/MUC16 to mesothelin mediates cell adhesion. J Biol Chem 2004;279(10):9190-9198.
[20] Hassan R, Laszik ZG, Lerner M, et al. Mesothelin is overexpressed in pancreaticobiliary adenocarcinoma but not in normal pancreas and chronic pancreatitis. Am J Clin Pathol 2005;124(6):838-845.
[21] Marincola FM, Jaffee EM, Hicklin DJ et al. Escape of human solid tumors from T-cell recognition:molecular mechanisms and functional significance. Adv Immunol. 2000;74:181-273.
[22] Menon AG, Fleuren GJ, Alphenaar EA, et al. A basal membrane-like structure surrending tumor nodules may prevent intraepithelial leucocyte infiltration in colorectal cancer. Cancer Immunol Immunother. 2003;52(2):121-6.
[23] Zang X, Allison JP. The B7 family and cancer therapy:costimulation and coinhibition. Clin Cancer Res. 2007;13(18 Pt 1):5271-9.
[24] Groh V, Wu J, Yee C, et al. Tumor-derived soluble MIC ligands impair expression of NKG2D and T-cell activation. Nature, 2002;419(6908):734-8.

[25] Gabrilovich DI, Chen HL, Girgis KR, et al. Production of vascular endothelial growth factor by human tumors inhibits the functional maturation of dendritic cells. Nat Med. 1996;2(10):1096-103

[26] Wang T, Niu G, Kortylewski M, et al. Regulation of the innate and adaptive immune responses by Stat-3 signaling in tumor cells. Nat Med. 2004;10(1):48-54.

[27] Woo EY, Yeh H, Chu CS, et al. Cutting edge:Regulatory T cells from lung cancer patients directly inhibit autologous T cell proliferation. J Immunol. 2002; 168(9):4272-6.

[28] Ungefroren H, Voss M, Jansen M, et al. Human pancreatic adenocarcinomas express Fas and Fas ligand yet are resistant to Fas-mediated apoptosis. Cancer Res 1998, 58(8):1741-1749.

[29] Bennett MW, O'Connell J, O'Sullivan GC, et al. The Fas countattack in vivo:apoptotic depletion of tumor-infiltrating lymphocytes associated with Fas ligand expression by human esophageal carcinomas. J Immunol 1998, 160(11):5669-5675.

[30] Ibrahim R, Frederickson H, Parr A, et al. Expression of FasL in squamous cell carcinomas of the cervix and cervical intraepithelial neoplasia and its role in tumor escape mechanism. Cancer 2006, 106(5):1065-1077.

[31] Ohta T, Elnemr A, Kitagawa H, et al. Fas ligand expression in human pancreatic cancer. Oncol Rep 2004;12(4):749-754.

[32] Dunn GP, Old LJ, Schreiber RD. The three Es of cancer immunoediting. Annu Rev Immunol. 2004;22:329-60.

[33] Shimizu J, Yamazaki S, Sakaguchi S. Induction of tumor immunity by removing CD25+CD4+ T cells:a common basis between tumor immunity and autoimmunity. J Immunol. 1999;163(10):5211-8.

[34] Savage ND, de Boer T, Walburg KV, et al. Human anti-inflammatory macrophage induced Foxp3-GITR CD25+ regulatory T cells, which suppress via membrane-bound TGFbeta-1. J Immunol. 2008;181(3):2220-6.

[35] Valzasina B, Piconese S, Guiducci C, et al. Tumor-induced expansion of regulatory T cells by conversion of CD4+CD25+-lymphocytes is thymus and proliferation independent. Cancer Res. 2006;66(8):4488-95.

[36] Moo-Young TA, Larson JW, Belt BA, et al. Tumor-derived TGF-beta mediates conversion of CD4+Foxp3+ regulatory T cells in a murine model of pancreas cancer. J Immunother. 2009;32(1):12-21.

[37] Liyanage UK, Moore TT, Joo HG, et al. Prevalence of regulatory T cells is increased in peripheral blood and tumor microenvironment of patients with pancreas or breast adenocarcinoma. J Immunol. 2002;169(5):2756-2761

[38] Hiraoka N, Onozato K, Kosuge T, et al. Prevalence of FOXP3+ regulatory T cells increases during the progression of pancreatic ductal adenocarcinoma and its premalignant lesions. Clin cancer Res. 2006;12(18):5423-5434.

[39] Yamamoto M, Kamigaki T, Yamashita K, et al. Enhancement of anti-tumor immunity by high levels of Th1 and Th17 with a combination of dendritic cell fusion hybrids and regulatory T cell depletion in pancreatic canxer. Oncol Rep. 2009;22(2):337-43.

[40] Tan MC, Goedegebuure PS, Belt BA, et al. Disruption of CCR5-dependent homing of regulatory T cells inhibits tumor growth in a murine model of pancreatic cancer. J Immunol 2009;182(3):1746-55.
[41] Leao IC, Ganesan P, Armstrong TD, et al. Effective depletion of regulatory T cells allows the recruitment of mesothelin-specific CD8+ T cells to the antitumor immune response against a mesothelin-expressing mouse pancreatic adenocarcinoma. Clin Transl Sci. 2008, 24;1(3):228-239.
[42] Gabrilovich DI, Nagaraj S. Myeloid-derived suppressor cells as regulators of the immune system. Nat Rev Immunol. 2009;9(3):162-74.
[43] Delano MJ, Scumpia PO, Weinstein JS, et al. MyD88-dependent expansion of an immature GR-1+CD11b+ population induces T cell suppression and Th2 polarization in sepsis. J Exp Med. 2007;204(6):1463-74.
[44] Goedegubuure P, Mitchem JB, Porembka MR, et al. Myeloid-derived suppressor cells:general characteristics and relevance to clinical management of pancreatic cancer. Curr Cancer Drug Targets. 2011 May 23. (Epub ahead of print.)
[45] Gabitass RF, Annels NE, Stocken DD, et al. Elevated myeloid-derived suppressor cells in pancreatic, esophageal and gastric cancer are an independent prognostic factor and are associated with significant elevation of the Th2 cytokine interleukin-13. Cancer Immunol Immnuother. 2011 Jun 5. (Epub ahead of print)
[46] Zhao F, Obermann S, von Wasielewski R, et al. Increase in frequency of myeloid-derived suppressor cells in mice with spontaneous pancreatic carcinoma. Immunology 2009;128(1):141-9.
[47] Nagaraj S, Youn JI, Weber H, et al. Anti-inflammatory triterpenoid blocks immune suppressive function of MDSCs and improves immune response in cancer. Clin Cancer Res. 2010;16(6):1812-23.
[48] Diefenbach A, Jensen ER, Jamieson AM, et al. Rael and H60 ligands of the NKG2D receptor stimulate tumor immunity. Nature. 2001;413(6852):165-171). (49Sun JC, Lanier LL. Nature killer cells remenber:an evolutionary bridge between innate and adaptive immunity?Eur J Immunol. 2009;39(8):2059-2064.
[49] Funa K, Nilsson B, Jacobsson G, et al. Decreased natural killer cell activity and interferon production by leucocytes in patients with adenocarcinoma of the pancreas. Br J Cancer. 1984;50(2):231-233.
[50] Frankel TL, Burns W, Riley J, et al. Identification and characterization of a tumor infiltrating CD56(+)/CD16(-) NK cell subset with specificity for pancreatic and prostate cancer cell lines. Cancer Immunol Immunother. 2010;59(12):1757-69.
[51] Imai K, Matsuyama S, Miyake S, et al. Nature cytotoxic activity of peripheral-blood lymphocytes and cancer incidence:an 11-year follow-up study of a general population. Lancet, 2000;356(9244):1795-1799.
[52] Albertsson PA, Basse PH, Hokland M, et al. Nk cells and the tumour microenvironment:implications for NK-cell function and anti-tumour activity. Trends in Immunology. 2003;24(11):603-609.
[53] Hokland M, Kjaergaard J, Kuppen PJ, et al. Endogenous and adoptively transferred A-NK and T-LAK cells continuously accumulate within murine metastases up to 48h after inoculation. In Vivo. 1999;13(3):199-204.

[54] Bhat R, Dempe S, Dinsart C, et al. Enhancement of NK cell antitumor responses using an oncolytic parvovirus. Int J Cancer. 2011;128(4):908-919
[55] Trapani JA, Voskoboinik I. Infective, neoplastic, and homeostatic sequelae of the loss of perforin function in humans. Adv Exp Med Biol. 2007;601:235-242.
[56] Garnock-Jones KP, Keating GM, Scott LJ. Trastuzumab:a review of its use as adjuvant treatment in human epidermal growth factor receptor 2 (HER2)-positive early breast cancer. Drugs, 2010;70(2):215-239
[57] Winter MC, Hancock BW. Ten years of rituximab in NHL. 2009. Expert Opin Drug saf;8(2):223-235.
[58] Lanier LL:Nature killer cells:from no receptors to too many. Immunity 1997;6(4):371-378
[59] Ryschich E, Notzel T, Hinz U, et al. Control of T-cell-mediated immune response by HLA class I in human pancreatic carcinoma. Clin Cancer Res 2005;11(2 Pt 1):498-504.
[60] Dranoff G, Jaffee E, Lazenby A, et al. Vaccination with irradiated tumor cells engineered to secrete murine granulocyte-marcrophage colony-stimulating factor stimulates potent, specific, and long-lasting anti-tumor immunity. Proc Natl Acad Sci U S A;1993:90(8), 3539-3543.
[61] Laheru D, Lutz E, Burke J, et al. Allogeneic granulocyte macrophage colony-stimulating factor-secreting tumor immunotherapy alone or in sequence with cyclophosphamide for metastatic pancreatic cancer:A pilot study of safety, feasibility and immune activation. Clin Cancer Res 2008;14(5):1455-1463
[62] Rosenberg SA, Lotze MT, Muul LM, et al. A progress report on the treatment of 157 patients with advanced cancer using lymphokine-activated killer cells and interleukin-2 or high-dose interleukin-2 alone. N Engl J Med, 1987;316(15):889-897.
[63] Uggeri F, Caprotti R, De Grate L, et al. Short-term preoperative IL-2 immunotherapy in operable pancreatic cancer:a randomized study. Hepatogastroenterology. 2009;56(91-92):861-865
[64] Degrate L, Nobili C, Franciosi C, et al. Interleukin-2 immunotherapy action on innate immunity cells in peripheral blood and tumoral tissue of pancreatic adenocarcinoma patients. Langenbecks Arch Surg 2009;394(1):115-121.
[65] Del Vecchio M, Bajetta E, Canova S, et al. Interleukin-12:biological properties and clinical application. Clin Cancer Res. 2007;13(16):4677-4685.
[66] Kobayashi M, Fitz L, Ryan M, et al. Identification and purification of natural killer cell stimulatory factor(NKSF), a cytokine with multiple biologic effects on human lymphocytes. J Exp Med. 1989;170(3):827-845
[67] Trinchieri G. Interleukin-12:a proinflammatory cytokine with immunoregulatory functions that bridge innate resistance and antigen-specific adaptive immunity. Annu Rev Immunol. 1995;13:251-276.
[68] Tassi E, Braga M, Longhi R, et al. Non-redundant role for IL-12 and IL-27 in modulating Th2 polarization of carcinoembryonic antigen specific CD4 T cells from pancreatic cancer patients. PLoS One. 2009;4(10):e7234.
[69] Zaharoff DA, Hance KW, Rogers CJ, et al. Intratumoral immunotherapy of established solid tumors with chitosan/IL-12. J Immunother. 2010;33(7):697-705.

[70] Kimura M, Tagawa M, Yoshida Y, et al. Impaired in vivo tumor growth of human pancreatic carcinoma cells retrovirally transduced with GM-CSF gene. Anticancer Res. 1998;18(1A):165-170.
[71] Jaffee EM, Hruban RH, Biedrzycki B, et al. Noval allogeneic granulocyte-macrophage colony-stimulating factor-secreting tumor vaccine for pancreatic cancer:a phase I trail of safety and immune activation. J Clin Oncol 2001;19:145-156.
[72] Laheru D, Yeo C, Biedrzycki B, et al. A safety and efficacy trial of lethally irradiated allogeneic pancreatic tumor cells transfected with the GM-CSF gene in combination with adjuvant chemoradiotherapy for the treatment of adenocarcinoma of the pancreas. J Clin Oncol(meeting abstracts) 2007;25:3010.
[73] Lutz E, Yeo CJ, Lillemoe KD, et al. A lethally irradiated allogeneic granulocyte-macrophage colony stimulating factor-secreting tumor vaccine for pancreatic adenocarcinoma:A phase II trial of safety, efficacy, and immune activation. Ann Surg. 2011;253(2):328-335.
[74] Miyazawa M, Ohsawa R, Tsunoda T, et al. Phase I clinical trial using peptide vaccine for human vascular endothelial growth receptor 2 in combination with gemcitabine for patients with advanced pancreatic cancer. Cancer Sci. 2010;101(2):433-9.
[75] Gjertsen MK, Bakka A, Breivik J, et al. Ex vivo ras peptide vaccination in patients with advanced pancreatic cancer:results of a phase I / II study. Int J cancer 1996;65(4):450-453.
[76] Gjertsen MK, Buanes T, Rosseland AR, et al. Intradermal ras peptide vaccination with granulocyte-macrophage colony-stimulating factor as adjuvant:clinical and immunological responses in patients with pancreatic adenocarcinoma. Int J Cancer 2001;92(3):441-450.
[77] Abou-Alfa GK, Chapman PB, Feilchenfeldt J, et al. Targeting mutated K-ras in pancreatic adenocarcinoma using an adjuvant vaccine. Am J Clin Oncol. 2011;34(3):321-5.
[78] Toubaji A, Achtar M, Provenzano M, et al. Pilot study of mutant ras peptide-based vaccine as an adjuvant treatment in pancreatic and colorectal cancers. Cancer Immunol Immunother. 2008;57(9):1413-1420.
[79] Weden S, Klemp M, Gladhaug IP, et al. Long-term follow-up of patients with resected pancreatic cancer following vaccination against mutant K-ras. Int J Cancer. 2011;128(5):1120-1128.
[80] Ramanathan RK, Lee KM, Mckolanis J, et al. Phase I study of a MUC1 vaccine composed of different doses of MUC1 peptide with SB-AS2 adjuvant in resected and locally advanced pancreatic cancer. Cancer Immunol Immunother 2005;54(3):254-264.
[81] Lepisto AJ, Moser AJ, Zeh H, et al. A phase I / II study of a MUC1 peptide pulsed autologous dendritic cell vaccine as adjuvant therapy in patients with resected pancreatic and biliary tumors. Cancer Ther. 2008;6(B):955-964.
[82] Pecher G, Haring A, Kaiser L, et al. Mucin gene (MUC1) transfected dendritic cells as vaccine:results of a phase I / II trial. Cancer Immunol Immnuother 2002;51(11-12):669-673.

[83] Nordqvist C, editor. Therion reports results of phase 3 PANVAC-VF trial and announces plans for company sale. Medical News Today. 2006.
[84] Kondo H, Hazama S, Kawaoka T, et al. Adoptive immunotherapy for pancreatic cancer using MUC1 peptide-pulsed dendritic cells and activated T lymphocytes. Anticancer Res. 2008;28(1B):379-87.
[85] Thomas AM, Santarsiero LM, Lutz ER, et al. Mesothelin-specific CD8+ T cell responses provide evidence of in vivo cross-priming by antigen-presenting cells in vaccinated pancreatic cancer patients. J Exp Med 2004;200(3):297-306.
[86] Gaffney MC, Goedegebuure P, Kashiwagi H, et al. DNA vaccination targeting mesothelin combined with anti-GITR antibody induces rejection of pancreatic adenocarcinoma. AACR Meeting Abstracts 2006;2006:329-a.
[87] Hung CF, Calizo R, Tsai YC, et al. A DNA vaccine encoding a single-chain trimer of HLA-A2 linked to human mesothelin peptide generates anti-tumor effects against human mesothelin-expressing tumors. Vaccine. 2007;25(1):127-135.
[88] Adams GP, Weiner LM. Monoclonal antibody therapy of cancer. Nat Biotechnol 2005;23(9):1147-1157.
[89] Huang ZQ, Buchsbaum DJ, Raisch KP, et al. Differential responses by pancreatic carcinoma cell lines to prolonged exposure to erbitux (IMC-C225) anti-EGFR antibody. J Surg Res 2003;111(2):274-283.
[90] Morgan MA, Parsels LA, Kollar LE, et al. The combination of epidermal growth factor receptor inhibitors with gemcitabine and radiation in pancreatic cancer. Clin Cancer Res 2008;14(16):5142-5149.
[91] Xiong HQ, Rosenberg A, Lobuglio A, et al. Cetuximab, a monoclonal antibody targeting the epidermal growth factor receptor, in combination with gemcitabine for advanced pancreatic cancer: a multicenter phase II Trial. J Clin Oncol. 2004;22(13):2610-2616
[92] Kullmann F, Hollerbach S, Dollinger MM, et al. Cetuximab plus gemcitabine/oxaliplatin (GEMOXCET) in first-line metastatic cancer:a multicentre phase II study. Br J Cancer. 2009;100(7):1032-1036.
[93] Cascinu S, Berardi R, Labianca R, et al. Cetuximab plus gemcitabine and cisplatin compared with gemcitabine and cisplatin alone in patients with advanced pancreatic cancer:a randomised, multicentre, phase II trail. Lancet Oncol 2008;9(1):39-44.
[94] Philip P, Benedetti J, Corless CL, et al. Phase III study comparing gemcitabine plus cetuximab versus gemcitabine in patients with advanced pancreatic adenocarcinoma:Southwest Oncology Group-directed intergroup trial S0205. J Clin Oncol 2010;28(22):3605-3610.
[95] Bangard C, Gossmann A, Papyan A, et al. Magnetic resonance imaging in an orthotopic rat model:blockade of epidermal growth factor receptor with EMD72000 inhibits human panvreatic carcinoma growth. Int J Cancer 2005;114(1):131-138.
[96] Graeven U, Kremer B, Sudhoff T, et al. Phase I study of the humanised anti-EGFR monoclonal antibody matuzumab (EMD72000) combined with gemcitabine in advanced pancreatic cancer. Br J Cancer 2006;94(9):1293-1299.

[97] Saeki H, Yanoma S, Takemiya S, et al. Antitumor activity of a combination of trastuzumab (Herceptin) and oral fluoropyrimidine S-1 on human epidermal growth factor receptor2-overexpressing pancreatic cancer. Oncol Rep 2007;18(2):433-439.

[98] Kimura K, Sawada T, Komatsu M, et al. Antitumor effect of trastuzumab for pancreatic cancer with high HER2 expression and enhancement of effect by combined therapy with gemcitabine. Clin Cancer Res 2006;12(16):4925-4932.

[99] Larbouret C, Robert B, Navarro-Teulon I, et al. In vivo therapeutic synergism of anti-epidermal growth factor receptor and anti-HER2 monoclonal antibodies against pancreatic carcinomas. Clin Cancer Res 2007;13(11):3356-3362.

[100] Larbouret C, Robert B, Bascoul-Mollevi C, et al. Combined cetuximab and trastuzumab are superior to gemcitabine in the treatment of human pancreatic carcinoma xenografts. Ann Oncol. 2010;21(1):98-103.

[101] Gold DV, Modrak DE, Schutsky K, et al. Combined 90Yttrium-DOTA-Labeled PAM$ antibody radioimmunotherapy and gemcitabine radiosensitization for the treatment of a human pancreatic cancer xenograft. Int J Cancer 2004;109(4):618-626.

[102] Gulec SA, Cohen SJ, Pennington KL, et al. Treatment of advanced pancreatic carcinoma with 90Y-clivatuzumab tetraxetan:A phase I single-dose escalation trial. Clin Cancer Res. 2011;17(12): 4091-4100

[103] Qu CF, Li Y, Song YJ, et al. MUC1 expression in primary and metastatic pancreatic cancer cells for in virto treatment by (213)Bi-C595 radioimmunoconjugate. Br J Cancer 2004;91(12):2086-2093.

[104] Hassan R, Williams-Gould J, Steinberg SM, et al. Tumor-directed radiation and the immunotoxin SS1P in the treatment of mesothelin-expressing tumor xenografts. Clin Cancer Res 2006;12(16):4983-4988.

[105] Hassan R, Broaddus VC, Wilson S, et al. Anti-mesothelin immunotoxin SS1P in combination with gemcitabine results in increased activity against mesothelin-expressing tumor xenografts. Clin Cancer Res 2007;13(23):7166-7171

[106] Hassan R, Bullock S, Premkumar A, et al. Phase I study of SS1P, a recombinant anti-mesothelin immunotoxin given as a bolus I. V. infusion to patients with mesothelin-expressing mesothelinoma, ovarian, and pancreatic cancer. Clin Cancer Res 2007;13(17):5144-5149.

[107] Hassan R, Ebel W, Routhier EL, et al. Preclinical evaluation of MORAb-009, a chimeric antibody targeting tumor-associated mesothelin. Cancer Immun 2007;7:20

[108] Hassan R, Cohen SJ, Phillips M, et al. Phase I clinical trial of the chimeric anti-mesothelin monoclonal antibody MORAb-009 in patients with mesothelin-expressing cancer. Clin Cancer Res. 2010;16(24):6132-6138.

[109] Yang B, He Y, Sun DL, et al. Specific immune against pancreatic cancer induced by dendritic cells pulsed with mutant K-ras peptide. Zhonghua yi xue za zhi. 2008;88(28):1956-60.

[110] Mukherjee P, Ginardi AR, Madsen CS, et al. Mice with spontaneous pancreatic cancer naturally develop MUC-1-specific CTLs that eradicate tumors when adoptively transferred. J Immunol 2000;165(6):3451-3460.

[111] Yamaguchi Y, Ohta K, Kawabuchi Y, et al. Feasibility study of adoptive immunotherapy for metastatic lung tumors using peptide-pulsed dendritic cells-activated killer(PDAK) cells. Anticancer Res 2005;25(3c):2407-2415.
[112] Mukherjee P, Ginardi AR, Madsen CS, et al. MUC1-specific CTLs are non-functional with a pancreatic tumor microenvironment. Glycoconj J. 2001;18(11-12):931-42.
[113] Schmidt J, Ryschich E, Sievers E, et al. Telomerase-specific T-cells kill pancreatic tumor cells in virto and in vivo. Cancer 2006;106(4):759-764.
[114] Yokokawa J, Palena C, Arlen P, et al. Identification of novel human CTL epitopes and their agonist epitopes of mesothelin. Clin Cancer Res. 2005;11(17):6342-51.

8

An Overview on Immunotherapy of Pancreatic Cancer

Fabrizio Romano, Luca Degrate, Mattia Garancini, Fabio Uggeri, Gianmaria Mauri and Franco Uggeri
Department of Surgery, San Gerardo Hospital, University Of Milan Bicocca, Monza, Italy

1. Introduction

Pancreatic cancer is the fourth leading cause of cancer mortality in both men and women. Approximately 32,000 Americans each year will develop and also die from this disease . Despite aggressive surgical and medical management, the mean life expectancy is approximately 15–18 months for patients with local and regional disease, and 3–6 months for patients with metastatic disease 1-2. Even in case of radical surgery it is associated with a poor prognosis and a 5-year survival rate of less than 4%. Early detection methods are under development but do not yet exist in practice for pancreatic cancer. Therefore, most patients present with advanced disease that cannot be cured by surgery (pancreaticoduodenectomy). Clinically, pancreatic cancer is characterized by rapid tumor progression, early metastatization and unresponsiveness to most conventional treatment modalities. In a recent analysis using a database from 1973 to 2003 based on modeled period analysis, 5-year survival of pancreatic cancer patients was 7.1% and 10-year survival was below 5%3. The survival rate is apparently related to the disease stage with a low rate at 1.6–3.3% among patients with distant metastases. Curative resection remains the most important factor determining outcome for resectable tumors. However, the resection rate for pancreatic carcinoma is only 10% and the overall five-year survival rate after resection is still only 10 to 20%. Early diagnosis and effective treatment to control the advanced stages of disease may prolong the survival rate of pancreatic cancer. Otherwise pancreatic cancer remains a disease with high mortality despite numerous efforts that have been made to improve its survival rates.

In developing cancer immunotherapy, the following aims must be considered: (1) detection of immune response to autologous tumor cells, (2) identification of tumor antigens and analysis of the immune responses in patients, (3) analysis of tumor escape mechanisms and development of methods to overcome them, and (4) development of a more efficient immune intervention system by way of animal model experiments and clinical trials. Identification of tumor antigens in the first objective is important because it subsequently allows their use not only as targets for immunotherapy in a more immunogenic form but also enables quantitative and qualitative monitoring of immune responses to tumor cells during immunotherapy. In many animal tumors and in human melanoma, T cells play an important role in in vivo tumor rejection. Because of their expression of MHC class I, CD8+ T cells are integral in the eradication of most solid tumors. However, CD4+ T cells are also important in the induction and maintenance of final effectors, such as CD8+ T cells and macrophages, as well as for the accumulation of CD8+ T cells in tumor tissues. Thus, we are applying various methods to identify human tumor antigens recognized by T cells.

Immunotherapy has an advantage over radiation therapy and chemotherapy because it can act specifically against the tumor without damaging normal tissue. Immunotherapeutic approaches to PC have included the use of monoclonal antibodies 47, cytokines 8, vaccine 9 and lymphokine activated killer (LAK) cells (10).

2. Immune surveillance and tumour evasion

The extraordinary features of the immune system make it possible to discern self from non-self. However, most human cancers, and pancreatic cancer in particular, are known to be poorly immunogenic, as crucial somatic genetic mutations can generate pancreatic cancer proteins that are essentially altered self proteins. Furthermore, promising immunotherapeutic approaches that have been used for relatively immunogenic cancers such as melanoma have met with variable success[6]. These observations have revealed that for tumours to form and progress, they must develop local and/or systemic mechanisms that subsequently allow them to escape the normal surveillance mechanisms of the intact immune system. Immune-based therapies must therefore incorporate at least one agent against a pancreatic cancer target as well as one or more agents that will modify both local and systemic mechanisms of pancreatic-cancer-induced IMMUNE TOLERANCE.

It is now clear that both local characteristics of the tumour microenvironment as well as systemic factors are important for the immune evasion of tumours. For example, T-cell recognition of pancreatic tumours might be inhibited or suppressed due to the downregulation of human leukocyte antigen (HLA) CLASS I tumour-antigen complexes on tumour cells by a range of intracellular mechanisms[4, 7] — upregulation of immune-inhibition molecules[11, 12, 13, 14, 15, 16, 17], loss of immune-regulation signals[15, 16, 17, 18, 19, 20, 21, 22, 23, 24, 25, 26, 27, 28, 29, 30], defects in immune-cell tumour localization[31, 32, 33, 34, 35, 36, 37, 38, 39, 40, 41, 42, 43, 44, 45, 46, 47, 48, 49, 50, 51] and loss of co-stimulatory molecules[52, 53, 54, 55, 56, 57]. Such alterations within a tumour cell would not be unexpected, as they have unstable genomes. The local inflammatory reaction is also an important triggering event in the recruitment of professional ANTIGEN-PRESENTING CELLS (APCs) and effector cells, such as T cells and NATURAL KILLER (NK) CELLS, to the tumour site. However, pancreatic tumour cells express a range of proteins that inhibit pro-inflammatory cytokines and DENDRITIC CELL (DC) MATURATION[58, 59, 60].

In addition, the numbers of $CD4^{+}CD25^{+}$ T regulatory (T_{Reg}) CELLS — a subset of T cells that are known to be important in the suppression of self-reactive T cells (peripheral tolerance) — accumulate in pancreatic tumours[61, 62, 63]. Although these cells are thought to be activated during the immunization process, T_{Reg} cells seem to localize to tumour sites. Tumour production of the chemokine CCL22 probably attracts the T_{Reg} cells by interacting with the CCR4 receptor that is expressed by these cells[64].

Other important elements in regulating the T-cell recognition of pancreatic tumours are the inhibitory pathways, known as 'immunological checkpoints'. Immunological checkpoints serve two purposes. One is to help generate and maintain self-tolerance, by eliminating T cells that are specific for self-antigens. The other is to restrain the amplitude of normal T-cell responses so that they do not 'overshoot' in their natural response to foreign pathogens. The prototypical immunological checkpoint is mediated by the cytotoxic-T-lymphocyte-associated protein 4 (CTLA4) counter-regulatory receptor that is expressed by T cells when they become activated[15, 23]. CTLA4 binds two B7-FAMILY members on the surface APCs – B7.1 (also known as CD80) and B7.2 (also known as CD86) – with roughly 20-fold higher affinity than the T-cell surface protein CD28 binds these molecules. CD28 is a co-stimulatory receptor that is constitutively expressed on naive T cells. Because of its higher affinity, CTLA4 out-competes CD28 for B7.1/B7.2 binding, resulting in the downmodulation of T-cell responses[20].

A range of B7-family members interact with co-stimulatory and counter-regulatory inhibitory receptors on T cells. Two recently discovered B7-family members, B7-H1 (also known as PD-L1) and B7-DC (also known as PD-L2) also seem to interact with T-cell co-stimulatory and counter-regulatory inhibitory receptors[18, 29, 30]. PD-L1, which is upregulated on T cells when they become activated, seems to control a counter-regulatory immunological checkpoint when it binds PD-1 26,28,29. Activating receptors for B7-DC and B7-H1 have not yet been definitively identified. B7-DC is expressed on DCs, and is likely to have a co-stimulatory role in increasing activation of naive or resting T cells. In contrast to B7.1, B7.2 and B7-DC, B7-H1 is also expressed on several peripheral tissues and on many tumours, including pancreatic tumours[30].

Another new B7-family member, B7-H4, seems to mediate a predominantly inhibitory function in the immune system[14]. Recent data indicate that pancreatic tumours also express B7-H4 (D.L. and E.M.J., manuscript in preparation), and both B7-H1 and B7-H4 probably protect tumours from immune-system attack. Preclinical studies have already demonstrated that it is possible to downregulate B7-H1 signalling in mice, improving the antitumour response to vaccination[18]. Monoclonal antibodies that downregulate B7-H1 and B7-H4 are currently in clinical development. These antibodies will probably begin clinical testing in patients with pancreatic cancer within 2 to 3 years.

3. Cancer immunotherapy protocols

Clinical trials using various immunotherapies, active immunization with tumor antigens, or tumor cell–derived products, and adoptive immunotherapy using antitumor immune cells were conducted in various cancers, most extensively in melanoma, and tumor regression was observed in some patients. Active Immunization Immunizations with synthetic peptides, particularly MHC class I–binding epitopes, were performed in various trials. Since native epitopes have relatively low immunogenicity, various immunoaugmenting methods, including coadministration of adjuvants and cytokines [incomplete Freund adjuvant (IFA), IL-2, IL-12, or GM-CSF], were applied to achieve efficient immunization. Tumor regression in melanoma patients was observed in various clinical trials using melanocytespecific antigens such as MART-1 and gp100 and, in particular, the HLA high-binding modified peptide. Since CD4+ T cells appear to be directly and indirectly important in tumor rejection, combined immunization with both Th and CTL antigens is being attempted. Immunization with proteins containing multiple Th and CTL epitopes may be effective, although production of recombinant GMP-grade proteins is costly, and modifications such as particle formation may be required for effective presentation of MHC class I–restricted epitopes. To facilitate peptide immunization in melanoma, coadministration of the anti-CTLA4 antibody, which blocks regulatory T cells and negative feedback regulation of T-cell activation, was carried out. Although tumor regression along with autoimmune reactions was observed, augmentation of the immune response to the administered peptides was not observed in peripheral blood.[24] In pancreatic cancer, intradermal immunization with the mutated K-*ras* peptides and GM-CSF resulted in the induction of a memory CD4+ T-cell response and prolonged survival, compared with nonresponders.[15] Immunization with the MUC1 peptide and BCG resulted in augmented immune responses without tumor regression.[22] Immunization with recombinant viruses or plasmids containing tumor antigen cDNA (DNA immunization) rather than peptide/proteins may be applied. In melanoma clinical trials, a generation of neutralizing antibodies against viral proteins appeared to interfere with the induction of immune response to tumor antigens following immunization with recombinant adenovirus and vaccinia virus.[25] However, recent protocols using a recombinant fowlpox virus containing the modified gp100 cDNA or the ER signal sequence–conjugated gp100-epitope minimal gene demonstrated frequent induction of tumor reactive T cells.[26] Interestingly, tumor regression was observed in patients after subsequent administration of IL-2.

Intramuscular immunization with the recombinant gp100 plasmids appeared to be insufficient to induce an antitumor T-cell response.27 DC are the most potent professional APC that can process antigens for both MHC class I and II pathways and activate both naive CD4+ T cells and CD8+T cells in vivo. In murine studies, immunization with DC pulsed with tumor antigens resulted in better antitumor effects than direct peptide administration. In immunization trials using DC pulsed with tumor lysates or synthetic peptides, tumor regression was observed in patients with various cancers, including melanoma, prostate cancer, colon cancer, and B-cell lymphoma.[28] Although most clinical trials have used monocyte-derived DC, peripheral blood DC as well as CD34+ cell–derived DC have been used in some protocols.[29] Antigen loading on DC using various antigens including RNA, cDNA, recombinant virusand cell-penetrating peptide conjugated proteins has also been exploited. DC fused with tumor cells and leukemia clone- derived DC have also been used in clinical trials. K-ras- specific T cells were detected in pancreatic cancer patients following multiple intravenous infusions of peptide-pulsed antigen presenting mononuclear cells obtained by leukapheresis, although no therapeutic effect in patients was observed. In addition, no tumor regression was observed following immunization with DC transfected with MUC1 cDNA. A decrease in tumor marker was observed in a patient with a pancreatic neuroendocrine tumor, following immunization with DC pulsed with autologous tumor lysates. Intratumoral administration of immature DC following intraoperative irradiation is currently being conducted in Japan. Thus far, any antitumor effects observed in these DC-based clinical trials for pancreatic cancer are weak. Protocols for the optimal use of DC in immunotherapy, including the source of DC, kinds of tumor antigens, methods for maturation and antigen loading, site and schedule for administration, remain to be determined. Based on murine experiments, immunization with more immunogenic tumor cells that are modified using various techniques, including hapten conjugation, foreign antigen introduction, and transfection with various genes such as cytokines (eg, GM-CSF, IL-2, TNF-_, IFN-_, IL-4) have been employed in melanoma, prostate cancer, and lung cancer. Strong antitumor effects, however, were not observed in the reported clinical trials. In pancreatic cancer, vaccination with GM-CSF transduced allogeneic pancreatic cancer cell lines along with adjuvant radiation and chemotherapy following surgical excision demonstrated possible benefit in disease-free survival, which appeared to be associated with the increase of postvaccination DTH responses against autologous tumor cells.

4. Adoptive Immunotherapy with antitumor

4.1 Immune cells

Passive immunotherapy with large doses of activated antitumor lymphocytes was also employed since there was a possibility that active immunization would be insufficient to induce enough of an immune response to cause tumor regression in the immunosuppressed patient with a large tumor burden. Adoptive transfer of tumor-reactive T cells cultured from tumor-infiltrating lymphocytes, along with IL-2, resulted in a clinical response in melanoma patients.[65] Adoptive transfer of EBV-specific T cells resulted in regression of EBV-associated lymphoma. Intraportal infusion of in vitro MUC1-stimulated T cells was performed in pancreatic cancer, yielding preliminary results that indicate inhibition of liver metastasis. Although the clinical use of tumor-reactive T cells was previously limited due to the difficulty in generating tumor-reactive T cells for most cancers, it is now possible to generate these cells from the PBMC of cancer patients by in vitro stimulation, using the identified tumor antigens.[66] Tumor-reactive T cells from patients preimmunized with tumor antigens were generated more efficiently, which suggests that combined use of active and passive immunotherapies is ideal. One of the problems that arises from adoptive transfer of cultured T cells is the low efficiency of administered T cells in in vivo maintenance and accumulation in tumor tissues. However, it was recently reported that nonmyeloablative, lymphodepletive pre-treatment with cyclophosphamide and fludarabine resulted in extended persistence of administered tumor-reactive T cells in peripheral blood and tumor tissues and increased tumor regression, which may be due to suppression of patient immune responses or the need to make room for homeostatic proliferation of transferred lymphocytes.[67] Adoptive immunotherapy with IL- 2–activated PBMC, LAK (lymphokine activated killer) cells displayed some antitumor effects when locally administered (ie, by intrapleural or intraarterial infusion) for lung or liver cancer. Intraportal administration following intraoperative irradiation in pancreatic cancer patients is reported to result in possible prolongation of survival[68].

Adoptive immunotherapy involves harvesting the patient's peripheral blood T-lymphocytes, stimulating and expanding the autologous tumour-reactive T-cells using IL-2 and CD3-specific antibody, before subsequently transferring them back into the patient. Twelve patients with advanced pancreatic cancer who underwent resection, intraoperative radiotherapy and intraportal infusion of LAK cells with recombinant IL-2 had lower incidence of liver metastasis compared to controls (three of 12 vs ten of 15; $p<0.05$)69. There was no significant difference in overall survival, but more patients were alive three years later (36% vs none).

Telomerase—Telomerase is a reverse transcriptase that contains a RNA template used to synthesise telomeric repeats onto chromosomal ends. Activation of telomerase and its maintenance of telomeres play a role in immortalisation of human cancer cells, as telomeres shrink after each cell division [70]. Telomerase activity is found in 92-95% of pancreatic cancers [71-72], and is associated with increased potential of invasion and metastasis and poor prognosis [73-74]. Upregulation of telomerase may also be responsible for the development of chemotherapy resistance [75]. Adenovirus-mediated transduction of p53 gene inhibited telomerase activity in MIAPaCa-2, SUIT-2 and AsPC-1 cells, independent of its effect on apoptosis, cell growth and cycle arrest [76]. Antisense to the RNA component of telomerase seemed to increase susceptibility of Panc-1 cells to cisplatin [77]. Telomerase reverse transcriptase antisense oligonucleotide (hTERT-ASO) was found to inhibit the proliferation of BxPC-3 cells *in vitro* by decreasing telomerase activity and increasing apoptosis [78]. Adoptive transfer of telomerase-specific T-cells was studied in a syngeneic pancreatic tumour mouse model [79]. T-cells were produced *in vitro* by coculturing human lymphocytes with telomerase peptide-pulsed dendritic cells (DCs) or *in vivo* by injection of peptide with adjuvant into C57BL/6 mice. Animals treated with these T-cells showed significantly delayed disease progression.

MUC1—Adoptive transfer of MUC1-specific cytotoxic T-lymphocytes (CTLs) was able to completely eradicate MUC1-expressing tumours in mice [80]. Intraportal infusion of *In vitro* MUC1-stimulated T-cells was performed in patients with pancreatic cancer, with subsequent inhibition of liver metastasis [81]. In a study of eleven patients with lung metastases (from colorectal, pancreatic, breast, lung, or melanoma primaries), effector cells were generated *in vitro* using cultured DCs, synthetic peptide, peripheral blood lymphocytes, IL-2 and anti-CD3 antibody [82]. A partial response of the lung metastases was observed in a patient with pancreatic cancer who received these cells stimulated with MUC1.

4.2 Cytokines and immunomodulators

TNFerade—TNF-α is a multifunctional cytokine that has shown antitumour potency [83-85]. TNFerade Biologic (TNFerade) is a replication-deficient adenovirus carrying the gene for human TNF-α, regulated by a radiation-inducible promoter Early Growth Response (Egr-1). The latter would ensure maximal gene expression when infected tissue is irradiated 86. TNFerade was effective in combination with radiation in a number of human xenograft models, including glioma [87], prostate [88], oesophageal [89] and radiation-resistant laryngeal cancers [90]. The multicentre phase II/III Pancreatic Cancer Clinical Trial with TNFerade (PACT) is currently ongoing and involved patients with locally advanced pancreatic cancer. Patients were given radiotherapy, 5-FU with or without CT-guided transabdominal injection of TNFerade. Preliminary data of 51 patients revealed that the one-year survival increased from 28% to 70.5% with the addition of TNFerade, with MS of 335 and 515 days respectively[91].

Virulizin—Virulizin (Lorus Therapeutics Inc.) is a biological response modifier obtained from bovine bile [92]. It stimulates the expression of TNF-α and activates macrophages, which subsequently activates natural killer cells via IL-12 [93-94]. Evidence exists to show that it also induces the production of IL-17E with resulting eosinophilia [95].

In vivo studies showed that Virulizin significantly inhibited the growth of human pancreatic cancer xenografts (BxPC-3, SU [86.86] and MIAPaCa-2) in nude mice, as well as potentiated the antitumour effect of gemcitabine and 5-FU [96-97]. A phase III trial was conducted to study the effect of gemcitabine with or without Virulizin in 434 chemotherapy-naïve patients with advanced pancreatic cancer [341]. MS was not significantly better for the gemcitabine and Virulizin group compared to gemcitabine with placebo (6.3 vs 6 months). However for stage 3 patients who received Virulizin in a salvage setting, a significant difference in survival was demonstrated (10.9 vs 7.4 months, p=0.017).

4.3 IL-2

Pancreatic cancer could thus constitute a paradigmatic example of neoplasia where tumor-related variables and host immunosuppressive status have the same importance in determining an unfavourable prognosis. The severe suppression of anticancer immunity, which characterizes patients suffering from pancreatic cancer, is further aggravated by surgical treatment [98]. In fact, it is known that surgery may inhibit anticancer immunity by provoking a postoperative decline in the absolute number of circulating lymphocytes [99-101], which play a fundamental role in generating an effective anticancer immune reaction; this is fundamentally an IL-2-dependent phenomenon [102].

Surgery-induced immunosuppression could represent one of the main factors responsible for relapse in cancer patients treated by radical surgery, by possibly promoting the growth of micro-metastases, already existing at the time of the surgical removal of the tumor . Previous clinical studies have shown that the immunosuppressive status occurring during the postoperative period is particularly severe in patients with pancreatic cancer and this evidence could explain, at least in part, the high percentage of recurrences occurring in patients radically operated for cancer of the pancreas [103]. At present, the only molecule which has been proven to correct the lymphocytopenia is IL-2, representing the main growth factor for lymphocytes, including T lymphocytes and natural killer (NK) cells [104] and the stimulation of lymphocyte proliferation would constitute the main mechanism responsible for the antitumor activity of IL-2 in the immunotherapy of cancer [105]. Moreover, the preoperative administration of IL-2 for only few days prior to surgery was effective in preventing surgery-induced lymphocytopenia [106]. In addition, the abrogation of surgery-induced lymphocyte decline has been shown to improve the prognosis of patients with colorectal cancer in whether treated by radical or palliative surgery [107]. The therapeutic impact of IL-2 presurgical administration remains to be better defined in gastric cancer [108], despite its efficacy in preventing the postoperative lymphocytopenia. Finally, the prevention of postoperative lymphocyte decline by IL-2 presurgical immunotherapy was associated with clear lymphocyte and eosinophil intratumoral infiltration in colorectal cancer patients, which, in contrast, was less evident in patients with gastric carcinoma. Preliminary clinical studies have suggested that preoperative injection of IL-2 may also prevent surgery-induced lymphocytopenia in patients with pancreatic cancer [109]. According to previous investigations, IL-2 presurgical immunotherapy may also completely abrogate surgery-induced lymphocytopenia also patients with pancreatic carcinoma, as well as previously described for both colorectal and gastric carcinomas. Moreover, in agreement with the clinical results previously reported for colorectal cancer patients and in contrast to those more controversially reported in gastric cancer, this study would suggest that a preoperative immunotherapy with IL-2 may improve the clinical course of the pancreatic cancer in terms of both FFPP and OS. Therefore, particularly because of its unfavourable prognosis, presurgical immunotherapy with IL-2 could represent a simple but effective clinical strategy to improve the prognosis of pancreatic cancer patients undergoing macroscopical radical surgery.

4.4 Allogeneic antigen-specific immunotherapy

Allogeneic antigen-specific immunotherapies, nonmyeloablative SCT (minitransplant) and DLI (donor leukocyte infusion), are reported to have some antitumor effect [graft versus tumor (GVT)] on solid tumors, including RCC, breast cancer, and pancreatic cancer, in addition to haematological malignancies.[110]GVT effects were also observed in pancreatic cancer patients in minitransplant protocols conducted in Japan. Although the mechanisms of the antitumor effects, such as allogeneic responses to minor histocompatibility antigens (mHa), on hematological malignancies are well studied, they remain unclear with regard to solid tumors. One of the major problems in allogeneic treatment of the solid tumor is severe GVHD. Several strategies for the separation of GVT and GVHD have been developed for hematological malignancies. Whether this separation is possible for solid tumors, however, is unclear.

Was reported on the efficacy of adoptive immunotherapy (AIT) with cytotoxic T lymphocytes (CTLs), induced from autologous pancreatic tumors but not from AIT with LAK cells. Although these immunotherapies have a potential as alternative treatments for PC, the effects have been limited.

Pancreatic cancer cells present an enormous challenge, as they are naturally resistant to current chemotherapy and radiation therapy. In addition, known pancreatic cancer antigens have generated relatively weak immune responses. This is probably due to a combination of mutations in oncogenes such as *KRAS* and tumour-suppressor genes such as *TP53*, *CDKN2A*, *DPC4* (deleted in pancreas cancer 4), *BRCA2* and *ERBB2* (also known as HER2/neu), as well as overexpression of growth factors such as transforming growth factor-α (TGFα), interleukin-1 (IL-1), IL-6 and IL-8, tumour-necrosis factor-a (TNFα), or vascular endothelial growth factor (VEGF), their receptors, or constitutive expression of multidrug-resistant genes[2, 3, 4, 5]. Alternative therapeutic approaches are therefore urgently needed for this disease.

Immune-based therapies aim to recruit and activate T cells that recognize tumour-specific antigens. In addition, recombinant monoclonal antibodies are being designed to target tumour-specific antigens — these would kill tumour cells either by direct lysis or through delivery of a conjugated cytotoxic agent. Both approaches are attractive for the treatment of pancreatic cancer for several reasons. First, these immune-based therapies act through a mechanism that is distinct from chemotherapy or radiation therapy, and represent a non-cross-resistant treatment with an entirely different spectrum of toxicities. Second, through the genetic recombination of their respective receptors, the B cells and T cells of the immune system are capable of recognizing a diverse array of potential tumour antigens. In addition, both T and B cells can distinguish small antigenic differences between normal and transformed cells, providing specificity while minimizing toxicity. New insights into the mechanisms by which T cells are successfully activated and by which tumours evade immune recognition are driving the development of new combinatorial immunotherapy approaches. In addition, recent advances in gene-expression analysis have allowed for the identification of new pancreatic targets, including candidate tumour antigens that might serve as T-cell and antibody targets. These advances now make it possible to exploit the immune system in the fight against pancreatic cancer.

4.5 Targeting signalling molecules

By the time that patients are diagnosed with pancreatic cancer, the tumour has typically progressed and invaded adjacent structures. Perineural invasion, metastasis to lymph nodes and liver, and an intense DESMOPLASTIC STROMAL REACTION are commonly observed. A range of signalling pathways, including epidermal growth factor receptor (EGFR) and the PI3K–AKT–mTOR–S6K cascades, are known to mediate pancreatic tumour growth and progression[111]n addition, new blood-vessel formation (angiogenesis) is required for the growth of primary pancreatic tumours and is essential for metastasis. In pancreatic tumours, this process is probably regulated by fibroblast growth factor, platelet-derived endothelial-cell growth factor and VEGF family members. In fact, several pancreatic-cancer-associated genes have been linked to angiogenesis. DPC4 upregulates VEGF expression, and mutated KRAS expression is associated with increased micro-vessel density[112].

Monoclonal antibodies that target a range of these pathways have demonstrated efficacy in preclinical models[113-115]dition, monoclonal antibodies that target EGFR and VEGF receptor have been tested in patients with a range of cancers, including pancreatic cance[115,117]hough these antibodies have demonstrated only modest results as single agents, the pathways they affect are also candidate targets for immune intervention.

Preclinical evidence has also shown that specific inhibitors of these signalling pathways can also increase immune activation. For example, VEGF is a key inhibitor of pro-inflammatory cytokines as well as dendritic-cell maturation, and it can also directly inhibit T-cell development. So antibodies that block signalling by this growth factor can promote antitumour immune responses. Furthermore, downregulation of the ERBB-receptor-family members with drugs such as herceptin promotes tumour-antigen presentation by HLA class I molecules, improving the potential for T-cell recognition and lysis[118]onoclonal antibodies that target these signalling pathways are now being developed for clinical trials as agents that potentially synergize with other immune-based approaches, including vaccines.

4.6 Vaccines against pancreatic tumour antigens

To develop the ideal vaccine for pancreatic cancer, the following wish list would probably need to be fulfilled. First, specific cell-surface proteins must be identified that are that are crucial in the cancer growth or progression pathway and are unique to pancreatic cancer tumours. Second, these tumour-exclusive proteins should be shown to elicit a vigorous tumour-protein-specific immune response. Third, the best carrier to deliver the appropriate immunogenic tumour proteins should be identified. Fourth, molecules that are immune stimulatory as well as molecules that can abrogate the natural immune-inhibition signalling that is seen in pancreatic cancer should be identified to enhance the immune response. Fifth, additional synergistic immune help should be identified (for example, antibodies or *ex vivo* tumour-reactive T cells). Several proteins, such as carcinoembryonic antigen (CEA), mutated KRAS, mucin-1 (MUC1) and gastrin, have in fact been identified to be specifically overexpressed in most pancreatic cancers[119-125] antigens were identified over 10 years ago using various methods to analyse gene expression in cancer cells. Vaccines and antibodies designed to target these antigens have been tested in early-phase clinical trials[126-131]hese antigens are known to have weak inherent immune potential, various immune-modulating agents were co-administered, including granulocyte–macrophage colony-stimulating factor (GM-CSF), and interleukin-2 (IL-2). So far, a few studies have demonstrated post-vaccination immune responses to the relevant peptides or whole proteins. Significant clinical responses have not yet been observed. This might be due to the lack of pooling of the right antigens, to the existence of host mechanisms of immune tolerance, the inability of the relevant immune cells to effectively localize to the sites of disease, or a combination of these factors.

Vaccination involves administering an antigen that is unique for a particular type of tumour with the aim of stimulating tumour-specific immunity. Antigens could be delivered in the form of DNA or peptide, as well as tumour cells or antigen-pulsed DCs. Additional synergistic help is added to elicit a more vigorous and effective immune response, such as cytokines and immunostimulating adjuvants.

Whole-Cell—GM-CSF is one of a few cytokines that has shown significant antitumour effect *in vivo* [342]. It is an important growth factor for granulocytes and monocytes, and has a crucial role in the growth and differentiation of DCs, the most potent antigen-presenting cells (APCs) for triggering immune response. *In vivo* growth of AsPC-1 cells, retrovirally transduced with the GM-CSF gene, was inhibited and associated with increased survival of the nude mice, even in the mature T-cell-deficient condition 132. Jaffee et al. conducted a phase I study using allogeneic GM-CSF-secreting whole-cell tumour vaccine for pancreatic cancer 133. This is based on the concept that the localisation of GMCSF in the implanted tumour environment together with the shared tumour antigen expressed by the primary cancer would effectively induce an antitumour immune response. In this study two pancreatic cancer cell lines (PANC 10.05 and PANC 6.03) were used as the vaccine, both genetically modified to express GM-CSF. 14 pancreatic cancer patients who had undergone pancreaticoduodenectomy eight weeks prior were given variable doses of the vaccine intradermally. Three of the eight patients who received ≥10 × 107 vaccine cells developed postvaccination delayed-type hypersensitivity (DTH) responses associated with increased disease free survival time, and remained disease-free for longer than 25 months after diagnosis. Side effects were mainly limited to local skin reactions at the site of vaccination. In a recently completed phase II study of 60 patients with resected pancreatic adenocarcinoma, patients received five treatments of 2.5 × 108 vaccine cells, together with 5-FU and radiotherapy134. The reported MS was 26 months, with a one- and two-year survival of 88% and 76% respectively.

4.7 Peptide and DNA

- **Ras:** As described earlier, mutated ras is highly prevalent in pancreatic cancer. A phase II study was done using mutant ras peptide-based subcutaneous vaccine in 12 cancer patients (five with fully resected pancreatic and seven with colorectal cancers). Five out of 11 patients showed showed ≥1.5 fold increase in interferon-γ (IFN-γ) mRNA copies in peripheral blood mononuclear cells. The pancreatic cancer patients showed a disease-free survival of >35.2 months and post-vaccination survival of >44.4 months 135. Gjertsen et al tested an intradermal vaccine of APCs loaded *ex vivo* with synthetic ras peptide corresponding to the ras mutation found in the patient's tumour 136. In this phase I/II study of five patients with advanced pancreatic cancer, two of them showed induced immune response. They also studied ras peptide in combination with GM-CSF in a phase I/II trial involving 48 patients with pancreatic adenocarcinoma of variable stage 137. Peptide-specific immunity was induced in 58% of patients. Of patients with advanced disease, those who responded to treatment showed increased survival compared to non-responders (148 and 61 days respectively; p=0.0002).

As IL-2 is involved in T-cell-mediated immune response, a vaccine consisting of mutant ras peptide in combination with GM-CSF and IL-2 was tested in a phase II trial of 17 patients with advanced cancers (14 colorectal, one non-small cell lung and two pancreatic cancers) 138. Of the six patients with positive immune response (by means of IFN-γ mRNA copies), the MS and the median PFS were 39.9 and 17.9 months compared to 18.5 and 15.6 months for nonresponders, respectively. Grade III toxicities led to IL-2 dose reduction in three of the patients.

- **CEA and MUC1:** Carcinoembryonic antigen (CEA) glycoprotein is expressed at a low level in normal colonic epithelium but is overexpressed in many malignant diseases, including those of the colon, rectum, stomach and pancreas (85-90%) 139. Its serum level is sometimes used as a marker for the diagnosis of pancreatic cancer, with a sensitivity of 25-40% and a specificity of 70-90% 140-141.

To boost MUC1-specific immune response, a vaccine composed of MUC1 peptide and SBAS2 adjuvant was tested in a phase I study 142. There was an increase in the percentage of CD8+ T-cells and MUC1-specific antibody (some developed IgG). Hope for the CEA or MUC1 vaccine was nevertheless crushed when a phase III trial of 255 patients using PANVAC-VF (vaccine consisted of recombinant vaccinia and fowlpox viruses coexpressing CEA, MUC-1 and TRICOM) failed to improve overall survival compared to palliative chemotherapy or best supportive care.

- **Gastrin:** G17DT (Gastrimmune or Insegia) is an immunoconjugate of the amino-terminal sequence of gastrin-17 (G-17) linked by means of a spacer peptide to diphtheria toxoid. Given intramuscularly it induces the formation of antibodies that can neutralise both amidated-G-17 and the precursor glycine-extended G17 143. In a phase II study of 30 patients, 67% mounted an antibody response. A significantly higher response (82%) was achieved in those given the highest dose of 250µg compared to 46% in the 100µg group. MS was significantly higher (217 days) for the antibody responders compared to non-responders (121 days; p=0.0023).

When used as a monotherapy for patients with advanced pancreatic cancer unwilling or unsuitable to take chemotherapy, MS was 151 compared to 82 days in the placebo group (p=0.03) [360]. G17DT was subsequently tested in a phase III trial with or without gemcitabine in 383 untreated patients with locally advanced, recurrent or metastatic pancreatic adenocarcinoma. This unfortunately showed that the addition of G17DT did not improve overall survival or secondary endpoints Increasing -17 antibody titre levels in a subset of patients, however, were associated with increased survival.

- **Mesothelin:** Thomas and colleagues provided the first direct evidence, by using mesothelin epitopes, that pancreatic cancer-specific CD8+ T-cell response can be generated via crosspresentation by an approach that recruits APCs to the vaccination site 144. Gaffney et al studied the mesothelin DNA vaccine in combination with the anti-glucocorticoid-induced TNF receptor antibody (anti-GITR) in mice with syngeneic mesothelin-expressing pancreatic cancer 145. 50% of animals treated with mesothelin were tumour-free 25 days after tumour injection compared to 0% of non-treated mice. This increased to 94% with the addition of anti-GITR. The agonist anti-GITR served to enhance T-cell-mediated response of the vaccine 146-147.

- **Telomerase:** The telomerase peptide vaccine GV1001 was tested in a phase I/II study of 48 patients with unresectable pancreatic cancer 148. They received intradermal injection in combination with GM-CSF. Immune responses, as measured by DTH skin reaction and T-cell proliferation *in vitro,* were demonstrated in 24 of 38 evaluable patients, with the highest percentage (75%) in the intermediate dose group. MS for this group was significantly longer at 8.6 months, and one-year survival was 25%. GV1001 was given to patients in a phase I trial using imiquimod as an adjuvant149. Imiquimod acts by binding to Toll-like receptor 7 on immune cells, resulting in the production of cytokines such as IFN-α, IFN-β and IL-12. Immune response was found in up to six (46%) of 13 evaluable patients.
- **Survivin:** Survivin-specific CTLs were isolated from pancreatic cancer patients and these could lyse pancreatic carcinoma cell lines *in vitro* 150. Vaccination with survivin DNA prolonged survival in murine pancreatic and lymphoma tumour models, associated with slower tumour growth and increased lymphocyte infiltration . Survivin peptide was tested in a patient with gemcitabine refractory pancreatic cancer . Whilst on treatment he had complete remission of liver metastases after six months. However when he was weaned from the vaccination he developed recurrent disease. Vaccine-induced immune activity was detected by IFN-γ enzyme-linked immunospot (ELISPOT) assay.

Antigen-pulsed DCs—Antigen-specific T-cell responses are initiated by DCs. They capture antigens secreted or shed by tumour cells and present peptides in association with the MHC class I and II molecules. This results in the expression and upregulation of cytokines and costimulatory molecules which in turn stimulate CD4+ and CD8+ T-cells to mount an antitumour response. As such DCs that carry the tumour antigen of interest is an ideal adjuvant in cancer immunotherapy.

- **MUC1:** In a phase I/II trial, human autologous DCs transfected with MUC1 cDNA were used as a vaccine for ten patients with advanced breast, pancreatic or papillary cancer 151. Four patients showed a two- to ten-fold increase in the frequency of mucin-specific IFN-γ-secreting CD8+ T-cells, suggesting an immune response. In a phase 1b study, eight patients with pancreatic or biliary tumours were vaccinated with DCs pulsed with MUC1 152.

As discussed previously, monoclonal antibodies have so far been the most successful form of immunotherapy clinically. They are being used as diagnostic tools, prognostic indicators, and for the treatment of many cancers. Advantages include their specific targeting of tumour cells while sparing normal tissue, their relative ease of administration, and their low toxicity profile. The major disadvantages include the absence of T-cell activation, which therefore precludes T-cell-mediated cytotoxic killing and the generation of memory immune responses. In addition, a potential limiting factor in its use involves tumour heterogeneity. Specifically, all tumour cells within a proliferating mass might not express the antigen that is being targeted. Inhibitors to EGFR and to VEGF have been tested in combination with gemcitabine and are currently in Phase III trials either with other approaches have used dendritic cells as the carrier of the antigen of interest. To date, CEA and MUC1 antigens have been among the initial antigens tested, with mixed results153-154 se of adoptively transferred pancreatic-cancer-specific T cells has been proposed to be another opportunity to augment the immune response. Although this strategy has been promising preclinically, and has been used with some success in melanoma, there have not been any clinical trials in pancreatic cancer so far.

A current limitation to the development of vaccines for pancreatic cancer has been the inability to correlate *in vitro* measures of antitumour immunity with *in vivo* responses. Post-vaccination DTH responses to autologous tumour are a potential useful surrogate, but this approach is not ideal. At present, it is technically challenging to produce sufficient quantity and purity of autologous tumour material for testing, as tumours vary in their composition of tumour cells versus other cell types between patients. Although other biological end points, such as an antibody response or *in vitro* CYTOLYTIC T LYMPHOCYTE (CTL) ASSAY against a vaccine-delivered tumour antigen (or antigens), have been measured and provide important 'proof of concept' data, these end points have also not been demonstrated to be predictors of traditional clinical end points, including tumour response and survival benefit.

It is difficult to assess whether the lack of improved survival after immunotherapy is due to inefficient antigen delivery, which could result in ineffective immunization, inappropriate selection of antigen targets, or both. As discussed above, there are formidable barriers to inducing an antitumour immune response, even when the vaccine itself is potent enough to reduce significant cancer burdens in more immunogenic tumour systems. Effective immunization will therefore require the targeting of relevant pancreatic tumour antigens using optimized antigen-delivery systems with immune-stimulating cytokines, in sequence with other therapeutic interventions that alter immune checkpoints in the tumour microenvironment, such as inhibitors to regulatory molecules on T cells (for example, antibody to CD152/CTLA4).

5. New immunotherapy targets

The inability of previously tested antigens (including CEA, KRAS, MUC1 and gastrin) to induce immune-specific responses underscores the challenge to identify more relevant immunogenic targets. Indeed, these antigens were chosen only because they were overexpressed or had altered expression in pancreatic tumours, and not because they had been shown to be immunogenic. Therefore, there might be additional as-yet-unidentified antigens that might be more immunogenic for inducing effective immunity against pancreatic cancers. How will such new candidate pancreatic cancer antigens be discovered? Two methods are routinely used in an attempt to identify new targets. The first method, serological analysis of recombinant tumour cDNA expression libraries (SEREX), uses serum to screen phage-display libraries prepared from tumour cells to identify candidate antigen targets that have elicited both humoral and cell-mediated immune responses in cancer patients. This method has identified coactosin-like protein (an actin-filament-binding protein that interacts directly with 5-liopoxygenase and has an important role in cellular leukotriene synthesis) as a potential pancreatic cancer target antigen. This protein seems to be recognized by antibody and T-cell responses in patients with pancreatic cancer[155].

The second method uses tumour-specific T cells that have been isolated from patients with pancreatic cancer to screen cDNA libraries prepared from autologous tumour cells. This method requires the isolation and culture of tumour-specific T cells, along with tumour cells, from patients with pancreatic cancer and is a technically challenging approach. This approach has been most successful in identifying melanoma-associated antigens[156].

A relatively newer, more promising method of tumour-antigen identification is the use of the patient's lymphocytes to evaluate proteins that are found to be differentially expressed by pancreatic cancer[157-158] approach has several advantages. First, it allows for a rapid screen of a large number of candidate antigens but requires the isolation from patients of only a few lymphocytes, which are limited in availability. Second, this approach is not dependent on the availability of autologous tumour cells, which are difficult to isolate in large enough numbers for generating cDNA libraries. Third, this approach can be used to identify tumour antigens that are expressed by any HLA type, allowing for the generalization of this approach to most patients. Finally, this approach has the potential to rapidly identify 'immune relevant' antigens, as it uses immunized lymphocytes from patients vaccinated with a whole-tumour-cell vaccine approach who ideally have demonstrated clinical evidence of immune activation following vaccination. So this method provides the best insurance that the antigens identified are ones that the patient's immune system is reacting to after immunization.

As additional 'immune relevant' pancreatic tumour antigens are identified, the next significant challenge lies in developing strategies to improve the *in vivo* delivery of these antigens to APCs and thereby allow effective antigen processing and presentation, and subsequent activation of a potent antitumour immune response. DCs are now accepted as the most efficient APCs in B- and T-cell activation. Several clinical trials have tested *ex vivo* expanded and primed DCs as a vaccine approach. However, these studies have revealed the difficulty in reliably producing phenotypically mature DCs for clinical testing, as only mature DCs are capable of efficiently presenting antigens to T cells. If an antigen is not presented in the proper context by mature DCs, immune downregulation or tolerance can occur. It has been shown in animal models that immature DCs induce T-cell tolerance. As an alternative to DC-based delivery, recombinant viral- and bacterial-vector delivery systems are currently under development or are already undergoing clinical testing. The use of modified viral particles or targeted bacteria to deliver tumour antigens to the immune system is based on the innate ability of the agent to efficiently infect APCs *in vivo*. Early approaches have included viruses such as vaccinia [159,160] er, the use of immunogenic vectors in cancer patients who have been previously exposed to a similar vector often induces vigorous immune responses against the vector before effective priming against the tumour antigen can occur. As such, other viral particles and bacterial delivery systems are currently nearing or are already undergoing clinical development for the treatment of pancreatic cancer.

6. Future directions

The limitations of currently available therapy for pancreatic cancer are more clearly exposed as we begin to appreciate the molecular changes behind the complex transformation of normal pancreatic ductal cells into frank pancreatic cancers, and the mechanisms of pancreatic cancer resistance to traditional anticancer modalities. It is clear that the most effective therapy will require a combined approach incorporating the best targeted interventions taken from each respective modality. Preclinical models have already revealed the synergy between immunotherapy and other targeted therapeutics, such as inhibitors of VEGF and EGF signalling. These combinations are about to be tested in patients with pancreatic cancer.

Pancreatic cancer remains one of the most resistant cancers to traditional forms of therapy. Until techniques for early detection can be developed, most patients will continue to present with incurable disease. The pancreatic cancer research community is committed to developing new therapies for this disease. Pancreatic cancer patients and their families, through a number of national pancreatic cancer non-profit organizations such as Pancreas Cancer Action Network have organized to support this effort. It is crucial that we move forward with scientifically driven innovative therapies, as the empirical approaches have failed. Recent developments in the design of mouse models that recapitulate early pre-invasive genetic changes in *KRAS* activation, inactivation of *CDKN2A*, *TP53* and *SMAD4* tumour-suppressor genes should provide the opportunity to test such approaches in a timely manner[161,162].

7. References

[1] Evans, D. B., Abbruzzese, J. L. & Willett, C. G. in *Principles and Practice of Oncology* 6th edn (ed. DeVita, V. T.) 1126–1161 (J. B. Lippincott, Philadelphia, 2001).

[2] Li, D. *et al.* Pancreatic cancer. *Lancet* 363, 1049–1057 (2004).

[3] Spratlin, J. *et al.* The absence of human equilibrative nucleoside transporter 1 is associated with reduced survival in patients with gemcitabine-treated pancreas adenocarcinoma. *Clin. Cancer Res.* 10, 6956–6961 (2004).

[4] Laheru, D., Biedrzycki, B. & Jaffee, E. M. Immunologic approaches to the management of pancreatic cancer. *Cancer J.* 7, 324–337 (2001).

[5] Pardoll, D. & Allison, J. Cancer Immunotherapy: breaking the barriers to harvest the crop. *Nature Med.* 10, 887–892 (2004).

[6] Rosenberg, S. A., Yang, J. C. & Restifo, N. P. Cancer immunotherapy: moving beyond current vaccines. *Nature Med.* 10, 909–915 (2004).

[7] Restifo, N. P. *et al.* Molecular mechanisms used by tumors to escape immune recognition: immunogenetherapy and the cell biology of major histocompatibility complex class I. *J. Immunol.* 14, 182–190 (1993).

[8] Ganss, R. & Hanahan, D. Tumor microenvironment can restrict the effectiveness of activated antitumor lymphocytes. *Cancer Res.* 58, 4673–4681 (1998).

[9] Wang, T. *et al.* Regulation of the innate and adaptive immune responses by Stat-3 signaling in tumor cells. *Nature Med.* 10, 48–54 (2004).

[10] Ohm, J. E. & Carbone, D. P. VEGF as a mediator of tumor-associated immunodeficiency. *Immunol. Res.* 23, 263–272 (2001).

[11] Bellone, G. *et al.* Tumor-associated transforming growth factor βand interleukin-10 contribute to a systemic Th2 immune phenotype in pancreatic carcinoma patrients. *Am. J. Pathol.* 155, 537–547 (1999).

[12] Carreno, B. M. & Collins, M. BTLA: a new inhibitory receptor with a B7-like ligand. *Trends Immunol.* 24, 524–527 (2003).

[13] Sica, G. L. *et al.* B7-H4, a molecule of the B7 family, negatively regulates T cell immunity. *Immunity* 18, 849–861 (2003).
[14] Coyle, A. J. & Gutierrez-Ramos, J. C. The expanding B7 superfamily: increasing complexity in co-stimulatory signals regulating T cell function. *Nature Immunol.* 2, 203–209 (2001).
[15] Schwartz, R. H. T cell anergy. *Annu. Rev. Immunol.* 21, 305–334 (2003).
[16] Greenwald, R. J. *et al.* CTLA-4 regulates induction of anergy *in vivo. Immunity* 14, 145–155 (2001).
[17] Chen, L. Co-inhibitory molecules of the B7-CD28 family in the control of T cell immunity. *Nature Rev. Immun.* 4, 336–347 (2004).
[18] Schwartz, R. H. T cell anergy. *Annu. Rev. Immunol.* 21, 305–334 (2003).
[19] Walunas, T. L., Bakker, C. Y. & Bluestone, J. A. CTLA-4 ligation blocks CD28-dependent T cell activation. *J. Exp. Med.* 183, 2541–2550 (1996).
[20] Greenwald, R. J. *et al.* CTLA-4 regulates induction of anergy *in vivo. Immunity* 14, 145–155 (2001).
[21] Slavik, J. M., Hutchcroft, J. E. & Bierer, B. E. CD28/CTLA-4 and CD80/86 families: signaling and function. *Immunol. Res.* 19, 1–24 (1999).
[22] Greenfield, E. A., Nguyen, K. A. & Kuchroo, V. K. CD28/B7 co-stimulation: a review. *Crit. Rev. Immunol.* 18, 389–418 (1998).
[23] Najafian, N. & Khoury, S. J. T cell costimulatory pathways: blockade for autoimmunity. *Expert Opin. Biol. Ther.* 3, 227–236 (2003).
[24] Carreno, B. M. & Collins, M. The B7 family of ligands and its receptors: new pathways for co-stimulaton inhibition of immune responses. *Annu. Rev. Immunol.* 20, 29–53 (2002)
[25] Dong, H. & Chen, L. B7-H1 pathway and its role in the evasion of tumor immunity. *J. Mol. Med.* 81, 281–287 (2003).
[26] Okazaki, T., Iwai, Y. & Honjo, T. New regulatory co-receptors: inducible co-stimulator and PD-1. *Curr. Opin. Immunol.* 14, 779–782 (2002).
[27] Agata, Y. *et al.* Expression of the PD-1 antigen on the surface of stimulated mouse T and B lymphocytes. *Int. Immunol.* 8, 765–772 (1996).
[28] Khoury, S. J. & Sayegh, M. H. The roles of the new negative T cell costimulatory pathways in regulating autoimmunity. *Immunity* 20, 529–538 (2004).
[29] Liang, S. C. *et al.* Regulation of PD-1, PD-L1,PD-L2 expression during normal and autoimmune responses. *Eur. J. Immunol.* 33, 2706–2716 (2003)
[30] Ungefroren, H. *et al.* Immunological escape mechanisms in pancreatic carcinoma. *Ann. NY Acad. Sci.* 880, 243–251 (1999).
[31] Kornmann, M., Ishiwata, T., Kleef, J., Beger, H. G. & Korc, M. Fas and Fas-ligand expression in human pancreatic cancer. *Ann. Surg.* 231, 368–379 (2000).
[32] Elnemr, A. *et al.* Human pancreatic cancer cells express non functional Fas receptors and counterattack lymphocytes by expressing Fas ligand; a potential mechanism for immune escape. *Int. J. Oncol.* 18, 33–39 (2001).
[33] Von Bernstorff, W. *et al.* Pancreatic cancer cells can evade immune surveillance via nonfunctional Fas (APO-1/CD95) receptors and aberrant expression of Fas ligand. *Surgery* 125, 73–84 (1999).

[34] Ungefroren, H. *et al.* Human pancreatic adenocarcinomas express Fas and Fas ligand yet are resistant to Fas mediated apoptosis. *Cancer Res.* 58, 1741–1749 (1998).

[35] Elhalel, M. D. *et al.* CTLA-4. FasL induces alloantigen-specific hyporesponsiveness. *J. Immunol.* 170, 5842–5850 (2003).

[36] Ito, D. *et al.* Chronic exposure of transforming growth factor β1 confers a more aggressive tumor phenotype through down-regulation of p21 (WAF1/CIP1) in conditionally immortalized pancreatic epithelial cells. *Surgery* 136, 364–374 (2004).

[37] Sawai, H. *et al.* Interleukin-1α enhances integrin $\alpha_6\beta_1$ expression metastatic capability of human pancreatic cancer. *Oncology* 65, 167–173 (2003).

[38] Duda, D. G. *et al.* Restoration of SMAD4 by gene therapy reverses the invasive phenotype in pancreatic adenocarcinoma cells. *Oncogene* 22, 6857–6864 (2003).

[39] Masui, T. *et al.* Expression of IL-6 receptor in pancreatic cancer: involvement in VEGF induction. *Anticancer Res.* 22, 4093–4100 (2002).

[40] Bellone, G. *et al.* Tumor-associated transforming growth factor β and interleukin-10 contribute to a systemic Th2 immune phenotype in pancreatic carcinoma patrients. *Am. J. Pathol.* 155, 537–547 (1999).

[41] Wahl, S. M. & Chen, W. TGF-β: how tolerant can it be? *Immunol. Res.* 28, 167–179 (2003).

Blumberg, R. S. *et al.* Structure of the T cell antigen receptor: evidence for two CD3 ε subunits in the T cell receptor–CD3 complex. *Proc. Natl Acad. Sci. USA* 87, 7220–7224 (1990).

[42] Clevers, H. The T cell receptor/CD3 complex: a dynamic protein ensemble. *Annu. Rev. Immunol.* 6, 629–662 (199

[43] Gold, D. P. *et al.* Evolutionary relationship between the T3 chain of the T-cell receptor complex and the immunoglobulin supergene family. *Proc. Natl Acad. Sci. USA* 84, 7649–7653 (1987).

[44] Wegener, A. M. K. *et al.* The T cell receptor/CD3 complex is composed of at least two autonomous transduction modules. *Cell* 68, 83–95 (1992).

[45] Klausner, R. D. & Samelson, L. E. T cell antigen receptor activation pathways: the tyrosine kinase connection. *Cell* 64, 875–878 (1991)

[46] Irving, B. A. & Weiss, A. The cytoplasmic domain of the T cell receptor ξ chain is sufficient to couple to receptor associated signal transduction pathways. *Cell* 64, 891–901 (1991).

[47] Samelson, L. E., Patel, M. D., Weissman, A. M., Harford, J. B. & Klausner, R. D. Antigen activation of murine T cells induces tyrosine phosphorylation of a polypeptide associated with the T cell antigen receptor. *Cell* 46, 1083–1090 (1986).

[48] Siegel, J. N., Klausner, R. D., Rapp, U. R. & Samelson, L. E. T cell receptor engagement stimulates c-raf associated kinase activity via a protein kinase C dependent pathway. *J. Biol. Chem.* 265, 18472–18480 (1990).

[49] Schmielau, J., Nalesnik, M. A. & Finn, O. J. Suppressed T-cell receptor ξ chain expression and cytokine production in pancreatic cancer patients. *Clin. Cancer Res.* 7, S933–S939 (2001).

[50] Matzinger, P. Tolerance, danger, and the extended family. *Annu. Rev. Immunol.* 12, 991–1045 (1994).

[51] Jenkins, M. K. & Schwartz, R. H. Antigen presentation by chemically modified splenocytes induces antigen-specific T cell unresponsiveness *in vitro* and *in vivo*. *J. Exp. Med.* 165, 302–319 (1987).
[52] Loke, P. & Allison, J. P. Emerging mechanisms of immune regulation-the extended B7 family and regulatory cells. *Arthritis Res. Ther.* 6, 208–214 (2004).
[53] Sugamura, K., Ishii, N. & Weinberg, A. D. Therapeutic targeting of the effector T cell co-stimulatory molecule OX40. *Nature Rev. Immunol.* 4, 420–431 (2004).
[54] Lane, P. Role of OX40 signals in coordinating CD4 T cell selection, migration, and cytokine differentiation in T helper (Th)1 and Th2 cells. *J. Exp. Med.* 191, 201–206 (2000).
[55] Eliopoulos, A. G. & Young, L. S. The role of the CD40 pathway in the pathogenesis and treatment of cancer. *Curr. Opin. Pharmacol.* 4, 360–367 (2004).
[56] Ohm, J. E. *et al.* VEGF inhibits T cell development and may contribute to tumor induced immune suppression. *Blood* 101, 4878–4886 (2003).
[57] Sharma, S. *et al.* Tumor cyclooxygenase 2 dependent suppression of dendritic cell function. *Clin. Cancer Res.* 9, 961–968 (2003).
[58] Sombroek, C. C. *et al.* Prostanoids play a major role in the primary tumor-induced inhibition of dendritic cell differentiation. *J. Immunol.* 168, 4333–4343 (2002).
[59] Chen, W. *et al.* Conversion of peripheral $CD4^+CD25^-$ naïve T cells to $CD4^+CD25^+$ regulatory T cells by TGF-β induction of transcription factor Foxp3. *J. Exp. Med.* 198, 1875–1886 (2003).
[60] Piccirillo, C. A. & Shevach, E. M. Naturally occurring $CD4^+CD25^+$ immunoregulatory T cells: central players in the arena of peripheral tolerance. *Sem. Immunol.* 16, 81–88 (2004).
[61] Liyanage, U. K. *et al.* Prevalence of regulatory T cells is increased in peripheral blood tumor microenvironment of patients with pancreas or breast adenocarcinoma. *J. Immunol.* 169, 2756–2761 (2002).
[62] Curiel, T. J. *et al.* Specific recruitment of regulatory T cells in ovarian carcinoma fosters immune privilege and predicts reduced survival. *Nature Med.* 10, 942–949 (2004).
[63] Mendelsohn, J. & Baselga, J. The EGF receptor family as targets for cancer therapy. *Oncogene* 19, 6550–6565 (2000).
[64] Schwarte-Waldhoff, I., Volpert, O. V. & Bouck, N. P. SMAD4/DPC4-mediated tumor suppression through suppression of angiogenesis. *Proc. Natl Acad. Sci. USA* 97, 9624–9629 (2000).
[65] Nair, S. *et al.* Synergy between tumor immunotherapy and antiangiogenic therapy. *Blood* 102, 964–971 (2003).
[66] Gabrilovich, D. I. *et al.* Antibodies to vascular endothelial growth factor enhance the efficacy of cancer immunotherapy by improving endogenous dendritic cell function. *Clin. Cancer Res.* 5, 2963–2970 (1999)
[67] Xiong, H. Q. *et al.* Cetuximab, a monoclonal antibody targeting the epidermal growth factor receptor, in combination with gemcitabine for advanced pancreatic Cancer: a multicenter phase II Trial. *J. Clin. Oncol.* 22, 2610–2616 (2004).

[68] Kindler, H. L. *et al.* Bevacizumab plus gemcitabine in patients with advanced pancreatic cancer: Updated results of a multi-center phase II trial. *Proc. Am. Soc. Clin. Oncol.* 23, A4009 (2004)
[69] Walpoe, M. E. *et al.* Her-2/neu specific monoclonal antibodies collaborate with her-2/neu targeted granulocyte macrophage stimulating factor secreting whole cell vaccination to augment $CD8^+$ T cell effector function and tumor free survival in her-2/neu transgenic mice. *J. Immunol.* 171, 2161–2169 (2003).
[70] Kobari M, Egawa S, Shibuya K, Sunamura M, Saitoh K, Matsuno S. Effect of intraportal adoptive immunotherapy on liver metastases after resection of pancreatic cancer. Br J Surg 2000;87:43–48
[71] Hahn WC. Role of telomeres and telomerase in the pathogenesis of human cancer. J Clin Oncol 2003;21:2034–2043.
[72] Hiyama E, Kodama T, Shinbara K, Iwao T, Itoh M, Hiyama K, Shay JW, Matsuura Y, Yokoyama T. Telomerase activity is detected in pancreatic cancer but not in benign tumors. Cancer Res 1997;57:326–331.
[73] Myung SJ, Kim MH, Kim YS, Kim HJ, Park ET, Yoo KS, Lim BC, Wan Seo D, Lee SK, Min YI, Kim JY. Telomerase activity in pure pancreatic juice for the diagnosis of pancreatic cancer may be complementary to K-ras mutation. Gastrointest Endosc 2000;51:708–713.
[74] Sato N, Maehara N, Mizumoto K, Nagai E, Yasoshima T, Hirata K, Tanaka M. Telomerase activity of cultured human pancreatic carcinoma cell lines correlates with their potential for migration and invasion. Cancer 2001;91:496–504.
[75] Tang SJ, Dumot JA, Wang L, Memmesheimer C, Conwell DL, Zuccaro G, Goormastic M, Ormsby AH, Cowell J. Telomerase activity in pancreatic endocrine tumors. Am J Gastroenterol 2002;97:1022–1030.
[76] Sato N, Mizumoto K, Kusumoto M, Nishio S, Maehara N, Urashima T, Ogawa T, Tanaka M. Upregulation of telomerase activity in human pancreatic cancer cells after exposure to etoposide. Br J Cancer 2000;82:1819–1826.
[77] Kusumoto M, Ogawa T, Mizumoto K, Ueno H, Niiyama H, Sato N, Nakamura M, Tanaka M. Adenovirus-mediated p53 gene transduction inhibits telomerase activity independent of its effects on cell cycle arrest and apoptosis in human pancreatic cancer cells. Clin Cancer Res 1999;5:2140- 2147.
[78] Teng LS, Fahey TJ 3rd. Can inhibition of telomerase increase pancreatic cancer cell's susceptibility to chemotherapeutic reagents? Hepatobiliary Pancreat Dis Int 2002;1:155–160.
[79] Wang YF, Guo KJ, Huang BT, Liu Y, Tang XY, Zhang JJ, Xia Q. Inhibitory effects of antisense phosphorothioate oligodeoxynucleotides on pancreatic cancer cell Bxpc-3 telomerase activity and cell growth in vitro. World J Gastroenterol 2006;12:4004–4008.
[80] Schmidt J, Ryschich E, Sievers E, Schmidt-Wolf IG, Buchler MW, Marten A. Telomerase-specific T-cells kill pancreatic tumor cells in vitro and in vivo. Cancer 2006;106:759–764.
[81] Mukherjee P, Ginardi AR, Madsen CS, Sterner CJ, Adriance MC, Tevethia MJ, Gendler SJ. Mice with spontaneous pancreatic cancer naturally develop MUC-1-specific

CTLs that eradicate tumors when adoptively transferred. J Immunol 2000;165:3451–3460.
[82] Kawakami Y, Okada T, Akada M. Development of immunotherapy for pancreatic cancer. Pancreas 2004;28:320–325.
[83] Yamaguchi Y, Ohta K, Kawabuchi Y, Ohshita A, Okita R, Okawaki M, Hironaka K, Matsuura K, Toge T. Feasibility study of adoptive immunotherapy for metastatic lung tumors using peptidepulsed dendritic cell-activated killer (PDAK) cells. Anticancer Res 2005;25:2407–2415.
[84] Balkwill FR, Lee A, Aldam G, Moodie E, Thomas JA, Tavernier J, Fiers W. Human tumor xenografts treated with recombinant human tumor necrosis factor alone or in combination with interferons. Cancer Res 1986;46:3990–3993.
[85] Sato T, Yamauchi N, Sasaki H, Takahashi M, Okamoto T, Sakamaki S, Watanabe N, Niitsu Y. An apoptosis-inducing gene therapy for pancreatic cancer with a combination of 55-kDa tumor necrosis factor (TNF) receptor gene transfection and mutein TNF administration. Cancer Res 1998;58:1677- 1683.
[86] Schmiegel WH, Caesar J, Kalthoff H, Greten H, Schreiber HW, Thiele HG. Antiproliferative effects exerted by recombinant human tumor necrosis factor-alpha (TNF-alpha) and interferon-gamma (IFN-gamma) on human pancreatic tumor cell lines. Pancreas 1988;3:180–188.
[87] Rasmussen H, Rasmussen C, Lempicki M, Durham R, Brough D, King CR, Weichselbaum R. TNFerade Biologic: preclinical toxicology of a novel adenovector with a radiation-inducible promoter, carrying the human tumor necrosis factor alpha gene. Cancer Gene Ther 2002;9:951- 957.
[88] Staba MJ, Mauceri HJ, Kufe DW, Hallahan DE, Weichselbaum RR. Adenoviral TNF-alpha gene therapy and radiation damage tumor vasculature in a human malignant glioma xenograft. Gene Ther 1998;5:293–300.
[89] Chung TD, Mauceri HJ, Hallahan DE, Yu JJ, Chung S, Grdina WL, Yajnik S, Kufe DW, Weichselbaum RR. Tumor necrosis factor-alpha-based gene therapy enhances radiation= cytotoxicity in human prostate cancer. Cancer Gene Ther 1998;5:344–349.
[90] Gupta VK, Park JO, Jaskowiak NT, Mauceri HJ, Seetharam S, Weichselbaum RR, Posner MC. Combined gene therapy and ionizing radiation is a novel approach to treat human esophageal adenocarcinoma. Ann Surg Oncol 2002;9:500–504.
[91] Hallahan DE, Mauceri HJ, Seung LP, Dunphy EJ, Wayne JD, Hanna NN, Toledano A, Hellman S, Kufe DW, Weichselbaum RR. Spatial and temporal control of gene therapy using ionizing radiation. Nat Med 1995;1:786–791.
[92] Posner M, Chang KJ, Rosemurgy A, Stephenson J, Khan M, Reid T, Fisher WE, Waxman I, Von Hoff D, Hecht R Jr. Multi-center phase II/III randomized controlled clinical trial using TNFerade combined with chemoradiation in patients with locally advanced pancreatic cancer (LAPC). J Clin Oncol (Meeting Abstracts) 2007;25:4518.
[93] Du C, Feng N, Jin H, Lee V, Wang M, Wright JA, Young AH. Macrophages play a critical role in the anti-tumor activity of Virulizin. Int J Oncol 2003;23:1341–1346.
[94] Li H, Cao MY, Lee Y, Lee V, Feng N, Benatar T, Jin H, Wang M, Der S, Wright JA, Young AH. Virulizin, a novel immunotherapy agent, activates NK cells through

induction of IL-12 expression in macrophages. Cancer Immunol Immunother 2005;54:1115–1126.

[95] Li H, Cao MY, Lee Y, Benatar T, Lee V, Feng N, Gu X, Liu P, Jin H, Wang M, Der S, Lightfoot J, Wright JA, Young AH. Virulizin, a novel immunotherapy agent, stimulates TNFalpha expression in monocytes/macrophages in vitro and in vivo. Int Immunopharmacol 2007;7:1350–1359.

[96] Benatar T, Cao MY, Lee Y, Feng N, Gu X, Lee V, Jin H, Wang M, Der S, Wright JA, Young AH. Virulizin induces production of IL-17E to enhance antitumor activity by recruitment of eosinophils into tumors. J Clin Oncol (Meeting Abstracts) 2005;23:2537.

[97] Liu C, Ferdinandi ES, Ely G, Joshi SS. Virulizin-2gamma, a novel immunotherapeutic agent, in treatment of human pancreatic cancer xenografts. Int J Oncol 2000;16:1015–1020.

[98] Feng N, Jin H, Wang M, Du C, Wright JA, Young AH. Antitumor activity of Virulizin, a novel biological response modifier (BRM) in a panel of human pancreatic cancer and melanoma xenografts. Cancer Chemother Pharmacol 2003;51:247–255. KPMC Funders Group Author Man

[99] Akiyoshi T, Koba F, Arinaga S, Miyazaki S, Wada T and Tsuji H: Impaired production of interleukin-2 after surgery. Clin Exp Immunol *59*: 45-49, 1985.

[100] Akiyoshi T, Koba F, Arinaga S, Wada T and Tsuji H: *In vitro* effect of interleukin-2 on depression of cell-mediated immune response after surgery. Jpn J Surg *15*: 375-378, 1985.

[101] 100.Brivio F, Lissoni P, Tisi E, Barni S, Tancini G, Rescaldani R and Nociti V: Effect of a preoperative therapy with interleukin-2 on surgery-induced lymphocytopenia in cancer patients: Oncology *49*: 215-218, 1992.

[102] Brivio F, Lissoni P, Brivio O, Marsili MT, Alderi G and Lavorato F: Timing and schedule of perioperative immunotherapy with interleukin-2 in oncological surgery. J Emerg Surg Intensive Care *19*: 59-62, 1996.

[103] Grimm EA, Mazumder A, Zhang HZ and Rosenberg SA: Lymphokine-activated killer cell phenomenon. J Exp Med *155*: 1823-1841, 1982.

[104] Uggeri F, Caprotti R, De Grate L, Crippa S, Nobili C, Penati C, Romano F. Short term preoperative IL-2 immunotherapy in operable pancreatic cancer: a randomized study Hepatogastroenterology. 2009 May-Jun;56(91-92):861-5.

[105] Atzpodien J and Kirchner H: Cancer, cytokines, and cytotoxic cells: interleukin-2 in the immunotherapy of human neoplasms. Klin Wochenschr *68*: 1-11, 1990.

[106] Brivio F, Lissoni P, Barni S, Tancini G, Ardizzoia A and Erba L: Effect of preoperative course of interleumin-2 on surgical and immunological variables in patients with colorectal cancer. Eur J Surg *159*: 43-47, 1993.

[107] Brivio F, Fumagalli L, Lissoni P, Nardone A, Nespoli L, Fattori L, Denova M, Chiarelli M and Nespoli A: Preoperative immunoprophilaxis with interleukin-2 may improve the prognosis in radical surgery for colorectal cancer stage B, C. Anticancer Res *26*: 599-604, 2006.

[108] Cerea K, Romano F, Ferrari-Bravo A, Motta V, Uggeri F, Brivio F and Fumagalli L: Phase I-b study on prevention of surgeryinduced immunodeficiency with

preoperative administration of low-dose subcutaneous interleukin-2 in gastric cancer patients. J Surg Oncol *78*: 32-37, 2001.

[109] Brivio F, Lissoni P, Fumagalli L, Brivio O, Lavorato F, Rescaldani R, Conti A, Roselli MG, Maestroni G and Barni S: Preoperative neuroimmunotherapy with subcutaneous low-dose interleukin-2 and melatonin in patients with gastrointestinal tumors: its efficacy in preventing surgery-induce lymphocytopenia. Oncol Rep 2: 597- 599, 1995.

[110] Fumagalli L, Lissoni P, Di Felice G, Meregalli S, Valsuani G, Mengo S and Rovelli F: Pretreatment serum markers and lymphocyte response to interleukin-2 therapy. Br J Cancer *80*: 407-411, 1999.

[111] Mendelsohn, J. & Baselga, J. The EGF receptor family as targets for cancer therapy. *Oncogene* 19, 6550–6565 (2000).

[112] Schwarte-Waldhoff, I., Volpert, O. V. & Bouck, N. P. SMAD4/DPC4-mediated tumor suppression through suppression of angiogenesis. *Proc. Natl Acad. Sci. USA* 97, 9624–9629 (2000).

[113] Nair, S. *et al.* Synergy between tumor immunotherapy and antiangiogenic therapy. *Blood* 102, 964–971 (2003).

[114] Gabrilovich, D. I. *et al.* Antibodies to vascular endothelial growth factor enhance the efficacy of cancer immunotherapy by improving endogenous dendritic cell function. *Clin. Cancer Res.* 5, 2963–2970 (1999)

[115] Xiong, H. Q. *et al.* Cetuximab, a monoclonal antibody targeting the epidermal growth factor receptor, in combination with gemcitabine for advanced pancreatic Cancer: a multicenter phase II Trial. *J. Clin. Oncol.* 22, 2610–2616 (2004).

[116] Kindler, H. L. *et al.* Bevacizumab plus gemcitabine in patients with advanced pancreatic cancer: Updated results of a multi-center phase II trial. *Proc. Am. Soc. Clin. Oncol.* 23, A4009 (2004)

[117] Walpoe, M. E. *et al.* Her-2/neu specific monoclonal antibodies collaborate with her-2/neu targeted granulocyte macrophage stimulating factor secreting whole cell vaccination to augment CD8+ T cell effector function and tumor free survival in her-2/neu transgenic mice. *J. Immunol.* 171, 2161–2169 (2003).

[118] Hruban, R. H. *et al. K-ras* oncogene activation in adenocarcinoma of the pancreas. *Am. J. Path.* 143, 545–554 (1993).

[119] Gjertsen, M. K. *et al.* Vaccination with mutant ras peptides and induction of T-cell responsiveness in pancreatic carcinoma patients carrying the corresponding ras mutation. *Lancet* 346, 1399–1400 (1995).

[120] Finn, O.J. *et al.* MUC-1 epithelial tumor mucin-based immunity and vaccines. *Immunol. Rev.* 145, 61–89 (1995).

[121] Apostopopoulos, V. & McKenzie, I. F. Cellular mucins: targets for immunotherapy. *Crit. Rev. Immunol.* 14, 293–309 (1994).

[122] Hammarstrom, S. The carcinoembryonic antigen (CEA) family: structures, suggested functions and expression in normal and malignant tissues. *Semin. Cancer Biol.* 9, 67–81 (1999).

[123] Achtar, M. *et al.* Mutant ras vaccine in advanced cancers. *Proc. Am. Soc. Clin. Oncol.* 22, A677 (2003).

[124] Jaffee, E. M. *et al.* A novel allogeneic GM-CSF secreting tumor vaccine for pancreatic cancer: a phase I trial of safety and immune activation. *J. Clin. Oncol.* 19, 145–156 (2001).

[125] Morse, M. *et al.* Phase I study of immunization with dendritic cells modified with recombinant fowlpox encoding carcinoembryonic antigen (CEA) and the triad of costimulatory molecules CD54, CD58 and CD80 (rF-CEA(6D)-TRICOM) in patients with advanced malignancies. *Proc. Am. Soc. Clin. Oncol.* 23, A2508 (2004).

[126] Finn, O. J. *et al.* A phase Ib study of a MUC1 pulsed autologous dendritic cell vaccine as adjuvant therapy in patients with resected pancreatic or biliary tumors. *Proc. Am. Soc. Clin. Oncol.* 23, A2578 (2004).

[127] Marshall, J. L. *et al.* Phase I study of sequential vaccinations with fowlpox-CEA(6D)-TRICOM alone and sequentially with vaccinia-CEA(6D)-TRICOM, with and without granulocyte-macrophage colony stimulating factor, in patients with carcinoembryonic antigen-expressing carcinomas. *J. Clin. Oncol.* 23, 720–731 (2005).

[128] Gilliam, A. D. *et al.* Randomised double blind placebo controlled multi-centre group sequential trial of G17DT for patients with advanced pancreatic cancer unsuitable or unwilling to take chemotherapy. *Proc. Am. Soc. Clin. Oncol.* 23, A2511 (2004).

[129] Harris, J. C. *et al.* The biological and therapeutic importance of gastrin gene expression in pancreatic adenocarcinomas. *Cancer Res.* 64, 5624–5631 (2004).

[130] Laheru, D. A. *et al.* A feasibility study of a GM-CSF secreting irradiated whole cell allogeneic vaccine (GVAX) alone or in sequence with cytoxan for patients with locally advanced or metastatic pancreatic cancer. *Proc. Am. Assoc. Cancer Res.* A54 (2004).

[131] Takigawa, Y. *et al.* Anti-tumor effect induced by dendritic cell (DC) based immunotherapy against peritoneal dissemination of the hamster pancreatic cancer. *Cancer Lett.* 215, 179–186 (2004).

[132] Jaffee EM, Hruban RH, Biedrzycki B, Laheru D, Schepers K, Sauter PR, Goemann M, Coleman J, Grochow L, Donehower RC, Lillemoe KD, O'Reilly S, Abrams RA, Pardoll DM, Cameron JL, Yeo CJ. Novel allogeneic granulocyte-macrophage colony-stimulating factor-secreting tumor vaccine for pancreatic cancer: a phase I trial of safety and immune activation. J Clin Oncol 2001;19:145–156

[133] Kimura M, Tagawa M, Yoshida Y, Takenouchi T, Takenaga K, Azuma K, Yamaguchi T, Saisho H, Sakiyama S. Impaired in vivo tumor growth of human pancreatic carcinoma cells retrovirally transduced with GM-CSF gene. Anticancer Res 1998;18:165–170.

[134] Laheru D, Yeo C, Biedrzycki B, Solt S, Lutz E, Onners B, Tartakovsky I, Herman J, Hruban R, Piantadosi S, Jaffee E. A safety and efficacy trial of lethally irradiated allogeneic pancreatic tumor cells transfected with the GM-CSF gene in combination with adjuvant chemoradiotherapy for the treatment of adenocarcinoma of the pancreas. J Clin Oncol (Meeting Abstracts) 2007;25:3010.

[135] Toubaji A, Achtar MS, Herrin VE, Provenzano M, Bernstein S, Brent-Steel T, Marincola F, Khleif SN. Immunotherapeutic role of mutant ras peptide-based vaccine as an adjuvant in pancreatic and colorectal cancer. J Clin Oncol (Meeting Abstracts) 2005;23:2573. 346.

[136] Gjertsen MK, Bakka A, 136.Breivik J, Saeterdal I, Gedde-Dahl T 3rd, Stokke KT, Solheim BG, Egge TS, Soreide O, Thorsby E, Gaudernack G. Ex vivo ras peptide vaccination in patients with advanced pancreatic cancer: results of a phase I/II study. Int J Cancer 1996;65:450–453. [PubMed: 8621226]

[137] Gjertsen MK, Buanes T, Rosseland AR, Bakka A, Gladhaug I, Soreide O, Eriksen JA, Moller M, Baksaas I, Lothe RA, Saeterdal I, Gaudernack G. Intradermal ras peptide vaccination with granulocyte-macrophage colony-stimulating factor as adjuvant: Clinical and immunological responses in patients with pancreatic adenocarcinoma. Int J Cancer 2001;92:441–450.

[138] Achtar MS, Toubaji A, Herrin V, Gause B, Hamilton M, Berhens R, Grollman F, Bernstein S, Khleif S. Phase II clinical trial of mutant Ras peptide vaccine in combination with GM-CSF and IL-2 in advanced cancer patients. J Clin Oncol Meeting Abstracts) 2007;25:3067.

[139] Buanes T, Bernhardt S, Lislerud K, Gladhaug I, Moeller M, Eriksen JA, Gaudernack G. RAS peptide vaccination in resected pancreatic cancer patients - persistence of anti tumour response and long term survival. J Clin Oncol (Meeting Abstracts) 2007;25:4543.

[140] Lieberman SM, Horig H, Kaufman HL. Innovative treatments for pancreatic cancer. Surg Clin North Am 2001;81:715–739.

[141] Duraker N, Hot S, Polat Y, Hobek A, Gencler N, Urhan N. CEA, CA 19-9, and CA 125 in the differential diagnosis of benign and malignant pancreatic diseases with or without jaundice. J Surg Oncol 2007;95:142–147.

[142] Ozkan H, Kaya M, Cengiz A. Comparison of tumor marker CA 242 with CA 19-9 and carcinoembryonic antigen (CEA) in pancreatic cancer. Hepatogastroenterology 2003;50:1669- 1674.

[143] Banfi G, Bravi S, Ardemagni A, Zerbi A. CA 19.9, CA 242 and CEA in the diagnosis and followup of pancreatic cancer. Int J Biol Markers 1996;11:77–81.

[144] Garnett CT, Greiner JW, Tsang KY, Kudo-Saito C, Grosenbach DW, Chakraborty M, Gulley JL, Arlen PM, Schlom J, Hodge JW. TRICOM vector based cancer vaccines. Curr Pharm Des 2006;12:351–361.

[145] Marshall JL, Gulley JL, Arlen PM, Beetham PK, Tsang KY, Slack R, Hodge JW, Doren S, Grosenbach DW, Hwang J, Fox E, Odogwu L, Park S, Panicali D, Schlom J. Phase I study of sequential vaccinations with fowlpox-CEA(6D)-TRICOM alone and sequentially with vaccinia- CEA(6D)-TRICOM, with and without granulocyte-macrophage colony-stimulating factor, in patients with carcinoembryonic antigen-expressing carcinomas. J Clin Oncol 2005;23:720–731.

[146] Marshall JL, Hawkins MJ, Tsang KY, Richmond E, Pedicano JE, Zhu M, Schlom J. Phase I Study in Cancer Patients of a Replication-Defective Avipox Recombinant Vaccine That Expresses Human Carcinoembryonic Antigen. J Clin Oncol 1999;17:332.

[147] Ramanathan RK, Lee KM, McKolanis J, Hitbold E, Schraut W, Moser AJ, Warnick E, Whiteside T, Osborne J, Kim H, Day R, Troetschel M, Finn OJ. Phase I study of a MUC1 vaccine composed of different doses of MUC1 peptide with SB-AS2

adjuvant in resected and locally advanced pancreatic cancer. Cancer Immunol Immunother 2005;54:254–264.

[148] Nordqvist, C., editor. Therion reports results of phase 3 PANVAC-VF trial and announces plans for company sale. Medical News Today. 2006.

[149] Brett BT, Smith SC, Bouvier CV, Michaeli D, Hochhauser D, Davidson BR, Kurzawinski TR, Watkinson AF, Van Someren N, Pounder RE, Caplin ME. Phase II study of anti-gastrin-17 antibodies, raised to G17DT, in advanced pancreatic cancer. J Clin Oncol 2002;20:4225–4231.

[150] Gilliam AD, Topuzov EG, Garin AM, Pulay I, Broome P, Watson SA, Rowlands B, Takhar A, Beckingham I. Randomised, double blind, placebo-controlled, multi-centre, group-sequential trial of G17DT for patients with advanced pancreatic cancer unsuitable or unwilling to take chemotherapy. J Clin Oncol (Meeting Abstracts) 2004;22:2511.

[151] Shapiro J, Marshall J, Karasek P, Figer A, Oettle H, Couture F, Jeziorski K, Broome P, Hawkins R. G17DT+gemcitabine [Gem] versus placebo+Gem in untreated subjects with locally advanced, recurrent, or metastatic adenocarcinoma of the pancreas: Results of a randomized, double-blind, multinational, multicenter study. J Clin Oncol (Meeting Abstracts) 2005;23:LBA4012.

[152] Thomas AM, Santarsiero LM, Lutz ER, Armstrong TD, Chen YC, Huang LQ, Laheru DA, Goggins M, Hruban RH, Jaffee EM. Mesothelin-specific CD8(+) T cell responses provide evidence of in vivo cross-priming by antigen-presenting cells in vaccinated pancreatic cancer patients. J Exp Med 2004;200:297–306.

[153] Gaffney MC, Goedegebuure P, Kashiwagi H, Hornick JR, Thaker RI, Eberlein T, Hawkins WG. DNA vaccination targeting mesothelin combined with anti-GITR antibody induces rejection of pancreatic adenocarcinoma. AACR Meeting Abstracts 2006;2006:329

[154] Bernhardt SL, Gjertsen MK, Trachsel S, Moller M, Eriksen JA, Meo M, Buanes T, Gaudernack G. Telomerase peptide vaccination of patients with non-resectable pancreatic cancer: A dose escalating phase I/II study. Br J Cancer 2006;95:1474–1482.

[155] Kawakami, Y., Okada, T. & Akada, M. Development of immunotherapy for pancreas cancer. *Pancreas* 28, 320–325 (2004).

[156] Nakatsura, T. *et al.* Cellular and humoral immune responses to a human pancreatic cancer antigen, coactosin-like protein, originally defined by the SEREX method. *Eur. J. Immunol* 32, 826–836 (2002).

[157] Rosenberg, S. A. Progress in human tumour immunology and immunotherapy. *Nature* 411, 380–384 (2001)

[158] Boon, T., *et al.* Tumor antigens recognized by T lymphocytes. *Annu. Rev. Immunol.* 12, 337–365 (1994).

[159] Argani, P. *et al.* Discovery of new markers of cancer through serial analysis of gene expression (SAGE): prostate stem cell antigen (PSCA) is overexpressed in pancreatic adenocarcinoma. *Cancer Res.* 61, 4320–4324 (2001).

[160] Leach, S. D. Mouse models of pancreatic cancer: the fur is finally flying! *Cancer Cell* 5, 7–11 (2004).

[161] Hingorani, S. R. *et al.* Preinvasive and invasive ductal pancreatic cancer and its early detection in the mouse. *Cancer Cell* 4, 437–450 (2003).

[162] Olive, K. P. *et al.* Mutant p53 gain of function in two mouse models of Li–Fraumeni syndrome. *Cell* 119, 847–860 (2004).

9

Bacterial Immunotherapy -Antitumoral Potential of the Streptococcal Toxin Streptolysin S-

Claudia Maletzki[1], Bernd Kreikemeyer[2], Peggy Bodammer[3], Joerg Emmrich[3] and Michael Linnebacher[1]
[1]*Department of General, Vascular, Thoracic and Transplantation Surgery, Section of Molecular Oncology and Immunotherapy,*
[2]*Institute of Medical Microbiology, Virology and Hygiene,*
[3]*Division of Gastroenterology Department of Internal Medicine University of Rostock, Rostock, Germany*

1. Introduction

Chronic infections can lead to cancer. However, acute infection has beneficial effects often contributing to complete eradication of tumors. In the wake of this, bacteria and their related products were applied therapeutically for experimental immunotherapy. They exhibit direct antitumoral potential and are recognized by the host's immune system via Toll-like receptors (TLRs) finally promoting pro-inflammatory, often Th1-directed immune responses.

Recently, we described that local injection of live as well as lysed gram-positive Group A Streptococci (GAS) eradicates established pancreatic tumors in mice (Linnebacher et al., 2008; Maletzki et al., 2008). This antitumoral effect could be attributed to activation of immune response mechanisms including both the innate and even more important, the adaptive arm of the immune system. In the face of the vigorous immune attack induced by *S. pyogenes*, the identification of factors responsible for tumor disintegration might provide the basis for development of therapeutic approaches. Amongst other virulence factors delivered by *S. pyogenes*, the cytolysins Streptolysin O (SLO) and S (SLS) represent the most obvious therapeutically active candidates (Fraser & Proft, 2008; Hobohm et al., 2008; Nizet et al., 2008). SLO is an oxygen-labile, pore-forming toxin mediating cytolysis by disturbing the balance between influxes and effluxes across the cell membrane. While SLS is non-immunogenic in the natural course of infection and can clinically be identified by beta-haemolysis surrounding GAS colonies grown on blood agar. Besides their capacity to lyse erythrocytes, SLS also exerts cytolytic effects towards tumor cells and is by weight one of the most potent cytotoxins known (Ginsberg, 1999; Taketo & Taketo, 1966).

To address the question of the SLS contribution to the antitumoral effects observed in our previous studies, we performed a series of *in vivo* experiments in our murine syngeneic

Panc02 tumor model using different strategies of SLS-inactivation. Endpoints of the study were survival and tumor response. In a first series of experiments, a vital mutant strain, unable to produce SLS (ΔsagA) was injected into tumor-carrying mice. This ΔsagA mutant has been described to exhibit reduced cytotoxicity. *In vitro* and in a nude mouse model *in vivo*, effects were induced by minimal inflammation and lesser necrotic skin lesions than the isogenic wildtype strain (Datta et al., 2005). However, to circumvent the potential risk of unpleasant side effects of live bacteria such as systemic toxicity, another microbial preparation of SLS-inactivated bacteria (by heating) was employed. Our *in vivo* data show that local application of SLS-negative agents attenuates the antitumoral effects. Moreover, potent immune responses are only marginally induced, most likely because of reduced tumor cell impairment after infection, finally leading to an inhibition of vigorous antitumoral activity.

In summary, when comparing with our earlier findings on using *S. pyogenes* as an active immunotherapeutic compound, the present data imply SLS as major antitumoral molecule both directly by acting on tumor cells and indirectly by activating the immune system.

2. Material & methods

2.1 Cell culture & mice

All cell lines (Panc02, EL4, CMT-93, and MC3T3-E1) were maintained in DMEM/HamsF12 supplemented with 10% fetal calf serum (FCS), L-glutamine (2mmol/l) and antibiotics. All media and supplements were from PAA unless stated otherwise (Cölbe, Germany). Female 8–10-week-old C57Bl/6N mice were purchased from Charles River Inc. (Sulzfeld, Germany). Animals were exposed to cycles of 12 h light/12 h darkness and received standard food and water ad libitum. Upon approval by the local animal welfare committee, experiments were performed in accordance with the German legislation on protection of animals and the "Guide for the Care and Use of Laboratory Animals".

2.2 Bacteria, toxin and culture conditions

Bacteria (*S. pyogenes* serotype M49 strain 591; the ΔsagA mutant isogenic to strain 591 is a kind gift from Victor Nizet: A detailed description of how this mutant was generated can be found in (Datta et al., 2005)) were cultured in Todd-Hewitt (TH) broth or on TH agar (Oxoid Unipath, Wesel, Germany), both supplemented with 0.5 % yeast extract (THY) overnight to mid-log phase. Concentration was adjusted on the basis of an optical density reading at 600 nm and on plating analysis. Heat-inactivation of bacteria was obtained by one-hour incubation in a water bath at 75 °C. Inactivation was confirmed by plating samples on sheep blood agar followed by over night incubation at 37 °C and 5 % CO_2. The purified toxin SLS (originally obtained from Sigma Aldrich, Munich, Germany) was dissolved in sterile PBS and supplemented with complete cell culture medium before treatment of cells.

2.3 Hemolysis assay for SLS activity

Hemolytic activity of SLS was determined by hemoglobin release from whole blood cells after 4 and 24 h incubation with bacteria or their related products. Briefly, whole blood of healthy donors was seeded in 96-well plates and supplemented with microbia. Following the incubation time, cell-free supernatants were transferred into a new 96-well plate and absorption was measured on a plate reader at 340 nm. Hemolytic activity was quantified by setting values of untreated cells as 1 and all other data were given as x-fold increase.

2.4 Cellular cytotoxicity assays

Toxicity of bacteria towards tumor cells was quantified using a cytotoxicity detection kit (Roche, Mannheim, Germany) according to the manufacturer's instructions. Quantification was performed by subsequent measurement on a plate reader at 492 nm.

For detection of apoptosis, activity of Caspase 3 was analyzed using the BD ApoAlert Caspase Assay plate system according to the manufacturer's instructions (BD Biosciences, Heidelberg, Germany). Cells were trypsinized and subsequently lysed. Quantification of Caspase 3 activity was performed by fluorometric detection on a Cytofluor 2300 (Millipore, Schwalbach, Germany, ex/em: 380/460 nm).

2.5 Pancreatic tumor model & treatment regimen

Under brief ether anaesthesia $1*10^6$ Panc02 were injected subcutaneously (s.c.) into the right hind leg. Tumor growth was routinely controlled at least twice a week and tumor volume was estimated according to the formula: $V= width^2 * length * 0.52$. After tumor establishment animals were subdivided into experimental groups. All treatments were performed by local, intratumoral application of bacterial preparations each dissolved in 50 µl of phosphate-buffered saline (PBS) according to the following treatment regimen: One group was given heat-inactivated *S. pyogenes* (8×10^7 cfu, four injections once a week, n=6). The second group received a single injection of the SLS-mu (ΔsagA). For control, mice were administered equivalent volumes of solvent alone (vehicle-treated controls, saline, n=6) or left without treatment (control, n=6). Tumor carrying mice (treatment, control) were sacrificed at day 28 or when they became moribund before the tumor volume reached 2000 mm^3. At the end of each experiment, tumors as well as spleens, mesenteric lymph nodes, and blood samples were removed from selected animals for further analysis. For visualization of tumor-infiltrating leukocytes, frozen sections of resected tumor tissues (6 µm) were stained by the As-D chloroacetate esterase (As-D) technique. Numbers of leukocytes/mm^2 were determined in blinded counts by positive staining and morphology in 20 consecutive high power fields (HPF).

2.6 Phenotyping of lymphocyte subpopulations by flow cytometry

Leukocytes from treated and non-treated animals were labeled using the following FITC-conjugated rat anti-mouse monoclonal antibodies (mAbs): CD3, CD19, NK1.1 (1 µg, Immunotools, Friesoythe, Germany), and Phycoerythrin (PE)-conjugated rat anti-mouse mAbs: CD4, CD8 (Miltenyi Biotec, Bergisch Gladbach, Germany). Afterwards, erythrocytes were lysed using FACS Lysing Solution (BD Pharmingen, Heidelberg, Germany). Negative controls consisted of blood lymphocytes stained with the appropriate isotypes (BD Pharmingen). Samples were analyzed on a FACSCalibur Cytometer (BD Biosciences). Data analysis was performed using CellQuest software (BD Biosciences) and gating on total leukocytes (Mounting View, BD Biosciences). Relative numbers are given.

2.7 ELISPOT assay for Interferon-γ–secreting lymphocytes

IFN-γ-specific, mAb (Mabtech, Hamburg, Germany) -coated, 96-well microtiter plates were filled with 1 x 10^4 target cells/well (Panc02, EL4, CMT-93, MC3T3-E1, and peripheral blood mononuclear cells (PBMC)) and incubated for 2 h. Splenocytes (10^5) were given to the targets and co-cultured overnight. Finally, bound antibody was visualized by BCIP/NBT (KPL, Gaithersburg, Maryland, USA), and spots were counted using a dissection microscope (Zeiss, Oberkochen, Germany). Presented are the numbers of IFN-γ-secreting cells per 10^5 effector cells corrected for background levels counted in the absence of target cells, which usually was between 10–50 spots/10^5 cells. Target cells without effector cells showed no background level.

2.8 LDH cytotoxicity assay

The colorimetric CytoTox-One Homogeneous Membrane Integrity Assay (Promega, Madison, WI) was used evaluating lactate dehydrogenase (LDH) release from lysed cells. Experiments were performed as described before (Maletzki et al., 2008).

2.9 Bio-plex protein array system

A panel of serum cytokines was measured in duplicate using the Bio-Plex Protein Array system (BioRad, Munich, Germany), according to the manufacturer's instructions. With the Bio-Plex cytokine assay kit in combination with the Bio-Plex Manager Software, serum IFN-γ, TNF-α, IL-6, IL-10, GM-CSF (granulocyte macrophage colony stimulating factor), and G-CSF (granulocyte-colony stimulating factor) levels were assessed. Values of the respective serum cytokine levels of untreated control mice were set as 1, and all other data were given as x-fold increase.

2.10 Statistical analysis

All values are expressed as mean ± SEM. After proving the assumption of normality, differences between saline and treated animals were determined by using the unpaired Student's *t*-test. If normality failed, the nonparametric Mann-Whitney *U*-Test was applied. Similarly, differences between treated and non-treated cell *in vitro* were calculated by using the nonparametric Mann-Whitney *U*-Test. Data were recruited from experiments which had been done in triplicates and replicated at least three times. The tests were performed by using Sigma-Stat 3.0 (Jandel Corp, San Rafael, CA). The criterion for significance was set to $p < 0.05$.

3. Results

3.1 In vitro analysis

First, activity of SLS from different bacterial preparations was analyzed in a simple hemoglobin release assay (Figure 1). As expected, the purified toxin mediated substantial lysis of erythrocytes within a few hours. In contrast, lysis was completely absent post infection with the ΔsagA strain or the heat-inactivated form of the M49wt, thereby confirming inactivation of the toxin. As a control, vital M49 bacteria and the lysate, used in our previous studies (Maletzki et al., 2008), were employed. Both preparations mediated nearly complete lysis of erythrocytes.

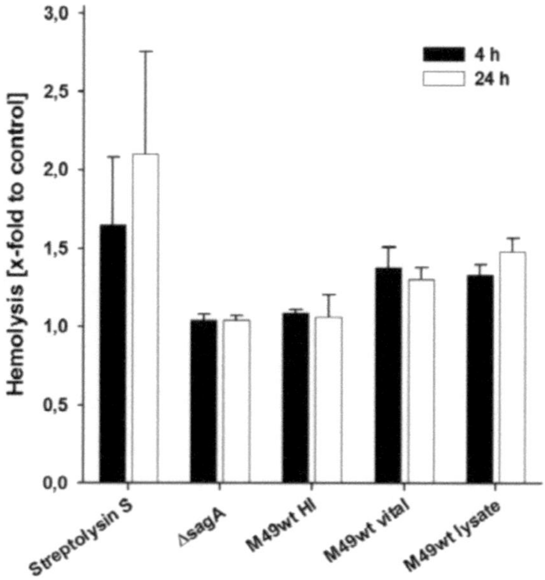

Fig. 1. Lytic activity of different bacterial preparations towards erythrocytes in whole blood samples. Following treatment with increasing concentrations of bacteria, cell-free supernatants were harvested and absorption was measured on a plate reader at 340 nm. Lytic activity was quantified by setting values of untreated cells as 1, and all other data were given as x-fold increase. Results show data from at least three separate experiments each performed with two healthy volunteer's blood samples. Values are given as the mean±SEM.

In order to elucidate, if SLS also directly damages tumor cells, we applied the purified toxin in LDH release experiments. In particular, Panc02 tumor cells were treated with three increasing concentrations (25, 50, and 100 U/ml) for six hours. These analyses revealed a dose-dependent increase in cell damage with a maximum of up to 65% (100 U/ml). To a minor part, these effects could be attributed to the induction of apoptosis as the activity of the effector caspase 3 slightly increased after treatment with the 100 U/ml doses of SLS (Figure 2).

In line with these findings, a ΔsagA strain of *S. pyogenes* mediated no significant growth inhibition or killing activity at a multiplicity of infection of 25 for four and six hours (Figure 2). Also, activity of Caspase 3 was not altered post infection.

3.2 SLS-deficient preparations of S. pyogenes have minor antitumoral potential

To further clarify the antitumoral potential of the toxin SLS a series of *in vivo* experiments using two different preparations of inactivated SLS was performed (Figure 3a). Panc02 tumors established subcutaneously in C57Bl/6 mice were infected with the ΔsagA strain (10^7 cfu). The intratumoral administration of ΔsagA did not affect pancreatic carcinoma growth within the first three weeks. Palpable tumors continued to grow and reached an average size of 723.8 ± 95.8 mm^3, which was comparable to tumor sizes of control animals (saline: 841.4 ± 96.3 mm^3). Thereafter, tumors in the infection group became frequently ulcerous and necrotized. This finally resulted in about 40 % reduced tumor volumes compared to saline-treated animals (day 28: 689.2 ± 119.8 mm^3 vs. saline: 1228.1 ± 220.2 mm^3, $p < 0.05$).

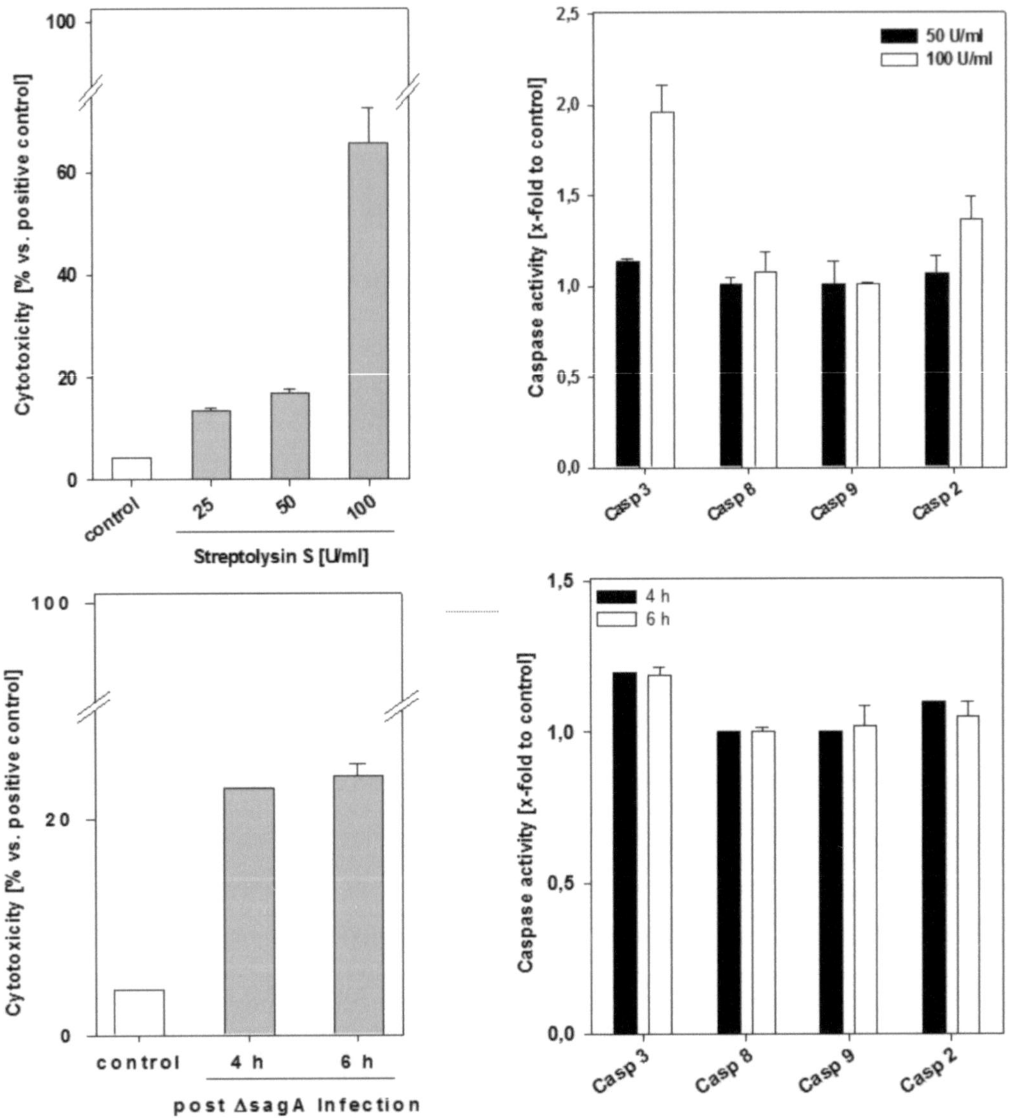

Fig. 2. ***In vitro* analysis on direct effects of SLS on tumor cells.** (A) Quantitative analysis of SLS cytotoxicity towards Panc02 cells as assessed by either LDH release or caspase activity following a 6 h incubation period. These analyses revealed a dose-dependent increase in cell damage. (B) Quantitative analysis of the ΔsagA effects on Panc02 tumor cells. Infection with the ΔsagA strain mediated no significant cytotoxicity, detected by LDH release. Results show data from three separate experiments. Values are given as the mean±SEM. $^{*}p<0.05$ vs. control, *U*-Test.

To validate these findings, tumor-carrying animals were repeatedly treated with a bacterial preparation which was preheated to inactivate SLS. Similar to what has been observed after i.t. infection with the ΔsagA strain, injection of heat-inactivated streptococci mediated no significant alteration of Panc02 tumor growth until day 14 post start of therapy. However, when comparing to controls, tumors showed a trend towards growth retardation, suggesting only reduced but not completely abolished antitumoral potential of the heat-inactivated bacteria. Hence, the final tumor volume at day 28 was significantly lower than in saline-treated mice (693.2 ± 63.0 mm^3 vs. 1154.5 ± 277.1 mm^3, $p < 0.05$).

3.3 Survival

Animals were sacrificed at day 28 post start of therapy. Infection with the ΔsagA strain was well tolerated by most animals, with only one animal displaying signs of systemic bacterial infection (i.e. weight loss, ataxia). Because of the severity of infection, this animal was euthanized and related data excluded. As expected, the heat-inactivated bacterial preparation had no negative impact on survival (Figure 3b).

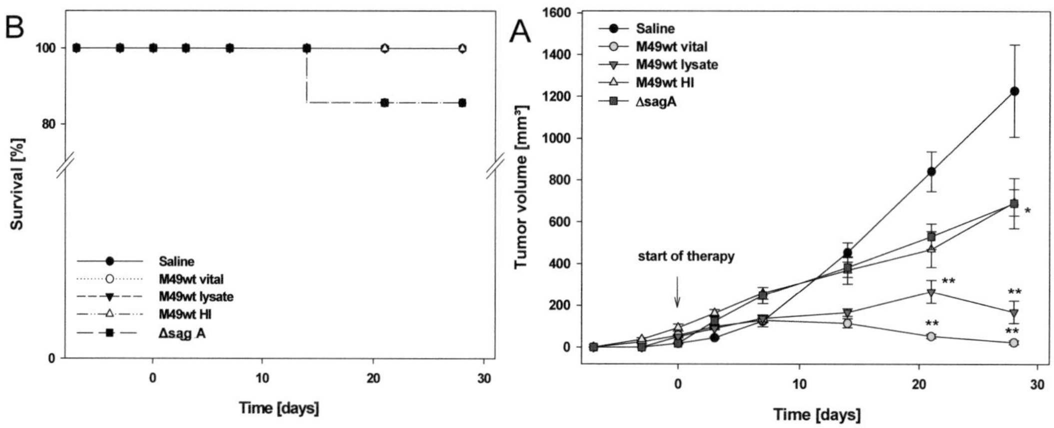

Fig. 3. **Data of *in vivo* analysis of Panc02-tumor carrying C57Bl/6N mice.** (A) Tumor growth kinetics and (B) survival curve after i.t. application of bacteria. Treatment regimens comprised the vital SLS-deficient ΔsagA strain (1 x 10^7 cfu,), which is isogenic to the M49 wildtype and heat-inactivated preparations of the M49 wildtype (8 x 10^7 cfu, four injections once a week, n=6). Control mice were administered equivalent volumes of solvent alone (saline, n=6) or left without treatment (tumor, n=6). Animals were sacrificed at day 28 or when they became moribund before the tumor volume reached 2000 mm^3. Tumor growth was only at later stages affected and when comparing with our previous studies on using vital as well as lysed wild type bacteria, to a lesser extend (graphical presentation adopted from Linnebacher et al., 2008 and Maletzki et al., 2008). *$p<0.05$ vs. saline, **$p<0.001$ vs. saline *U*-Test.

3.4 Gross findings & hematological alterations post ΔsagA infection

To further validate the potential of SLS to influence tumor growth, we analyzed systemic parameters of animals treated with ΔsagA in more detail. Analysis of blood samples from ΔsagA infected animals revealed no alteration regarding the number of circulating leukocytes. However, thrombocyte as well as hematocrit levels were found to be decreased post infection (Figure 4a). Similarly, activities of the plasma enzymes ASAT and LDH were reduced, while levels of ALAT were not affected by bacteria (Figure 4b). In this case, the infection-mediated decrease in blood LDH activities might correlate with the retardation of tumor growth observed *in vivo*.

As these data indicated an inflammatory reaction in the ΔsagA treated animals, we subsequently determined plasma cytokine levels from infected and non-infected animals (Figure 4c). Analysis of the neutrophile chemotaxis polypeptide G-CSF and the GM-CSF showed slight increases post infection which were, however not statistically significant. Levels of both cytokines displayed 2-fold rises post infection ($p=0.256$ vs. saline (G-CSF) and $p= 0.007$ vs. saline (GM-CSF), *t*-test). A similar pattern was seen for IL6 ($p=0.62$), while the Th1 cytokines TNF-α and IFN-γ showed no alterations at all.

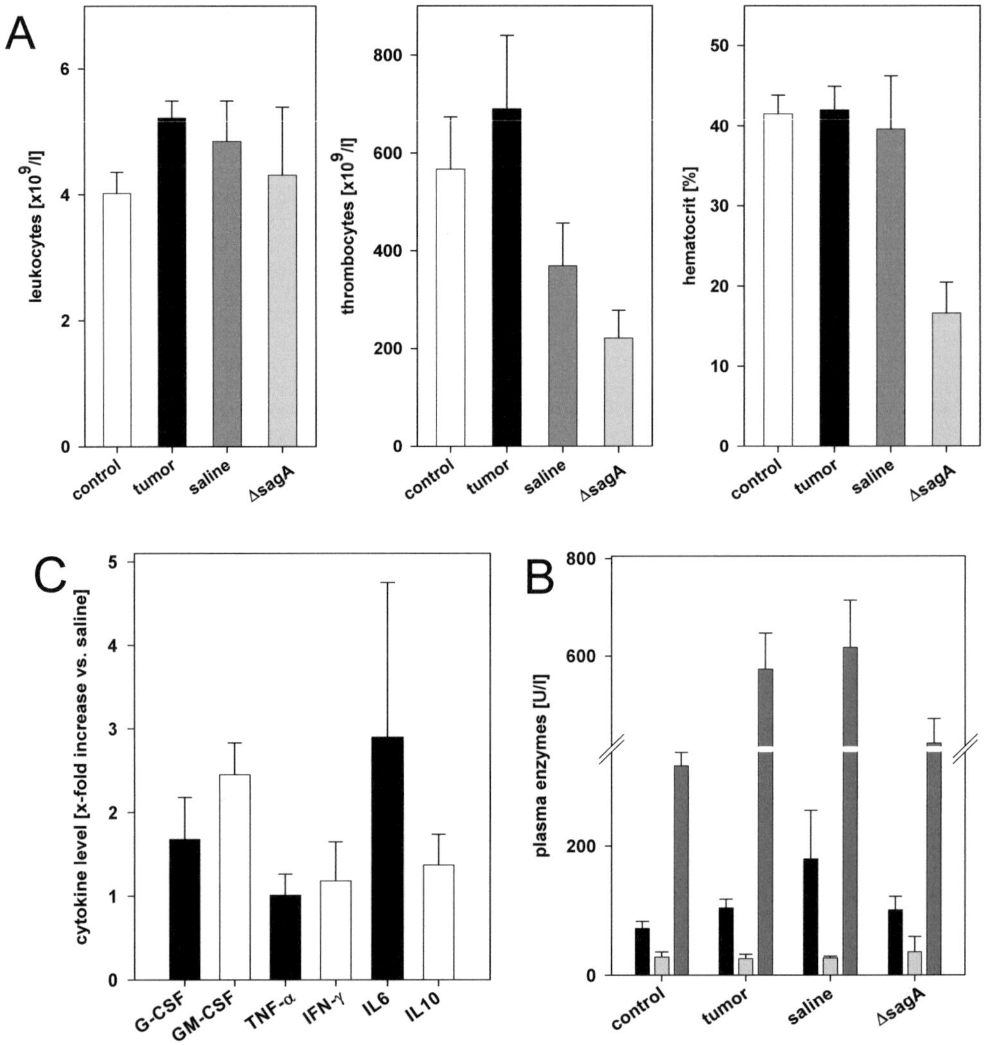

Fig. 4. **Assessment of systemic blood parameters.** (A) Numbers of leukocytes, thrombocytes, and hematocrit levels as well as (B) plasma enzyme activities of ALAT, ASAT and LDH from ΔsagA-infected and control animals at day 28. (C) Levels of Th_1 and Th_2 cytokines in serum of treated and untreated mice. Mice received a single i.t. infection of the ΔsagA strain (1x 10^7 cfu). Control animals received equivalent volumes of PBS (saline) or no injection (tumor). Values are given as the mean±SEM. *U*-Test.

3.5 Flow cytometric phenotyping of circulating leukocytes

Next, flow cytometric phenotyping of circulating leukocytes was performed. As shown in Table 1, we observed higher numbers of circulating NK cells in animals treated with the ΔsagA strain (34.6 ± 7.1% vs. saline 16.5 ± 2.7%). Similarly, levels of $Gr1^+$ granulocytes were also raised (32.5 ± 4.6% vs. saline 25.0 ± 3.0%). Regarding the number of T cells, no significant differences were obtained between the infection and control groups. Likewise, numbers of circulating $CD19^+$ pre B cells showed no alteration after therapy with values remaining similar to controls. Thus, in our experimental system, microbial therapy with SLS-deficient or heat-inactivated *S. pyogenes* preparations seemed to affect exclusively the innate arm of the immune system.

	Control	Tumor	Saline	ΔsagA
$CD3^+CD4^+$	19.5 ± 1.9	15.7 ± 1.4	8.6 ± 1.4	14.1 ± 0.9
$CD3^+CD8^+$	10.9 ± 0.7	9.5 ± 1.3	6.9 ± 1.7	10.3 ± 0.5
$CD19^+$	56.5 ± 1.9	42.2 ± 4.1	31.4 ± 2.5	41.6 ± 4.2
$NK1.1^+$	14.8 ± 2.6	15.8 ± 1.8	16.5 ± 2.7	34.6 ± 7.1
$Gr1^+$	9.5 ± 2.4	19.8 ± 3.1	25.0 ± 3.0	32.5 ± 4.6

Values are given as mean ± SEM. ΔsagA-infected animals (n=7); saline-treated animals (n=6); tumor control animals (n=7); *U*-Test.

Table 1. Flow cytometric phenotyping of whole blood in control groups (control, tumor, saline) and post infection with the ΔsagA strain (% positive cells).

3.6 Analysis of antitumoral immune responses

Despite raised levels of infiltrating granulocytes, especially in the boundary areas of treated tumors (Figure 5a), we did not observe any significant difference in the number of $CD4^+$ and $CD8^+$ lymphocytes infiltrating tumors between control and treatment groups (data not shown).

In a first series of experiments, reactivity against syngeneic tumor cell lines was tested in ELISpot assays using lymph node derived lymphocytes as effector cells from control as well as ΔsagA-treated animals. Surprisingly, recognition of tumor cells was restricted to the syngeneic colorectal carcinoma cell line CMT-93. Other tested cells (i.e. Panc02, EL4) did not induce release of IFN-γ from lymphocytes of ΔsagA treated animals (Figure 5b).

In a more functional cytotoxicity assay, splenocytes were used as effectors. Again, Panc02 tumor cells were only ineffectively lysed by immune cells from infected mice (22.1 ± 2.5 % vs. saline 6.7 ± 1.7 %). Similar results were obtained with the non-cancerous MC3T3-E1 fibroblasts and with PBMCs (Figure 5c), indicating only little specific killing activity of effector cells. In contrast, we again observed most lytic activity against the syngeneic tumor cell line CMT-93 (35.8 ± 12.7 % vs. saline: 22.2% ± 7.5 %) and additionally against EL4 (38.6 ± 11.4 % vs. saline: 18.2% ± 3.0 %).

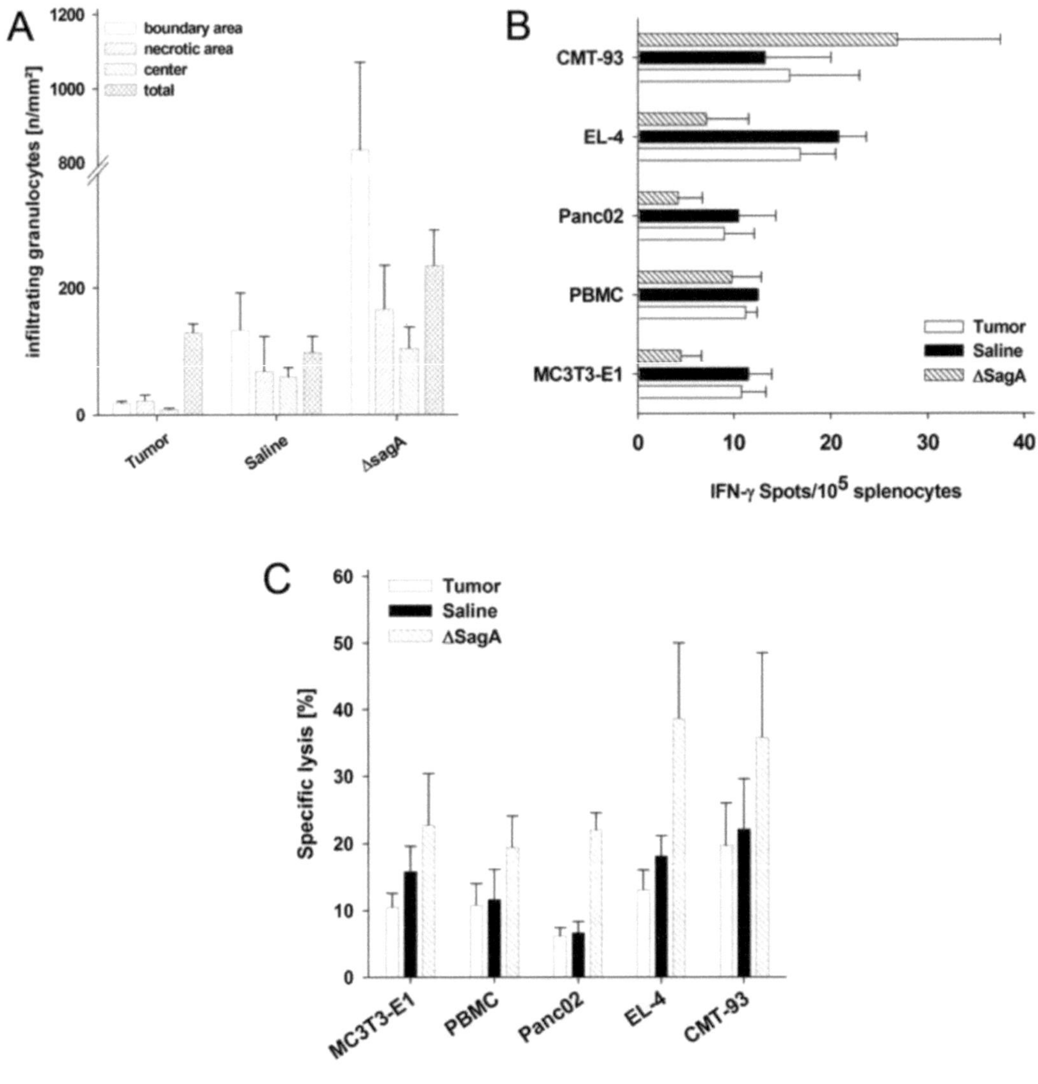

Fig. 5. **Data of immune responses from Panc02 tumor-carrying mice.** (A) Quantitative analysis of tumor-infiltrating As-D chloroacetate esterase-positive leukocytes shown as number of positive cells per mm². Leukocytes were found especially in boundary areas, and minor in the center of treated tumors. (B) Quantitative analysis of IFN-γ ELISpot assay. Reactivity of splenocytes against tumor targets was tested after co-incubation overnight at an E:T cell ratio of 30:1. Splenocytes from infected animals at 28 days after i.t. bacterial infection showed a marginally higher reactivity against target cells than those from control animals. (C) Quantitative analysis of cytotoxicity using LDH release assay. Lymphocytes were isolated from mesenteric lymph nodes and co-cultured with targets for 24 h at an E:T ratio of 30:1. Lymphocytes from infected animals at 28 days after i.t. bacterial infection lysed syngeneic tumor cell lines EL4 and CMT-93, but only to a minor extend Panc02 cells. Experiments were performed in triplicates. Values are given as the mean±SEM. $^{*}p<0.05$ vs. saline, *U*-Test.

4. Discussion

Different observations indicate that exposure by vaccination or infection to pathogen-associated molecular patterns (PAMP) can have beneficial effects on neoplastic diseases (Hobohm et al., 2008). PAMP recognizing TLRs serve as a first line of defense for the immune system, inducing soluble and cellular mediators of innate immunity and initiating key steps of the adaptive immune response. In recent years, manipulating the immune response via TLR stimulation has gained therapeutic and/or prophylactic value for cancer. In particular, administration of the synthetic TLR9 agonist CpG-ODN is being developed for cancer vaccines and cancer therapy, due to its described capacity to stimulate Th_1-like innate and adaptive anti-tumor responses in numerous preclinical models (Krieg 2007; Jacobs et al., 2010). Another potent inducer of tumor-directed cellular immune responses is the TLR7 agonist imiquimod. In recent years, several studies proved enhancement of antigen-specific T cell activation followed by tumor eradication (Rechtsteiner et al., 2005; Prins et al., 2006; Xiong & Ohlfest, 2011). Very recently, we provided evidence for tumor growth control by avitalized gram-positive bacteria. In these experiments, therapeutic application of avitalized bacteria effectively delayed tumor growth accompanied by increased numbers of tumor-infiltrating immune cells mainly belonging to the innate arm of the immune system (Klier et al., 2011).

In line with this, we previously observed that treatment with *S. pyogenes* leads to pancreatic tumor reduction or even cure by the orchestrated induction of innate and subsequent adaptive antitumoral immune responses (Linnebacher et al., 2008; Maletzki et al., 2008). However, little is known about the nature of active components responsible for this success. We hypothesized, that bacterial toxins are the most obvious candidate molecules to explain the antitumoral activity of *S. pyogenes*. Here, we explored the potential of the streptococcal-elaborated oxygen-stable cytolysin Streptolysin S. In agreement with previous data referring to the broad cytolytic spectrum of SLS, we were able to confirm that it also efficiently kills tumor cells and in particular Panc02 mouse pancreatic carcinoma cells. To a minor part, these effects could be attributed to the induction of caspase-dependent apoptosis. In a first series of *in vivo* experiments, the SLS-deficient mutant *S. pyogenes* strain ΔsagA showed only impaired antitumoral activity. This strain has been described to exhibit strongly reduced epithelial cell killing compared with SLS-producing wildtype strains (Datta et al., 2005; Lin et al. 2009). Moreover, minimal evidence of necrosis and tissue injury is seen post infection with SLS-negative bacteria in murine models of skin lesions (Datta et al., 2005). Similarly, local infection with the ΔsagA strain exhibited antitumoral potential only at later time-points post infection in our syngeneic murine Panc02 tumor model. This therapeutic success was significantly weaker than what we observed in our earlier studies using vital as well as lysed preparations of *S. pyogenes*. The hypothesis that SLS is a major antitumoral-acting molecule could be further substantiated in a second series of *in vivo* experiments. The application of streptococci depleted of active SLS by heating also resulted only in reduced antitumoral activity even after repetitive local treatments.

However, despite incomplete eradication of tumors, we want to strengthen the fact, that both preparations led to therapeutic responses as detected by significant reduction in tumor volumes. Thus, other factors are likely to contribute to the antitumoral effects of living and lysed *S. pyogenes* (e.g. M-Protein, superantigens, lipoteichoic acid) (Chau et al., 2009). Moreover, these findings hint towards a significant contribution of the immune system in partial control of tumor growth.

To understand the underlying immunological effects evoked by an inflammatory reaction in the ΔsagA treated animals, leading to reduced but not completely abolished antitumoral potential, *ex vivo* analyses were performed. Our observations imply an ongoing inflammatory response including systemic production of Th1 cytokines such as G-CSF and GM-CSF as well as raised levels of circulating NK cells and granulocytes. Functional analyses revealed recognition of syngeneic tumor cells as detected by IFN-γ release from lymphocytes obtained from infected animals. However, these effects were rather supposed to be mediated by activated NK cells than by tumor antigen specific T cells. This finding is additionally supported by the lymphocytes' killing activity especially towards the syngeneic tumor cell lines EL4 and CMT-93, but only marginally towards Panc02 cells.

To explain our findings, we propose that intratumoral injection of SLS-deficient streptococcal preparations leads to minor tumor cell damage driven by cytotoxic activity of other bacterial components. This triggers a comparably weak local inflammatory reaction followed by negligible systemic activation of the immune system. Thus, few specific antitumoral effector cells will be activated which can not totally control tumor growth whereas NK cells are the main effector type population mediating some degree of tumor growth control. The question, whether SLS may be an interesting molecule for tumor therapy will be addressed in ongoing trials.

5. Conclusion

Based on our previous findings on *Streptococcus pyogenes*-mediated eradication of established pancreatic murine tumors, we here elucidated the impact of the cytolytic toxin Streptolysin S on tumors *in vitro* and *in vivo*. We were able to show that direct exposure of the toxin to tumor cells results in a dose-dependent increase in cell damage. Contrary, the SLS-deficient ΔsagA strain showed only minor cytolytic potential. *In vivo*, a single i.t. injection of the ΔsagA strain affected pancreatic carcinomas only at later time points. This hints towards -at least partial- growth control of tumors by SLS, since comparable effects were observed following repetitive local applications of SLS-inactivated (by heating) bacteria. This finding is further supported by the histologic observation of ΔsagA-infected tumors. Those tumors showed slight increases in infiltrating granulocytes. Moreover, we found that recognition and killing of tumor cells was not restricted to Panc02 cells, but also detectable towards other syngeneic tumor entities. Taken together, we here provide clear evidence of strong antitumoral effects of SLS. However, in terms of the delayed, but significant impact on tumor growth *in vivo*, other factors are likely to contribute to the strong antitumoral effects of wildtype *S. pyogenes*.

6. Acknowledgment

We kindly thank Prof. Victor Nizet for providing the *S. pyogenes* strain ΔsagA.

7. References

Chau TA, McCully ML, Brintnell W, An G, Kasper KJ, Vinés ED, Kubes P, Haeryfar SM, McCormick JK, Cairns E, Heinrichs DE, Madrenas J. (2009). Toll-like receptor 2 ligands on the staphylococcal cell wall downregulate superantigen-induced T cell activation and prevent toxic shock syndrome. *Nat Med.* 15: 641-8.

Craft N, Bruhn KW, Nguyen BD, Prins R, Lin JW, Liau LM, Miller JF. 2005. The TLR7 agonist imiquimod enhances the antimelanoma effects of a recombinant Listeria monocytogenes vaccine. *J Immunol.* 175: 1983–1990.

Datta V, Myskowski SM, Kwinn LA, Chiem DN, Varki N, Kansal RG, Kotb M, Nizet V. 2005. Mutational analysis of the group A streptococcal operon encoding streptolysin S and its virulence role in invasive infection. *Mol Microbiol.* 56: 681-95.

Fraser JD, Proft T. The bacterial superantigen and superantigen-like proteins. *Immunol Rev.* 2008 Oct; 225: 226-43. Review.

Ginsburg I. 1999. Is streptolysin S of group A streptococci a virulence factor? *APMIS.* 107: 1051-9.

Hobohm U, Stanford JL, Grange JM. 2008.Pathogen-associated molecular pattern in cancer immunotherapy. *Crit Rev Immunol.* 28: 95-107.

Jacobs C, Duewell P, Heckelsmiller K, Wei J, Bauernfeind F, Ellermeier J, Kisser U, Bauer CA, Dauer M, Eigler A, Maraskovsky E, Endres S, Schnurr M. 2010. An ISCOM vaccine combined with a TLR9 agonist breaks immune evasion mediated by regulatory T cells in an orthotopic model of pancreatic carcinoma. Int J Cancer. 19. [Epub ahead of print]

Krieg AM. 2007.Development of TLR9 agonists for cancer therapy. *J Clin Invest.* 117: 1184-94. Review.

Lin A, Loughman JA, Zinselmeyer BH, Miller MJ, Caparon MG. 2009.Streptolysin S inhibits neutrophil recruitment during the early stages of Streptococcus pyogenes infection. *Infect Immun.* 77: 5190-201.

Linnebacher M, Maletzki C, Emmrich J, Kreikemeyer B. 2008.Lysates of S. pyogenes serotype M49 induce pancreatic tumor growth delay by specific and unspecific antitumor immune responses. *J Immunother.* 31: 704-13.

Maletzki C, Linnebacher M, Kreikemeyer B, Emmrich J. 2008. Pancreatic cancer regression by intratumoural injection of live Streptococcus pyogenes in a syngeneic mouse model. *Gut.* 57: 483-91.

Nizet V, Beall B, Bast DJ, Datta V, Kilburn L, Low DE, De Azavedo JC. 2008. Genetic locus for streptolysin S production by group A streptococcus. *Infect Immun.* 68: 4245-54.

Prins RM, Craft N, Bruhn KW, Khan-Farooqi H, Koya RC, Stripecke R Miller JF, Liau LM. 2006. TheTLR-7 agonist, imiquimod, enhances dendritic cell survival and promotes tumor antigen-specific T cell priming: relation to central nervous system antitumor immunity. *J Immunol.* 176: 157–164.

Rechtsteiner G, Warger T, Osterloh P, Schild H, Radsak MP. 2005. Cutting edge: priming of CTL by transcutaneous peptide immunization with imiquimod. *J Immunol.* 174: 2476–2480.

Taketo Y, Taketo A. 1966.Cytolytic effect of streptolysin S complex on Ehrlich ascites tumor cells. *J Biochem.* 60: 357-362.

Xiong Z, Ohlfest JR. (2011) Topical imiquimod has therapeutic and immunomodulatory effects against intracranial tumors. *J Immunother.* 34: 264-269.

Klier U, Maletzki C, Göttmann N, Kreikemeyer B, Linnebacher M. (2011) Avitalized bacteria mediate tumor growth control via activation of innate immunity. *Cell Immunol.* 269: 120-127.

10

Anesthesia and Pain Management: Techniques and Practice

Maurizio Marandola and Alida Albante
"Sapienza" University – Policlinico Umberto I, Rome, Italy

1. Introduction

Surgery for pancreatic cancer (PC) is widely viewed as a complex procedure associated with considerable perioperative morbidity and mortality. Many aspects of surgery for pancreatic cancer, such as the extent of resection, the value of vascular resection, the use of laparoscopy and the importance of treatment at high-volume centers are currently under debate. PC is the fourth leading cause of cancer related mortality in the United States with an estimated 42500 new cases and 35000 deaths from the disease each year (Jemal, 2009). Analysis of overall survival shows that the prognosis of PC is still quite poor despite the fact that 1-year survival has increased from 15.2% to 21.6% and 5-year survival has increased from 3% to 5% (ShaibYH et al., 2006). Surgery is the only chance of cure and the presence of negative resection margins of the primary tumor represent the strongest prognostic factor. Preoperative staging modalities include the combination of several imaging techniques such as computed tomography (CT scan), magnetic resonance imaging (MRI), endoscopic ultrasounds (EUS), staging laparoscopy and laparoscopic ultrasound which aim to identify patients with resectable disease. There is consensus that patients with distant metastases (liver, lung, peritoneum) or local invasion of the surrounding organs (stomach, colon, small bowel) are usually not surgical candidates. A decision analysis demonstrated that the best strategy to assess tumor resectability was based on CT as an initial test and the use of EUS to confirm the results of resectability by CT (Delbecke et al., 1999). Laparoscopic ultrasonography (LUS) has been introduced as an additional procedure to increase the detection of intrahepatic metastases, identify enlarged and suspicious lymph nodes and to evaluate local growth in the vascular structures (Tilleman et al., 2004). The routine use of staging laparoscopy and LUS in patients with radiographically resectable PC remains controversial as imaging modalities has significantly improved, thus reducing the risk of discovering non resectable disease at the time of surgery. Surgery for the PC can be considered an high-risk surgery. This term is rarely explicitly defined in scientific articles. There seems to be a common understanding among surgeons and anesthesiologists of what major surgery means. It can be defined as a surgical procedure that is extensive, involves removal of whole or parts of organs and/or is life-threatening. It has also been defined as a surgical procedure with >1 mortality (Ghaferi et al., 2009). One possibility of evaluating the perioperative risk is the use of 1 of several risk scores. The American Society of Anesthesiologists score is widely used and easy to apply, but excludes age from its risk analysis (Kullavanijaya et al., 2001). Age is securely one of the most important, if not the single most predictive, risk factors for morbidity and mortality after major surgery, including major pancreatic surgery (Riall et al., 2008).

2. Preanesthetic considerations

Patients undergoing pancreatic surgey require a complete history and physical examination. Coexisting medical illnesses may complicate the surgical and anesthetic course. The objectives of the preanesthetic evaluation include establishing a doctor-patient relationship, becoming familiar with the surgical illness and coexisting medical conditions, developing a management strategy for perioperative anesthetic care and obtaining informed consent for the anesthetic plan.

2.1 History of smoking

The risk of PC in smokers ranks second to lung cancer and is proportionate to the frequency, duration and cumulative smoking dose (Lynch et al., 2009; Neugut et el., 1995). The patients who smoke have an increased risk of intra- and postoperative complications, particularly of a pulmonary or cardiovascular nature, compared with nonsmoking patients (Bluman et al., 1998; Myles et al., 2002). As carbon monoxide (CO) preferentially binds to hemoglobin in place of oxygen, the short-term effects of cigarette smoking include elevated blood CO levels that result in a 3% to 12% reduction of oxygen availability in the periphery (Pearce & Jones, 1984). Moreover, nicotine stimulates a surgical stress response with increase in heart rate, arterial blood pressure and peripheral vascular resistance. Postoperative pulmonary complications are an important part of the risk of surgery and prolong the hospital stay by an average of one to two weeks. A careful history taking and physical examination are the most important parts of preoperative pulmonary risk assessment. One should seek a history of exercise intolerance, chronic cough or dyspnea. The physical examination may identify

PREOPERATIVE
Encourage cessation of cigarette smoking for at least 8 wk
Treat airflow obstruction in patients with chronic obstructive pulmonary disease or asthma
Administer antibiotics and delay surgery if respiratory infection is present
Begin patient education regarding lung-expansion maneuvers
INTRAOPERATIVE
Limit duration of surgery to less than 3 hr
Use spinal or epidural anesthesia
Use laparoscopic procedures when possible
Substitute less ambitious procedure for upper abdominal or thoracic surgery when possible
POSTOPERATIVE
Use deep-breathing exercises or incentive spirometry
Use continuous positive airway pressure
Use epidural analgesia
Use intercostal nerve blocks

Table 1. Risk-Reduction strategies

decreased breath sounds, dullness to percussion, wheezes, rhonchi and a prolonged expiratory phase that can predict an increase in the risk of pulmonary complications (Lawrence et al., 1996). The value of routine preoperative pulmonary testing remains controversial. There is consensus that such testing should be performed selectively in patients undergoing no-lung resection. It has been suggested that an increased risk of pulmonary complications is associated with a forced expiratory volume in one second (FEV_1) or forced vital capacity (FVC) of less than 70 percent of the predicted value or a ratio of FEV_1 to FVC of less than 65 percent (Gass & Olsen, 1986). A partial pressure of arterial carbon dioxide ($PaCO_2$) greater than 45 mmHg can't be considered as a risk factor for pulmonary complications. Several strategies can be adopted in the perioperative period reducing the risks of complications (Table 1).

2.2 Diabetes

Nearly 80% of PC patients have either frank diabetes or impaired glucose tolerance. Diabetes is usually diagnosed either concomitantly or during the two years preceding the diagnosis (Gullo et al. 1994; Permet et al. 1993). The link between abnormal glucose and PC exists only for type II diabetes. Better glycaemic control in diabetic patients undergoing major surgery has been shown to improve perioperative mortality and morbidity. Diabetics are at increased risk of myocardial ischaemia, cerebrovascular infarction and renal ischaemia because of their increased incidence of coronary artery disease, arterial atheroma and renal parenchymal disease. Increased mortality is found in all diabetics undergoing surgery and type I diabetics are particularly at risk of post-operative complications. Increased wound complications are associated with diabetes and anastomotic healing is severely impaired when glycaemic control is poor (Treiman, 1994; Verhofstad & Hendriks, 1996; Zacharias & Habib, 1996). Type 2 diabetics not receiving insulin and undergoing minor surgery usually can be managed satisfactory without insulin. However, diabetic patients scheduled for major surgery, who are receiving hypoglicaemic medication or who have poor glycaemic control, should be established on insulin therapy preoperatively. Continuous i.v. infusion of insulin is a better option than intermittent s.c. bolus regimens and may be associated with improved outcome. The immediate perioperative problems facing the diabetic patient are: a) surgical induction of the stress response with catabolic hormone secretion; b) interruption of food intake, which will be prolonged in PC surgery; c) circulatory disturbances associated with anesthesia and surgery, which may alter the absorption of subcutaneous insulin. Surgery evokes the "stress response", that is the secretion of catecholamines, cortisol, growth hormone and, in some cases, glucagone. These hormones oppose glucose homeostasis, as they have anti-insulin and hyperglicaemic effects. Although diabetics need increased insulin during the perioperative period, requirements for glucose and insulin in this period are unpredictable and close monitoring is essential, especially in the unconscious or sedated patients. The main concern for the anesthetist in the perioperative management of diabetic patients has been the avoidance of harmful hypoglicaemia; mild hyperglicaemia has tended to be seen as acceptable. High-dose opiate anesthetic techniques produce not only haemodinamic, but also hormonal and metabolic stability. Abolition of the catabolic hormonal response to surgery will abolish the hyperglicaemia seen in normal patients and may be of benefit in the diabetic patients. Tight metabolic control in the perioperative period is imperative and is a goal which is attainable in most patients. IV infusion of insulin is the standard therapy for the perioperative management of diabetes, especially in type 1 diabetic patients and patients with type 2 diabetes undergoing major procedure (Clement et al., 2004). Institutions around the world use a variety of insulin infusion algorithms that can be implemented by nursing staff. Recently, several insulin infusion protocols have been reported in the literature. Two main methods of insulin delivery have been used either combining insulin with glucose and potassium in the same bag (GIK regimen) or giving insulin separately with an infusion pump. The GIK is initiated at a rate of 100 mL/h in a solution of 500 mL of 10% dextrose, 10 mmol of potassium, and 15 U of insulin. Adjustments in the insulin dose are made in 5 U increments according to blood glucose measurements performed at least every 2 hours. The combined GIK infusion is efficient, safe and effective but does not permit selective adjustment of insulin delivery without changing the bag. Separate continuous glucose and insulin infusions are used more frequently than the glucose-potassium-insulin infusion (Coursin et al., 2004; Furnary et al., 2003; Goldberg et al., 2004; Rehman & Mohammed, 2003). A proposed regimen for separate IV insulin infusion for perioperative diabetes management is shown in Table 2.

I) Initiating continuous insulin infusion (CII):
Prepare solution: 1 unit (U) per 1 mL of 0.9% normal saline.
Start continuous insulin infusion (CII) when blood glucose level ≥140 mg/dL (x 2).
Patients with known diabetes treated with insulin can start CII when blood glucose ≥70 mg/dL.
Initial rate: divide blood glucose level (mg/dL) by 100, then round to nearest 0.5 U

II) Insulin infusion rate change:

BloodGlucose (mg/dL)	instructions:
>200	↑rate by 2 U/h
>160–200	↑rate by 1.0 U/h
>120–160	↑rate by 0.5 U/h
80–120	No change in rate
60–80 If <10%	lower blood glucose, rate by 1 U/h, Check BG within 30 min If >10% lower blood glucose, 2 rate by 50%, Check BG within 30 min
< 60	Stop infusion (give IV dextrose 12.5 g IV bolus), Check blood glucose within 30 min. When blood glucose>100 mg/dL, restart infusion at 50% of previous rate

III) Patient monitoring:
Check capillary blood glucose every hour until it is within goal range for 2 hours, and then decrease to every 2 hours.
Hourly monitoring may be indicated for critically ill patients even if they have stable blood glucose.
If a patient is eating, hourly blood glucose monitoring is necessary for at least 3 hours after eating.
Decrease insulin infusion rate by 50% if nutritional therapy (e.g. total parenteral nutrition or tube feeds) are discontinued or significantly reduced.

Table 2. Continuous insulin infusion (CII) protocol

2.3 Nutritional status

Malnurished patients who require major operations are predisposed to infectious complications and poor outcome. A low preoperative body mass index (BMI, kg/m^2) may be regarded as an overall indicator of the size of the patient's reserves; a BMI<20 kg/m^2 is an accepted indicator of malnutrition. However, it has been recognized that acutely malnourished patients may still have a normal or even elevated BMI. Serum protein markers such as albumin (for evaluating long-term nutritional status) and prealbumin (for evaluating acute responses to nutritional support) have been shown to be useful additional measurements for assessing nutritional status. Low albumin levels have been identified as an independent risk factor for postoperative morbidity and mortality (Gibbs et al., 1999). It should be emphasized that, although preoperative enteral or parenteral nutritional support clearly benefits surgical cancer patients, a systematic review showed that "preventive" administration of parenteral support in non-malnourished patients did not positively influence outcome and may even be potentially harmful for certain patient subgroups (Koretz et al., 2001). More recently, the concept of immunonutrition has evolved, in which enteral formulas are supplemented with arginine and glutamine, nucleotides or omega-3 fatty acids in an attempt to positively modulate the immune system, but the benefits of immunonutrition remain debatable. Where as perioperative nutrition in the malnourished patient can improve postoperative outcome, immunonutrition seems to attenuate the inflammatory response and interferes with certain immune functions in selected patient groups.

2.4 Patient with jaundice

Jaundice results from an abnormally high bilirubin in the blood whose origin may be difficulty in eliminating; it's then an obstructive jaundice. This is the most symptom in patients with periampullary cancer (located near the Vater's ampulla) or cancer of the pancreatic head. It can be considered a risk factor for postoperative complications. [8, 9] Many studies demonstrate that it could be associated with a higher incidence of insufficient postoperative renal function, but also of sepsis, haemorrhage, of liver failure and risk of mortality from about 16% (Jiang & Puntis, 1997). Jaundice causes a retention of acids and bile salts. In the long term, may cause ascending cholangitis and secondary hepatocellular damage. In case of interruption of bile flow, bile acids and salts can't inhibit the phenomenon of translocation and endotoxemia caused by gram-negative from the digestive tract. These bacteria will then multiply and, for a phenomenon of translocation, can contribute to the dissemination of endotoxins into the systemic circulation then creating a pro-inflammatory state with production of cytokines by activated macrophages and a subsequent risk of multiple organ failure, including the appearance of coagulation disorders. Since surgery in patients with jaundice is thought to increase the risk of postoperative complications, preoperative biliary drainage was introduced to improve the postoperative outcome. In several experimental studies preoperative biliary drainage reduced morbidity and mortality after surgery (Van der Gaag et al., 2009). In a multicentre, randomized trial, Van der Gaag et al compared preoperative biliary drainage with surgery alone for patients with cancer of the pancreatic head and they found that endoscopic preoperative drainage with placement of a plastic stent did not have a beneficial effect on the surgical outcome and early surgery without preoperative drainage did not increase the risk of complications (Van der Gaag, 2010). The preoperative oral administration of bile salts or lactulose has been proposed in order to reduce the risk of endotoxemia by blocking bacterial translocation phenomenon from the gut. The effectiveness of this practice has not been validated. Anti-inflammatory and antibiotic prophylaxis should be avoided. In severe cases, a preoperative hemodiafiltration session can address the surgery with more serenity.

2.5 The general physical examination

The physical examination should be thorough but focused. Special attention is directed toward evaluation of the airway, heart, lungs and neurologic status.

2.5.1 Vital signs and head and neck

Height and wheight are useful in estimating drug dosages and determining volume requirements and the adequacy of perioperative urine output. Ideal body weight should be calculated in obese patients to help determine proper drug dosages and ventilator settings (e.g. tidal volume). Blood pressure should be recorded in both arms and any disparity noted (significant differences may imply disease of the thoracic aorta or its major branches). At same time should be observed and noted the respiration rate and oxygen saturation. One should evaluate maximal mouth opening, the size of the tongue, the ability to visualize the posterior pharyngeal structures and Mallampati classification. A thyromental distance shorter or longer than three fingerbreadth may be a sign of a difficult intubation.

2.6 Laboratory studies

A routine laboratory screening tests are necessary to evaluate a recent hematocrit/ hemoglobin level, the platelet activity and the coagulation status before surgery. An ECG should be obtained in any patient with risk factors for coronary artery disease (CAD). It can also detect new dysrhythmias and be useful to evaluate the stability of known abnormal rhythms. A chest radiography should be obtained in all patients to evaluate the cardiovascular image and to document any tracheal deviation or cervical masses.

3. Anaesthetic management

General anesthesia with mechanical ventilation is the rule. Spinal anesthesia is impractical owing to the length of the operation. However, epidural analgesia could, in theory, be used as the sole anesthetic technique. It's our belief that the length of surgery, insertion of central lines and the high likelihood of conversion to general anesthesia make epidural alone unsatisfactory. Epidural analgesia may be beneficial post-operatively in reducing venous thromboembolic events, the incidence of respiratory failure and in providing superior analgesia in comparison with opioids. However, there may be clotting abnormalities perioperatively leading to an increased risk of neurological complications. Epidural can make assessment of the patient's volume status more difficult and, with large fluid shifts occurring in this group, a period of hypovolemia could be worsened by concomitant vasodilatation secondary to the epidural analgesia. A balance of these risks needs to be addressed before embarking on an epidural anesthesia technique. It's our practice to routinely use epidural analgesia as a part of combined general and regional technique in these patients. Postoperative analgesia is then provided by a catheter left in place in epidural space. The choice of anesthetics must consider the interference pharmacokinetic: benzodiazepines should be avoided for premedication; propofol are the preferred induction agent; morphine should be used with caution in patients with hepatic or renal function (accumulation); muscle relaxants not metabolized by hepatobiliary system (atracurium, *cis*-atracurium) are to be used in the first intent with adequate monitoring. The antibiotic prophilaxis (Enterobacteriaceae and Staphylococcus) is essential in this surgery. Fluid and volume therapy is an important cornerstone of treating critically ill patients in the operating room. New findings concerning the vascular barrier, its physiological functions and its role regarding vascular leakage have lead to a new view of fluid and volume administration. Avoiding hypervolemia, as well as hypovolemia, plays a pivotal role when treating patients both perioperatively and in the intensive care unit. The postoperative phase may be studded with complications: sepsis, hepatic dysfunction, coagulation and metabolic disorders, renal and pulmonary failure and, in addition to the typical risks associated with abdominal surgery, some specific to the Whipple procedure, the two most common are pancreatic fistula and delayed gastric emptying (Buchler et al., 2003). Therefore the recovery in the postanesthesia care unit (PACU) is necessary for these fragile patients.

3.1 Pharmacology of anesthetics

3.1.1 Benzodiazepines

Pre-, intra-and postoperative use of benzodiazepines (BZP) is widely not recommended because of their hepatic metabolism that exposed to an increased half-life, an extension the duration of action and delayed recovery. In premedication for anxiolysis, with the exception of jaundiced patients, midazolam 0.1-0.4 mg/Kg is indicated; after i.v. administration, the onset of central nervous system effects occurs in 2 to 3 minutes. BZP enhance inhibitory neurotransmission by increasing the affinity of $GABA_A$ receptors for GABA . Effects are terminated by redistribution, the metabolism is tipically hepatic and renal the elimination. Administration of a BZP to a patient receveing the anticolvulsivant valproate may precipitate a psychotic episode.

3.1.2 Induction agents

Thiopental has no longer the place it has had for very many years. In addition, its use was largely dissuaded in the presence of hepatobiliary disease because of its hepatic metabolism (cytochrome P450). Thiopental is metabolized to pentobarbital, an active metabolite with a longer half- life. Its use therefore exposed to delayed awakening. Similar to propofol, barbiturates facilitate inhibitory neurotransmission by enhancing $GABA_A$ receptor function. They also inhibit exicitatory neurotransmission via glutamate and nicotinic acetylcholine receptors. Absolutely contraindicated in patient with acute intermittent porphyria, variegate porphyria and hereditary coproporphyria (barbiturates induce porphyrin synthetic enzymes such as δ-aminolevulinic acid synthetase). Ketamine for its variable pharmacokinetics in the presence of extrahepatic biliary obstruction and postoperative hallucinatory effects has a limited use in clinical practice. Propofol is the agent of choice, not only for the induction, but also for sedation in patients requiring postoperative ventilatory support. It has a short action effect and the rapid metabolism is not influenced in the presence of liver failure. It is prepared as a 1% isotonic oil-in water emulsion, which contains egg lecithin, glycerol and soybean oil. Bacterial growth is inhibited by ethylenediaminetetraacetic acid (EDTA), diethylenetriaminepentaacetic acid (DPTA), sulfite, or benzyl alcohol depending on the manufacturer (don't use opened propofol after 6 hours to prevent inadvertent bacterial contamination). Mode of action: facilitation inhibitory neurotransmission by enhancing the function of $GABA_A$ receptors in the central nervous system; the modulation of glycine receptors, N-etyl-D aspartate receptors, cannabinoid receptors and voltage-gated ion channels may also contribute to propofol's actions. After the infusion it can be observed dose-dependent decreases in preload, afterload and contractility that lead to decrease in blood pressure and cardiac output. Hypotension may be marked in hipovolemic, elderly, or hemodynamically compromised patients. Heart rate is minimally affected and baroreceptor reflex is blunted. Adverse effects are: venous irritation, lipid disorders, myoclonus and hiccups, "propofol infusion syndrome".

3.1.3 Opioids

Morphine and its derivatives are essential for the perioperative period (commonly used in general anesthesia) and are frequently used to ensure postoperative analgesia. Opioids, including morphine and fentanyl, have been accused to increase the bile ducts tone and to determine a spasm of Oddi's sphincter. However, the consequences in clinical practice are limited: the pressure is most often in the bile duct within normal limits and the delay of the bile's drainage in the duodenum is not significant. Opioids differ in their potencies, pharmacokinetics and site effects. The mode of action is due to the interaction with specific receptors in the brain, spinal cord and peripheral neurons (Kumamoto et al., 2011). After i.v. administration, the onset of action is within minutes for the fentanyl derivatives; due to their lower lipid solubility hydromorphone and morphine may take from 20 to 30 minutes for their peak effect. Elimination is primarily by the liver and depends on hepatic blood flow. In patients with renal failure, the accumulation of morphine -6- glucuronide, the active metabolite, may cause prolonged narcosis and respiratory depression. Fentanyl is metabolized by hydrolysis and N-dealkylation and its metabolites are excreted in the urine. Function liver in the normal range is necessary to plasma clearance in case of repeated injections. The pharmakocinets of alfentanil is also changed, with a longer duration of action and an initial effect over pronounced. The sufentanil phamacokinetics is not altered even in cases of moderate hepatic insufficiency. The short duration of action of remifentanil (context-insensitive half-time) and especially its extrahepatic metabolism (by non specific esterases in tissues, primarily skeletal muscle) are purely an advantage (Dershwitz et al., 1996). Opioids exert emetogenic effects and represent a significant cause of patient discomfort. Nausea and vomiting can occur because of the direct stimulation of the chemoreceptor trigger zone, of the vestibular apparatus, inhibition of gut motility (Porreca & Ossipov, 2009).

3.1.4 Halogenated

Inhalation agents represent a basic drug used in modern balanced anesthesia. Actually the most important halogenated in the clinical use are sevoflurane and desflurane. They were developed in the late 1960s and tested in clinical practice much later. Sevoflurane was not immediately introduced to the USA because of its fluorine release and its reaction with absorbed carbon dioxide. After several years of clinical application, no renal failure was observed and appropriate studies on compound A did not show any renal effects in human. Desflurane is largely appreciated for its high stability. Less than 0.02% of desflurane is metabolized, thus, plasma fluorine levels are very low. The very low solubility of desflurane allows for a surprisingly rapid emergence from anesthesia. Nitrous oxide has a controversial role in the modern anesthesia. For one and a half centuries it has played a relevant role in general anesthesia. Many of the side effects of nitrous oxide correlate with its physical properties. Its ability to diffuse into air filled cavities increases the likelihood of pneumothorax, air emboli and pressure in the cuff of the endotracheal tube. Nitrous oxide diffusion causes an increase in the middle ear pressure and distension of the bowel, possibly resulting in increases in postoperative nausea and vomiting. The results of a questionnaire proposed by the Association of Anesthesist of Great Britain and Ireland indicate that 49% of anesthesist had reduced their use of nitrous oxide (Henderson et al., 2002). According to Baum, nitrous oxide should not be used routinely as a carrier gas and the safer mixture of oxygen/medical air is able to replace this old anesthetic with some economical advantages (Baum, 2004). The combination of halogenated agents with short acting opioids results in the possibility of limiting the clinical application of nitrous oxide. Attempts to replace nitrous oxide with other gases has led to an increase in studies on xenon. This inert gas does not undergo metabolic biotransformation and has no direct negative environmental effects. Xenon has a very low solubility in the blood and its potency is higher when compared to nitrous oxide solubility (Hecker et al., 2004). Xenon cannot be synthesized and the available amount is very low. Consequently, at present, the cost of compound may be a limiting factor for the clinical use. The pharmacokinetic advantages of inhalation anesthetics are unique. By increasing or decreasing their inspired concentration, it is possible to increase or decrease their concentration in the blood and tissues, allowing for rapid changes in anesthesia depth and providing a simple method for inducing, maintaining and reversing general anesthesia. The flexibility of inhalation anesthesia cannot be reproduced with modern intravenous hypnotics or opioids. Furthermore, it is important to underline the protective effects of inhalation agents on several different organs.

3.1.5 Neuromuscolar blocking drugs

Non depolarizing blockade is produced by reversible competitive antagonism of Ach at the α subunits of the AChRs. The principal pharmacologic effect is to interrupt transmission of synaptic signaling at the neuromuscular junction. The neuromuscular blocking agents in biliary excretion (e.g. vecuronium) should be avoided in favor of those metabolized by way of Hoffman (atracurium, *cis*-atracurium). In all cases, the use of a monitoring of neuromuscular blockade is obviously essential (Chiu & White, 2000; Murphy & Szokol,2004).

3.2 Monitoring

Standard monitoring for general anaesthesia involves oxygenation (analyzer and pulse oximetry), ventilation (capnography and minute ventilation), circulation (ECG with ST-segment analysis, blood pressure and perfusion assessment) and temperature if necessary. Additional monitoring may be added such as invasive arterial and venous pressure monitoring, trans esophageal echocardiography (TEE), neuromuscular blockade and central nervous system monitoring. Automated noninvasive blood pressure is the most common noninvasive method of measuring blood pressure in the operating room for minor surgery. Invasive blood pressure (IBP) monitoring is imperative in the pancreatic surgery; there is potential for rapid swings in blood pressure and acid-base balance often needs managing (acidosis is common). IBP uses an indwelling arterial catheter coupled through fluid-filled tubing to a pressure transducer. The transducer converts pressure into a electrical signal to be displayed. Generally the catheter size is 18 to 20 gauge for adults. The radial artery is the most common site. Other locations include ulnar, brachial, axillary, femoral and dorsal pedis arteries. The procedure should be perfomed aseptically. Local anesthetic may be used to raise a skin wheal if the patient is awake. For catheter insertion it can be used the Seldinger technique. The modified Allen test has been recommended to assess the relative patency and contribution of the radial and ulnar arteries to the blood supply to the hand, but the results are unreliable. Central venous catheter (CVC) is essential; ultrasound guidance can be useful in the patients that have had multiple previous cannulation. The central venous pressure (CVP) and cardiac output (CO) are monitored by CVC. CVP is measured by coupling the intravascular space to a pressure transducer using a fluid-filled tubing. Pressure is monitored at the level of the vena cava or the right atrium. The normal CVP is 2 to 6 mmHg. Positive- pressure ventilation affects both cardiac output and venous return. According to the Starling rule, the transmural pressure, which is the difference between the atrial pressure and extracardiac pressure, correlates with the cardiac output. At low level of PEEP, the CVP increases with increased PEEP, at high levels of PEEP (over 15 cmH_2O), CVP increases as the cardiac output is depressed because of impaired right ventricular output. Common locations include internal jugular and subclavian vein. Multiple lumen catheters are directly inserted and are available with one to four lumens to provide access for multiple drugs, pressure monitoring and blood sampling. Temperature may be measured continuously; the limitation of more external methods of temperature determination is that they may not reflect changes in the core body temperature, especially in the presence of vasoconstriction. Oropharyngeal temperature monitoring is preferred in any lengthy laparotomy, which has potential for blood loss and perioperative clotting abnormalities. Ventilation is assessed by end- tidal carbon dioxide measurements and spirometry. Capnometry and capnography are often used as synonyms, as both analyze and record carbon dioxide, with the latter including a waveform. Capnography not only evaluates respiration but also confirms of endotracheal intubation and its diagnostic of pathologic conditions. Neuromuscular blockade is utilized, above all for patients with co-existing renal failure. The adductor pollicis response to ulnar nerve stimulation at the wrist is most often used, because it is easily accessible, and the results are not confused with direct muscle activation. Cutaneous electrodes are placed at the wrist over the ulnar nerve and attached to a battery-driven pulse generator, which delivers a graded impulse of electrical current at a specified frequency. For maximal twitch response, the negative pole (active) should be placed distally over the ulnar nerve at the wrist. Evoked muscle tension can be estimated by feeling for thumb adduction or measured by using a force transducer attached to the thumb. After administration of a neuromuscular blocking drug (NMBD), the developed tension and twitch height decrease with the onset of blockade. Foley catheter is the rule in all patient ones, necessary for fluid management and the control of the renal functionality.

3.3 Conduct of anaesthesia

The primary goals of general anesthesia are to maintain the health of the patient while providing amnesia, hypnosis (lack of awareness), analgesia and immobility. Secondary goals may vary depending on the patient's medical condition and the surgical procedure. Perioperative planning involves the integration of preoperative, intraoperative and postoperative care. Flexibility, the ability to anticipate problems before they occur and the ability to execute contingency plans are skills that define the expert anesthetist. An anesthetic plan developed prior to entering the operating room helps the anesthetist marshal appropriate resources and anticipate potential difficulties. Important elements to consider in the anesthetic plain include: risk assessment (ASA classification), specific homeostatic challenges, intravenous access, monitoring, airway management, medications, perioperative analgesia, postoperative transport and disposition. Preoperative medications is realized with midazolam 0.1-0.4 mg/Kg (except cases of jaundice) for anxiety control. It is also important to consider aspiration prophylaxis; drugs to neutralize gastric acid and decrease gastric volume are used: metoclopramide 10 mg and ranitidine 50 mg usually. Induction of anesthesia produces an unconscious patient with depressed reflexes who is dependent on the anesthetist for maintenance of homeostatic mechanisms and safety. The patient's position for induction is usually supine, with extremities resting comfortably on padded surface in a neutral anatomic position. The head should rest comfortably on a firm support, which is raised in a "sniff" position. Routine pre-induction administration of oxygen minimizes the risk of hypoxia developing during induction of anesthesia. High flow (8 to 10 L/minute) oxygen should be delivered via a face mask placed gently on the patient's face. Commonly, for the induction of anesthesia, we use propofol 4-6 mg/Kg, a non- depolarizing neuromuscular blocking agent (cis–atracurium 0,15 mg/Kg is the usual choice) and sufentanil 0.1-0.5 mcg/Kg. Hypertensive patients may have an exaggerated pressor response to laryngoscopy. To obtund this response, opioids or β-blockers can be used. Tracheal intubation is performed with laryngoscopy usually. An appropriate ETT size depends on the patient's age, body habitus. Proper placement of the ETT needs to be verified by the detection of carbon dioxide in end-tidal or mixed expiratory gas as well as inspection and auscultation of the stomach and both lung fields during positive-pressure ventilation. Tidal volumes of 8-10 ml/ Kg and a respiratory rate of 10 to 12 breaths/minute are set and low level PEEP is beneficial. For the maintenance of anesthesia we use normally a mixture of oxygen and air (40%/60%) and an halogenated (sevoflurane or desflurane) with a continuous infusion of sufentanil until the end of operation. The infusion of sufentanil generally is continued in the PACU to better adapt the patient to the mechanical ventilation. If we decide for a blended anesthesia, before the induction of anesthesia, we perform a thoracic epidural anesthesia (T8-T10) with the patient in sitting position.

3.4 Epidural anaesthesia / analgesia

The epidural space is surrounded by the outer surface of the dura mater and the bony and ligamentous walls of the spinal canal and extends from the foramen magnum to the sacral hiatus. The cross-sectional area of the epidural space becomes smaller cranially, as the theca and its contents tend to occupy a greater proportion of space. Hence, a given volume of drugs affects a greater number of segments the more cranially it is introduced. The epidural space contains nerve roots, fat, spinal arteries and lymphatics, as well as a valveless venous system that communicates directly with both the intracranial sinuses via the basovertebral veins and the general circulation via the azygos vein. Dorsal and ventral spinal nerve roots covered by dura mater pass across the epidural space and drugs within this space can act on any nerve that traverses it - whether it be motor, sensory or autonomic. Epidural analgesics may prevent the release of neurotransmitters from afferent pain fibres, block receptors to neurotransmitters released by primary afferent pain fibres or interrupt the transmission of pain-related information in the dorsal horn of the spinal cord. Drugs introduced into the epidural space also have the potential to pass into the brain and the general circulation depending on their pharmacokinetics. Epidural analgesia was originally achieved with local anaesthetic agents but, more recently, with opioids or a combination of local anaesthetics and opioids. This combination has a synergistic action that allows the concentration of each drug to be reduced, thereby limiting unwanted effect produced by higher concentrations. Ketamine, midazolam or clonidine has also been used in combination with local anaesthetics and opioids to obtain the best intra- and post-operative pain control. Local anaesthetics penetrate axonal membranes within the epidural space and bind to sodium channels in nerves. This inhibits sodium conductance and reduces action potential depolarization, thereby reducing nerve stimulus propagation. The drawback is that the effect is non selective, involving both autonomic and somatic nerves. Thinner nerve fibres are affected by lower local anaesthetic concentrations than thicker fibres, suggesting that neuronal block is a function of diameter. With increasing local anesthetic concentration, the thinner C fibres (pain and autonomic fibres) are blocked first, followed by B fibres (preganglionic sympathetic fibres) and finally the largest A fibres (touch, pressure sensation and motor fibres). Epidural analgesia aims to produce a differential nerve block, affecting predominantely nociceptive fibres with few motor effects. Opioids act on opioid receptors that are widespread throughout the nervous system, but more concentrated in the medullary dorsal horn of the spinal cord and the periaqueductal grey matter of the brain. Opioid receptors belong to the family of guanine nucleotide-binding protein receptors. They exist as three principle types (OP1, OP2 and OP3) and opioids acting at these receptors have the advantage of selectively blocking pain without affecting motor function or the sense of touch. Epidural opioids act mainly on presynaptic and postsynaptic receptors in the substantia gelatinosa of the dorsal horn of the spinal cord (Fotiadis et al., 2004). The combination of thoracic epidural analgesia (TEA) and general anesthesia has become a widespread anesthetic technique for the perioperative treatment of patients undergoing major abdominal surgery. The neuraxial application of local anesthetics and opioids provides superior pain relief, reduced hormonal and metabolic stress, enhanced normalization of gastrointestinal function and thus a shortened postoperative recovery time, facilitating mobilization and physiotherapy. TEA is currently thought to mitigate this effect by blocking nociceptive afferent nerves and thoracolumbar sympathetic efferent routes. In a very recent cohort study Van Lier F. et al. (Van Lier et al., 2011) demonstrated that epidural analgesia reduces postoperative pneumonia in patients with chronic obstructive pulmonary disease (COPD) undergoing major abdominal surgery. Among the long-acting local anesthetics, the S-enantiomer, ropivacaine, is gaining increasing preference for continuous epidural analgesia. Ropivacaine has lower central nervous system and cardiac toxicity and a less frequent incidence of motor block (differential block) during mobilization than bupivacaine (Macias et al., 2002). Panousis et al. evaluated the effect of different epidurally administered concentrations of ropivacaine on inhaled anesthetic, fluid and vasopressor requirement and hemodynamic changes. They concluded that ropivacaine 0.5% compared with a ropivacaine 0.2 % concentration led to a greater inhaled anesthetic-sparing effect at the same levels of IV fuid supply and vasopressor support (Panousis et al., 2009). In a critical appraisal published on 2008, Pratt WB et al. concluded that although it may provide more effective initial pain control, epidural analgesia does not necessarily improve the critical outcome as after pancreatoduodenectomy. The Authors explained it with the high propensity for rapid fluid shifts and excessive blood loss during this operation, which may negate the proposed benefits of administering analgesic medications by epidural infusion and they reinforced these results considering the frequent need to terminate epidural infusions because of hemodynamic compromise or inadequate analgesia. Spinal epidural hematoma (SHE) after epidural analgesia is a rare but serious complication. Most cases of SHE after epidural block are attributed to a bleeding tendency or anticoagulant therapy. Placement of an epidural catheter may cause SHE more often than expected, but most SEHs remain asymptomatic (Inoue, 2002). The incidence of significant spinal bleeding (paraplegia requiring laminectomy) has been estimated at 1:1,000,000 in patients without clinically apparent coagulation disorders. Vandermeulen et al. found spinal bleeding immediately after removal of the epidural catheter in 15 of the 32 cases that he reviewed. Spontaneous SHE has been reported in a few cases (Skilton, 1998; Vandermeulen, 1994). The maximum incidence of clinically important spinal bleeding after epidural catheter blocks without specific additional risk factors probably list between 1:190,000-200,000. Approximately 60-80% of all clinically important spinal bleeding is associated with haemostatic disorders or a blood tap. Removal of an epidural catheter should be considered a significant risk factor for spinal bleeding because 30-60% of clinically important spinal hematomas occurs after catheter removal (Tryba, 1998). A practical approach to the patients with anticoagulant/antiaggregant therapy is reported in Table 3, according to the last guidelines of the European Society of Anaesthesiology.

Where central neural block is contraindicated (e.g systemic sepsis, in anti-coagulated patients), or where epidural catheterization is technically impossible, bilateral paravertebral nerve blocks (PVB) is a suitable alternative. The paravertebral space is a potential space, which is turned into a temporary cavity by fluid. Anaesthesia occurs because of direct penetration of local anesthetic (LA) into the neurological structures contained within the PVB (anterior and posterior ramus of the intercostals nerve, sympathetic chain, rami comunicantes, sinu-vertebral nerve). The spinal nerve, lacking both an epineurvium and part of the perinervium and with only a thin membranous root sheath is easily penetrated by LA and hence easily and efficiently blocked (Karmaker, 2001). We recommend the use of levobupivacaine or ropivacaine for bilateral blocks. Good preservation of postoperative pulmonary function has been demonstrated, particularly in thoracotomy, which is a significant benefit over epidural analgesia (Davies et al., 2006). The incidence of complications such as pneumothorax and hypotension is low. For bilateral PVB a variety of techniques, including loss of resistance, nerve stimulators and ultrasound, have been used. Potential or relative contraindications to the use of PVB are: coagulation disordes, tumor in the PVB and empyema. The relationship of regional anaesthesia to wound healing, chronic postoperative pain, and cancer recurrence rates with this and other block is important.

	Time before puncture/catheter manipulation or removal	Time after puncture/catheter manipulation or removal	Laboratory tests
Unfractionated heparins (for prophylaxis, ≤ 15 000 IU per day)	4-6 h	1 h	Platelets during treatment for more than 5 days
Unfractionated heparins (for treatment)	i.v. 4–6 h s.c. 8–12 h	1 h 1 h	aPTT, ACT, platelets
Low-molecular-weight heparins (for prophylaxis)	12 h	4 h	Platelets during treatment for more than 5 days
Low-molecular-weight heparins (for treatment)	24h	4h	Platelets during treatment for more than 5 days
Fondaparinux (for prophylaxis, 2.5mg per day)	36-42h	6-12h	(anti-Xa, standardised for specific agent)
Rivaroxaban (for prophylaxis, 10mg q.d.)	22-26 h	4–6 h	(PT, standardised for specific agent)
Apixaban (for prophylaxis, 2.5mg b.i.d.)	26-30 h	4–6 h	?
Dabigatran (for prophylaxis, 150–220 mg)	Contraindicated according to the manufacturer	6 h	?
Coumarins	INR ≤1.4	after catheter removal	INR
Hirudins (lepirudin, desirudin)	8-10 h	2-4 h	aPTT, ECT
Argatrobanc	4 h	2 h	aPTT, ECT, ACT
Acetylsalicylic acid	None	None	
Clopidogrel	7 days	after catheter removal	
Ticlopidine	10 days	after catheter removal	
Ticagrelor	5 days	6 h after catheter removal	
Cilostazolc	42 h	5 h after catheter removal	
Prasugrel	7-10 days	6 h after catheter removal	
NSAIDs	None	None	

ACT, activated clotting time; aPTT, activated partial thromboplastin time; b.i.d., twice daily; ECT, ecarin clotting time; INR, international normalised ratio; IU, international unit;
i.v., intravenously; NSAIDs, non-steroidal anti-inflammatory drugs; s.c., subcutaneously; q.d., daily.
All time intervals refer to patients with normal renal function. Prolonged time interval in patients with hepatic insufficiency.

Table 3. Recommended time intervals before and after neuraxial puncture or catheter removal (Gogarten et al., 2010)

3.5 Postoperative care

3.5.1 Postoperative I.V. analgesia

In patients with epidural catheter the analgesia can be continued with a volumetric or elastomeric pump with a rate infusion of 5-8 ml/h, by using local anesthetics alone or in combination with opioids. Generally we use ropivacaine 2mg/ml and sufentanil 5 mcg/ml. In patients where was impossible the positioning of an epidural catheter the postoperative analgesia is performed with NSAIDs or opioids or mixture of them. Several protocols are reported in literature for IV analgesia, but generally morphine is the leader drug. The patient controlled analgesia (PCA) is the best route of administration with a primary dose of 2-10 mg and a rescue dose of 0.5-2 mg with a lock-out of 5-10 minutes (Miaskowski, 2005). A specific role have the COX-2 inhibitors. Parecoxib (40-80 mg) is disposable for intravenous administration (Nussmeier et al, 2006).

3.6 Pain and inoperable pancreatic cancer

Pancreatic diseases such as cancer can cause clinically significant pain in the upper abdomen, which may radiate to the back. Pain management for pancreatic cancer patients is one of the most important aspects of their care, as it is one of the most weakening symptoms. The best therapy involves adequate therapy with constant assessment. The current management of pancreatic pain follows the WHO three-step ladder for pain control, starting with non-opioid analgesics such as nonsteroidal anti-inflammatory drugs (NSAIDs) and progressing to increasing doses of opioid analgesics (WHO, 2008). For pain that does not respond to drugs, or when oral or topical medication leads to unacceptable side effects such as nausea, constipation, somnolence, confusion, dependence and addiction, an alcohol nerve block can be indicated. This provides pain relief by acting directly on the nerves (celiac plexus) that carry painful stimuli from the diseased pancreas to the brain. Pancreatic cancer causes severe pain in 50% to 70% of patients. This kind of pain is multi-factorial (pancreatic duct obstruction and hypertension, neural invasion) and it is often difficult to treat (Staatas 2001). Different mechanisms perpetuate pancreatic pain: infiltration of nerve sheaths and neural ganglia, increased ductal and interstitial pressure and gland inflammation. Pancreatic pain is generally transmitted through the celiac plexus, a neural structure located in the upper abdomen, near the emergence of the celiac trunk from the aorta. Celiac plexus neurolysis was first described by Kappis (1919) and is done at the level of the L1 vertebral body, with the patient in the prone position. There are a number of variations on the technique (Giménez, 1993). It has been described in the literature since the 1950s but the first prospective study was published in 1990 and the first randomized in 1992. Celiac plexus neurolysis can be done surgically under fluoroscopic guidance or under computed tomography (CT) guidance. The target for celiac axis destruction are the splanchnic nerves and/or celiac ganglia. The splanchnic nerves cross the diaphragm, enter the abdominal cavity and form the celiac plexus. The celiac ganglia are located around the celiac artery anterior to the aorta, in varying positions, from T12 to L2. They can be reached percutaneously by different routes, with one needle through the anterior approach (under CT or ultrasound guidance) or with one or two needles through the posterior approach. During abdominal surgical procedures for pancreatic cancer chemical splanchnicectomy can be achieved by injecting the neurolytic solutions directly into the junction area of the splanchnic nerves with the celiac ganglia in the retroperitoneal area. With the advent of endoscopic ultrasonography (EUS) new therapeutic applications for endoscopy have been developed and a needle can now be guided safely in the celiac plexus (Puli, 2009). The celiac plexus is destroyed by alcohol injected under the guidance of real-time endosonography. First, using a linear array echo-endoscope, the region of the celiac ganglia is located from the lesser curve of the stomach, following the emergence of the celiac trunk from the aorta. The anterior approach avoids the retro-crural space and minimizes the risk of neurologic complications such as paraesthesia or paralysis. Anyway, although statistical evidence is minimal for the superiority of pain relief over analgesic therapy, the fact that CPB causes fewer adverse effects than opioids is important for patients.

4. Conclusion

Pancreatic ductal adenocarcinoma (90% of pancreatic cancers) remains a devastating disease. For a select group in which complete resection is possible, surgery prolongs survival. Pancreaticoduodenectomy, the "Cadillac" of abdominal operations, is a major surgery with significant morbidity and mortality. The pancreatico-enteric anastomosis has been the Achilles' heel of this operation. Adequate nutritional support, reduction of invasiveness, shorter operation times, combined regional/general anesthesia, and target-controlled fluid management are options for reducing postoperative morbidity. In recent decades, diagnostic modalities and the surgical and palliative treatments of PC have clearly progressed, although the overall prognosis has barely changed. The management of patient affected by PC is complex and requires exepertise in many fields. Multidisciplinary teams are necessary to optimize the overall care. The anesthesiologist plays a crucial role in the perioperative management of such patients and for patient with unresectable PC (anesthesia and analgesia). Careful patient selection, individualized preoperative evaluation and optimization go a long way in improving the short-term and long-term outcomes of these patients. In the future new protocols are necessary for pain control, adjuvant strategies, palliative measures in patients with pancreatic cancer.

5. References

Baum, J.A. (2004). The carrier gas in anaesthesia: nitrous oxide/oxygen, medical air/oxygen and pure oxygen. *Curr Opin Anaesthesiol* Vol. 17, No. 6, pp. 513-6, ISSN 0952-7907

Bluman, L.G., Mosca, L., Newman, N. & Simon, D.G. (1998). Preoperative smoking habits and postoperative pulmonary complications. *Chest,* Vol. 113, pp. 883-9, ISSN 0012-3692

Buchler, M.W. et al. (2003). Changes in morbidity after pancreatic resection : toward the end of completion pancreatectomy. Arch Surg, Vol. 138,No. 12, pp. 1310-1314, ISSN 0004-0010

Chiu, J.W.& White, P.F. (2000). The pharmacoeconomics of neuromuscular blocking drugs. J Anaesth, Vol.90, pp. S19-S23, ISSN 0003-2999

Clement, S., Braithwaite, S.S., Magee, M.F., et al. (2004). Management of diabetes and hyperglycemia in hospitals. *Diabetes Care,* Vol. 27, pp. 553–597, ISSN 0149-5992

Coursin, D.B., Connery, L.E. & Ketzler, J.T.(2004). Perioperative diabetic and hyperglycemic management issues. *Crit Care Med,* Vol. 32, pp. S116–S125, ISSN 0090-3493

Davies, R.G., Myles, P.S. & Graham, J.M. (2006). A comparison of the analgesic efficacy and site effects of paravertebral epidural blockade for thoracotomy- a systematic review and meta-analysis of randomized trials. *Br j Anaesth,* Vol. 96, No. 4, pp. 418-26, ISSN 0007-0912

Delbeke D., Rose, D.M., Chapman, W.C., Pinson, C.W., Wright, J.K., Beauchamp, R.D., Shyr Y. & Learch, S.D. (1999). Optimal interpretation of FDG PET in the diagnosis, staging and management of pancreatic carcinoma. *J Nucl Med,* Vol. 40, No. 11, pp. 1784-1791, ISSN 0161-5505

Dershwitz, M., Hoke, J.F., Rosow, C.E., Michalowski, P., Connors, P.M., Muir, K.T et al. (1996). Pharmacokinetics and pharmacodynamics of remifentanil in volunteer subjects with severe liver disease. *Anesthesiology,* Vol. 84, No.4, pp. 812-20, ISSN 0003-3022

Fotiadis, R.J., Badvie, S., Weston, M.D. & Allen-Mersh T.G. (2004). Epidural analgesia in gastrointestinal surgery. *British Journal of Surgery,* Vol. 91, No.7, pp. 828-841, ISSN 0007-1323

Furnary, A.P., Gao, G., Grunkemeier, G.L. et al.(2003). Continuous insulin infusion reduces mortality in patients with diabetes undergoing coronary artery bypass grafting. *J Thorac Cardiovasc Surg,*Vol. 125, No. 5, pp. 1007–1021, ISSN 0022-5223

Gass, G.D. & Olsen, G.N. (1986). Preoperative pulmonary function testing to predict postoperative morbidity and mortality. *Chest,* Vol. 89, No. 1, pp. 127-35, ISSN 0012-3692

Ghaferi, A.A., Birkmeyer, J.D. & Dimik, J.B. (2009). Variation in hospital mortality associated with inpatient surgery. *N Engl J Med* Vol. 361, No. 14, pp. 1368-75, ISSN 1533-4406

Gibbs, J., Cull,W., Henderson,W., Daley, J., Hur, K. & Khuri, S.F.(1999). Preoperative serum albumin level as a predictor of operative mortality and morbidity : results from the National VA Surgical Risk Study. *Arch Surg,* Vol.134, No. 1, pp.36-42, ISSN 0004-0010

Giménez, A., Martínez-Noguera, A., Donoso, L., Catalá, E. & Serra, R.(1993). Percutaneous neurolysis of the celiac plexus via the anterior approach with sonographic guidance. *AJR Am J Roentgenol,* Vol. 161, No. 5,pp. 1061-3, ISSN 0361-803X

Gogarten, W., Vandermeulen, E., Van Aken, H., Kozek, S., Van Llau, J. & Samama, C.M. (2010). Regional anaesthesia and antithrombotic agents: recommendations of the European Society of Anaesthesiology. *Eur J Anaesthesiol,* Vol. 27, No. 12, pp. 999–1015, ISSN 0265-0215

Goldberg, P.A., Siegel, M.D., Sherwin, R.S., et al. (2004). Implementation of a safe and effective insulin infusion protocol in a medical intensive care unit. *Diabetes Care,* Vol. 27, No. 2, pp. 461–467, ISSN 0149-5992

Gullo, L., Pezzilli, R. & Morselli-Labate, A.M. (1994). Diabetes and the risk of pancreatic cancer. *N Engl J Med,* Vol. 331, No. 2, pp. 81-84, ISSN 0028-4793

Hecker K, Baumert, J.H., Horn, N. & Rossaint, R. (2004). Xenon, a modern anaesthesia gas. *Minerva Anestesiol,* Vol.70, No. 5, pp. 255-60, ISSN 0375-9393

Henderson, K.A., Raj, N. & Hall, J.E. (2002). The use of nitrous oxide in anaesthetic practice: a questionnaire survey. Anaesthesia, Vol. 57, No. 12, pp. 1155-8, ISSN 0003-2409

Inoue, K. et al. (2002). Spontaneous resolution of epidural hematoma after continuous epidural analgesia in a patient without bleeding tendency. *Anesthesiology,* Vol. 97, No. 3, pp. 735-7, ISSN 0003-3022

Jemal A. et al. (2009). Cancer statistics, 2009.*CA Cancer J Clin*, Vol. 59, No. 4, pp. 225-249, ISSN 0007-9235

Jiang, W.G .& Puntis MC. (1997). Immune dysfunction in patients with obstructive jaundice, mediators and implications for treatments. *HPB Surg*, Vol.10, No. 3, pp. 129-42, ISSN 0894-8569

Karmaker, M.K. (2001). Thoracic paravertebral block. *Anesthesiology*, Vol. 95, No. 3, pp. 771-80, ISSN 0003-3022

Koretz, R.L., Lipman,T.O. & Klein, S. (2001). AGA technical review on parenteral nutrition. *Gastroenterology*, Vol. 121, No. 4, pp. 970-1001, ISSN 0016-5085

Kullavanijaya, P., Treeprasertsuk, S., Thong-Nham, D., Kladcharoen, N., Mahachai, V. & Suwanagool, P. (2001). Adenocarcinoma of the pancreas: the clinical experience of 45 histopathologically proven patients, a 6 year study. *J Med Assoc Thai*, Vol. 84, No 5,. pp. 640-647, ISSN 0125-2208

Kumamoto, e., Mizuta, K. & Fujita, T. (2011). Opiod actions in primary- afferent fibers-involvement in analgesia and anestesia. *Pharmaceuticals*, Vol. 4, (January 2011), pp. 343-365, ISSN 1424-8247

Lawrence, V.A., Dhanda, R., Hilsenbeck, S.G. & Page, P.G. (1996). Risk of pulmonary omplications after elective abdominal surgery. *Chest*, Vol. 110, No.3, pp. 744-50, ISSN 0012-3692

Lynch, S.M., Vrieling, A., Lubin, J.H., Kraft, P., Mendelson, J.B., Hartge, P., Canzian, F., Steplowski, E., Arslan, A.A., Gross,M.,Helzlsouer, K., Jacobs,E.J., La Croix,A., Petersen, G., Zheng, W., Albanes,D., Amundadottir, L., Bingham, S.A., Boffetta, P., Boutron-Ruault, M.C., Chanock, S.J., Clipp,S., Hoover, R.N., Jacobs, K. *et al.* (2009). Cigarette smoking and pancreatic cancer : a pooled analysis from the pancreatic cancer cohort consortium. *Am J Epidemiol* Vol. 170, No. 4,pp. 403-413, ISSN 0002-9262

Macias, A., Monedero, P., Adame, M., Torre, T., Fidalgo, I. & Hidalgo, F. (2002). A randomized, double-blinded comparison of thoracic epidural ropivacaine, ropivacaine/ fentanyl, or bupivacaine / fentanyl for postthoracotomy analgesia. *Anesth Analg*, Vol. 95, No. 5, pp. 1344-50, ISSN 0003-2999

Miaskowski, C. (2005). Patient-controlled modalities for acute postoperative pain management. *J Perianesth Nurs*,Vol. 20, No. 4,pp. 255-67, ISSN 1089-9472

Murphy, G.S. & Szokol, J.W. (2004). Monitoring neuromuscular blockade. *Int Anesthesiol Clin*, Vol.42, No.2, pp.25-40, ISSN 0020-5907

Myles, P.S., Iacono, G.A., Hunt, J.O., Fletcher, H., Morris, J., McIlory, D. & Fritschi, L. (2002). Risk of respiratory complications and wound infection in patients undergoing ambulatory surgery : smokers versus nonsmokers. *Anesthesiology*, Vol. 97, No. 4, pp. 842-7, ISSN 0003-3022

Nussmeier, N.A., Whelton, A.A., Brown, M..T, Joshi, G.P., Langford, R.M., Singla, N.K., Boye, M.E. & Verburg, K.M (2006). Anesthesiology,Vol. 104, No. 3, pp. 255-67, ISSN 0003-3022

Neugut, A.I., Ahsan, H. & Robinson, E. (1995). Pancreas cancer as a second primary malignancy. A population- based study. *Cancer*, Vol. 76, No. 4, pp. 589-592, ISSN 0008-543X

Panousis,P., Heller, A.R., Koch, T. & Litz, R. (2009). Epidural ropivacaine concentrations for intraoperative analgesia during major upper abdominal surgery : A prospective, randomized, double-blinded, placebo-controlled study. *Anesthesia & analgesia*, Vol.108, No. 6, (June 2009), pp. 1971-6, ISSN 0003-2999

Pearce, A.C. & Jones, R.M. (1984). Smoking and anesthesia : preoperative abstinence and perioperative morbidity. *Anesthesiology*, Vol. 61, No. 5, pp. 576-84, ISSN 0003-3022

Permet, J., Ihse, I., Jorfeldt, L., von Schenck H et al. (1993). Pancreatic cancer is associated with impaired glucose metabolism. *Eur J Surg*, Vol. 159, No. 2, pp. 101-107, ISSN 1102-4151

Puli, S.R. et al. (2009). US-guided celiac plexus neurolysis for pain due to chronic pancreatitis or pancreatic cancer pain: A meta-analysis and systematic review. *Digestive Diseases Science*, Vol. 54, No. 11, pp. 2330-7, ISSN 0163-2116

Riall, T.S., Reddy, D.M., Nelson, W.H. & Goodwin, J.S. (2008). The effect of age on short-term outcomes after pancreatic resection : a population-based study. *Ann Surg*, Vol. 248, No. 3, pp. 459-67, ISSN 0003-4932

Rehman, H.U. & Mohammed, K. (2003). Perioperative management of diabetic patients. *Curr Surg*, Vol.60, No. 6, pp. 607–611, ISSN 0149-7944

Shaib Y.H., Davila J.A. & El-Serag H.B. (2006). The epidemiology of pancreatic cancer in the United States: changes below the surface. *Aliment pharmacol Ther*, Vol. 24, No. 1, pp. 87-94, ISSN 0269-2813

Skilton, R.W.H. & Justice, W. (1998). Epidural hematoma following anticoagulant treatment in a patient with an indwelling epidural catheter. *Anesthesia*, Vol. 53, No. 7, pp. 691-701, ISSN 0003-2409

Staatas, P.S. et al. (2001). The effects of alcohol celiac block, pain and mood on longevity in patients with unresectable pancreatic pain: A double-blind, randomized, placebo-controlled study. *Pain Medicine*, Vol. 2, No. 1, pp. 28-34, ISSN 1526-2375

Tilleman, E.H., Busch, O.R., Bemelman, W.A., van Gulik, T.M., Obertop, H. & Gouma, D.J. (2004). Diagnostic laparoscopy in staging pancreatic carcinoma: Developments during the past decade. *J Hepatobiliary Pancreat Surg*, Vol. 11, No. 1, pp. 11-16, ISSN 0944-1166

Treiman, G.S., Treiman RL, Foran RF et al. (1994). The influence of diabetes mellitus on the risk of abdominal aortic surgery. *Am Surg*, Vol. 60, No. 6, pp. 436-40, ISSN 0003-1348

Tryba, M. (1998). European practice guidelines: Thromboembolism prophylaxis and regional anesthesia. *Reg Anesth Pain Med*, Vol. 23 (Suppl. 2), pp. 178-82, ISSN 1098-7339

Van der Gaag, N.A., Kloek, J.J., de Castro, S.M., Busch, O.R., van Gulik, T.M. & Gouma, D.J. (2009). Preoperative biliary drainage in patients with obstructive jaundice : history and current status. *J Gastrointest Surg*, Vol. 13, No. 4, pp. 814-20, ISSN 1091-255X

Van der Gaag, N.A., Rauws, E.A.J., van Eijck, H.J., Bruno, M.J., van derd Harst, E., Kubben, F.J., Gerritsen, J., Greve, J.W., Gerhards, M.F. et al. (2010). Preoperative biliary drainage for cancer of the head of the pancreas. *N Engl J Med*, Vol. 362, No. 2, pp. 129-37, ISSN 0028-4793

Van Lier, F., Van der Geest, P., Hoeks, S., Van Gestel, Y., Hol, J., Sin, D., Stolker, R.J. & Poldermans, D. (2011). Epidural analgesia is associated with improved health outcomes of surgical patients with chronic obstructive pulmonary disease. *Anesthesiology*, Vol. 115, No. 2, pp. 315-21, ISSN 0003-3022

Vandermeulen, E.P., Van Haken, H. & Vermylen, J. (1994). Anticoagulants and spinal-epidural anesthesia. *Anesth Analg*, Vol. 79,No. 6, pp. 1165-77, ISSN 0003-2999

Verhofstad, H.J. & Hendriks, T. (1996). Complete prevention of impaired anastomotic healing in diabetic rats requires preoperative blood glucose control. *Br J Surg*, Vol. 83, No. 12, pp. 1717-21, ISSN 0007-1323

Zacharias, A.Z. & Habib, R.H. (1996). Factors predisposing to median sternotomy complications. *Chest*, Vol. 110, No. 5, pp. 1173-8, ISSN 0012-3692

WHO (2008). Scoping document for WHO treatment guideline on pain related to cancer, HIV and other progressive life-threatening illnesess in adult adopted in WHO steering group on pain guidelines, 14 October 2008. WHO Steereing Group on Pain Guidelines

11

Multi-Disciplinary Management of Metastatic Pancreatic Cancer

Marwan Ghosn*, Colette Hanna and Fadi El. Karak
Faculty of Medicine, Saint-Joseph University, Beirut, Lebanon

1. Introduction

Pancreatic cancer (PC) is a devastating disease with the worst mortality rate and an overall 5-year survival rate lower than 5% (2% in distant cases; 9% in regional cases and 22% in localized cases). Although accounting for only 3% of all cancers, this disease is the fourth leading cause of death and represents 6 - 7 % of all cancer related deaths. In males, the incidence ASR is 8.2 and 2.7 and the mortality ASR is 7.9 and 2.5 in more developed areas and less developed areas, respectively.

In females, the incidence ASR is 5.4 and 2.1 and the mortality ASR is 5.1 and 2.0 in more developed areas and less developed areas, respectively.

We noticed that the incidence and the mortality rates are very close (*Jemal et al. 2011*). Also, the death rate is increasing from 9.28 per 100,000 in 1991 to 9.48 in 2006 with an absolute change of 0.2 (2.1%). (*Jemal et al. 2010*).

In the United States, the overall incidence is about 8–10 cases per 100,000 persons/year and rises slowly over the years with 43 140 new cases in 2010.

Pancreatic cancer remains one of the most difficult to treat due to late initial diagnosis and to intrinsic resistance to conventional treatments. About 50% of patients have distant disease at the time of diagnosis (locally advanced stage) and in 40% the tumor has spread (metastatic stage).

2. Risk factors

Risk factors have been identified, molecular pathogenesis has been elucidated, but advances in early detection and efficient treatments remain rather disappointing despite tremendous efforts.

Studies results show that long-term diabetes, even though risk diminishes over time, remains a risk factor for PC independent of obesity and smoking with a latency period of more than 5 years. Type 3 diabetes mellitus is an effect, and therefore a harbinger, of pancreatic cancer in at least 30% of patients (*Magruder JT et al, 2011; Li D et al. 2011*).

---

* Corresponding Author

After a pooled analysis of 14 cohort studies, a review study noted that, coffee consumption was inversely associated with pancreatic cancer (RR, 0.82; 95% CI, 0.69-0.95) *(Yu X et al, 2011).*

Although there have not been a sufficient number of clinical trials, promising dietary factors to prevent pancreatic cancer include citrus fruits, flavonoids, curcumin, folate, and vitamin D. Phase II clinical trials of curcumin have shown encouraging chemoprotective effects in patients with pancreatic cancer and have determined that curcumin can be safely administrated to patients at oral doses up to 8 g/d.

Several flavonoids found in a variety of fruits and vegetables have also been shown to inhibit pancreatic cancer at various molecular targets including cell-cycle, Akt, NFkB, ERK, and many others. Currently, there is one on-going phase II clinical trial on the use of genistein in treating resectable pancreatic cancer patients. However, more clinical trials are needed to explore the efficacy and application of these factors in treating pancreatic cancer.

The use of citrus fruit extracts to treat pancreatic cancer has become of interest only in the past few years. Using citrus fruit extracts instead of individual compounds to treat pancreatic cancer is of great interest because it allows the use of low doses of multiple bioactive compounds and nutrients instead of large doses of single compounds, and therefore reducing the possibility of reaching toxic effects.

When comparing the inhibitory effects of different extraction methods of lime juice on pancreatic cancer, it was found that the methanol extract exhibited the highest inhibitory effect. Although the results from this study provide insight into the best options for extracting citrus fruits, more research needs to be conducted on various types of citrus fruits extracts and their mechanisms of action by which they affect pancreatic cancer.

Folate and vitamin D have good epidemiological evidence that shows that consumption of either of these nutrients leads to a reduced risk of pancreatic cancer. However, both of the nutrients have few experimental studies needed to help draw conclusions about either of their impacts on pancreatic cancer. *(Jodee Johnson et al. 2011).*

The pooled data of 6 studies involving a total of 2335 patients suggests an association between infection with H. pylori and the development of pancreatic cancer ((AOR 1.38, 95% CI: 1.08-1.75; P=0.009). *(Trikudanathan G et al, 2011)*

As is the case in other complex diseases, common, low-risk variants in different genes may act collectively to confer susceptibility to pancreatic cancer in individuals with repeated environmental exposures, such as smoking and red meat intake. Clarification of gene–gene and gene–environmental interaction is therefore indispensable for future studies. To address these issues, a rigorously designed molecular epidemiologic study with a large sample is desirable. *(Yingsong Lin et al, 2011.)*

3. Diagnosis

Pancreatic cancer is usually detected at an advanced stage and responds poorly to treatment.

Ductal adenocarcinoma and its variants account for over 90% of pancreatic malignancies. The presenting symptoms of the disease can include weight loss, jaundice, floating stools, pain, dyspepsia, nausea and depression. However, no early warning signs of pancreatic cancer have been established. As previously noted, long term diabetes is a risk factor thus diagnosis of pancreatic cancer should be considered in diabetic patients with continuous weight loss and abdominal symptoms. All patients for whom there is clinical suspicion of pancreatic cancer or evidence of dilated duct should undergo initial evaluation by dynamic-phase CT scan. Subsequent decisions regarding diagnostic management and resectability should involve multidisciplinary consultation with reference to appropriate radiographic studies to evaluate the extent of the disease *(Agarwal B et al, 2001. Johnson CD. 2010)*

The principles of diagnosis and staging are:

1. Decisions about diagnostic management and resectability should involve multidisciplinary consultation with reference to appropriate radiographic studies to evaluate the extent of disease. Resections should be done at institutions that perform a large number (15-20) of pancreatic resections annually.
2. Imaging should include specialized pancreatic CT scan. CT should be performed according to a defined protocol such as triphasic cross-sectional imaging and thin slices.
3. The role of PET/CT scan remains unclear. PET/CT may be considered after formal pancreatic CT protocol in high risk patients to detect extra-pancreatic metastases. It is not a substitute for high quality contrast enhances CT scan.
4. Endoscopic Ultrasound (EUS) may be complementary to CT for staging.
5. EUS directed fine needle biopsy is preferable to a CT-guided FNA in patients with resectable disease because of lower risk of peritoneal seeding with EUS FNA when compared with the percutaneous approach. Biopsy proof of malignancy is not required before surgical resection and a non diagnostic biopsy should not delay surgical resection when the clinical suspicion for pancreatic cancer is high.
6. Diagnostic staging with laparoscopy to rule out subradiologic metastases (especially for body and tall lesions) is used routinely in some institutions prior to surgery or chemoradiation or selectively in patients whoa re at higher risk for disseminated disease (borderline resectable disease, markedly elevated CA 19-9, large primary tumors or large regional lympnodes).
7. Positive cytology from washings obtained at laparoscopy or laparotomy is equivalent to M1 disease. If resection has been done for such a patient, they should be treated as for M1 disease.

The key advances are:

In 2010 new insights were added to the complex biology of pancreatic cancer offering new opportunities for early diagnosis and treatment.

The first comprehensive analysis of pancreatic tumors and their metastases describes the patterns of genomic instability and estimates the time from tumor initiation to metastatic spread to be at least 10 years *(Yachida, S. et al, 2010).*

Genome-wide association studies point towards multiple common disease alleles with small effects influencing pancreatic cancer risk *(Petersen, G. M. et al. 2010; Low, S. K. et al. 2010).*

The ESPAC-3 trial reported that gemcitabine did not result in improved overall survival compared with fluorouracil plus folinic acid in patients with resected pancreatic cancer *(Neoptolemos, J. P. et al. 2010).*

Superior values for diagnostic performance were shown for MIC-1, PAM4, OPN, HSP27, TPS, TSGF, and CAM17.1 as individual markers. Panels of biomarkers comprised CA 19-9, MCSF, CEA, SAA, Haptoglobin, TSGF, CA 242, and HSP27. Individually or in concerted form, sensitivity and specificity ranged from 77 to 100% and 84-100%, respectively. While these markers show high screening potential for pancreatic cancer, standardized validation studies using multiplex assays are required to pave the way for clinical routine application *(Bünger S et al, 2011).*

4. Treatment

There is consensus on the fact that surgical removal of the tumor represents the best option for pancreatic cancer treatment; to be resectable, tumors need to be small and strictly localized to pancreas without invasion into surrounding organs and evidence of metastasis. However, only 15–20% of all patients are candidates for potentially curative surgery. Depending on the tumor localization, pancreaticoduodenectomy, distal or total pancreatectomy can be performed. However, even with an optimal curative surgery, metastases often occur. Median survival time without evidence of recurrent disease is 21.2 months after resection.

Systemic therapy is used in the adjuvant setting and in the management of locally advanced unresectable and metastatic disease.

4.1 Neoadjuvant resectable / borderline resectable

No standard treatment regimen currently exists for neoadjuvant resectable or borderline resectable pancreatic cancer. Neoadjuvant therapy for patients with resectable tumors should ideally be conducted on a clinical trial. Generally, use similar paradigms as for locally advanced unresectable disease:

- Upfront 5-FU or Capecitabine based chemoradiation
- Upfront gemcitabine-based chemoradiation therapy
- Induction chemotherapy (2 to 4 cycles) followed by 5-FU or Gemcitabine based chemoradiation therapy.

Ideally, surgical resection should be atatempted 6 to 8 weeks following chemoradiation. Surgery can be performed after 8 weeks following chemoradiation however radiation induced fibrosis may potentially make surgery more difficult.

4.2 Chemoradiation therapy for locally advanced disease

Chemoradiation is a conventional option for the management of unresectable locorgeional pancreatic cancer, although the utility of chemoradiation in this population of patients is controversial.

4.3 Post-operative adjuvant treatment

Clinical trial preferred or Systemic Gemcitabine or 5-FU/Leucovorin before or after chemoradiation (fluoropyrimidine or gemcitabine based) or chemotherapy alone Gemcitabine (category 1) or 5-FU/Leucovorin (category 1) or Capeciatbine (Category 2B).

4.4 Chemotherapy for locally advanced and metastatic disease

The primary goals of treatment for advanced pancreatic cancer are palliation and improved survival. Although some effect on survival may be achieved, these benefits are usually limited to patients with adequate performance status (ECIG 0-2). Patients who present with very poor performance status may benefit from the administration of Gemcitabine, but comfort-directed measures are always paramount. Before initiating cytotoxic therapy, an open dialogue regarding the goals of treatment should take place, and adjunctive strategies should be discussed (including nonsurgical bypass, celiac block for pain; of note debilitated patients with advanced disease may have abrupt changes in clinical status. Therefore, if treatment is begun, it should proceed with close follow-up. Patients may experience sudden onset of bleeding or thromboembolism, rapidly escalating pain, biliary stent occlusion, cholangitis, or other infections. Moreover, clinically meaningful tumor progression may develop quickly, and tumor-related symptoms may be inappropriately attributed to chemotherapy or other causes. For instance, patients who complain of intractable nausea and vomiting may have gastric outlet obstruction rather than chemotherapy-induced emesis. Peritoneal carcinomatosis may manifest as ascites or in its more subtle form, as abdominal bloating, decreased oral intake and constipation.

Prior to approval of Gemcitabine, 5-FU was the most extensively evaluated agent for PC, either alone or in combination without survival advantage. Gemcitabine, with or without Erlotinib, has been the standard chemotherapy in APC. The FDA approval in 1997 was based on the results of the randomized trial where Gemcitabine was compared to 5-FU in previously untreated patients. Patients treated with Gemcitabine had a median survival of 5.65 months, compared to 4.41 months ($p < 0.05$) in those treated with 5-FU. Twenty-four percent of patients treated with gemcitabine were alive at 9 months, compared to 6% of patients treated with 5-FU. In addition, more clinically meaningful effects on disease-related symptoms were seen with gemcitabine (23.8%) than with 5-FU (4.8%). *(Burris HA 3rd, Moore MJ, Andersen J et al. 1997).*

Platinum compounds have been widely evaluated. A pooled analysis of two randomized trials indicates that the combination of gemcitabine with a platinum analog such as oxaliplatin or cisplatin significantly improves progression-free (PFS) and overall survival (OS) when compared to gemcitabine alone (HR for PFS: 0.75 with p=0.0030; HR for OS: 0.64 with p=0.063 in favour of the GP combination). The benefit from combination therapy is predominantly detected in patients with a good performance status. *(V. Heinemann, Labianca R, Hinke A, Louvet C. et al. 2007).*

Among the numerous randomized phase III studies comparing gemcitabine as single agent to gemcitabine combined to a new agent, only the gemcitabine-erlotinib combination has shown a small, but statistical improvement in survival. A trend to better survival was also observed with a gemcitabine-capecitabine regimen. The use of low-weight heparin may be of value to reduce venous thromboembolic events

The various combinations of new generation drugs showed 13% - 28.7 % RR with the Gemcitabine/Oxaliplatin, 8.2% - 17.3% with Gemcitabine alone, 12.8 % with Gemcitabine/CPT-11, 16% - 23% with Gemcitabine/Capecitabine, 22% with Oxaliplatin/Capecitabine and 10% with Oxaliplatin and 5-FU, 12.9% with Cisplatin / Gemcitabine, 13 % with Bevacizumab/Gemcitabine, 8.6 % with Erlotinib/Gemcitabine and 12.5 % with Cetuximab/Gemcitabine and 31% with the Folfirinox regimen.

The addition of Cisplatin, Bevacizumab, Cetuximab to Gemcitabine did not improve survival compared with patients treated with Gemcitabine alone in APC patients. The OS ranged between 5.8 and 9 months (table 1).

(G. Stathopoulos, K. Syrigos, G. Aravantinos, et al. 2006; V. Heinemann, T. Hoehler, G. Seipelt et al. 2008; K. Song, Y. Do, H. Chang et al. 2008; M. Moore, D. Goldstein, J. Hamm et al. 2007; Hedy Lee Kindler et al. 2010; Philip A. Philip. 2010; Giuseppe Colucci et al. 2010; E. Popli, Y. Feng, J. Berlin et al. Phase III, 2009; Jürg Bernhard et al. 2008; J. C. Bendell, S. Britton, M. R. Green et al. 2011; P. E. Oberstein, M. Saif. First 2011).

Reference	Regimen	Clinical benefit	ORR	median PFS	median survival
Berlin et al. JCO 2002	5FU + Gem	23.8%	6.9%	3.4 mo	6.7 mo
	Gem	4.8%	5.6%	2.2 mo	5.4 mo
Colucci et al. JCO 2010	Gem + Cisplatin	15.1%	12.9%	3.8 mo	7.2 mo
	Gem	23.0%	10.1%	3.9 mo	8.3 mo
Louvet et al. JCO 2005	Gem + Oxaliplatin	38.2%	26.8%	5.8 mo	9 mo
	Gem	26.9%	17.3%	3.7 mo	7.1 mo
Poplin et al. JCO 2009	Gemox	ND	9.0%	2.7 mo	5.7 mo
	Gem fixed dose rate	ND	10.0%	3.5 mo	6.2 mo
	Gem	ND	6.0%	2.6 mo	4.9 mo
Heinemann et al Ann Oncol 2007	Gem + Platinum	ND	22.0%	24 weeks	36 weeks
	Gem	ND	14.0%	15 weeks	29 weeks
Ghosn et al. Am J Clin Oncol 2007	Gem + Oxaliplatin + 5FU/LV	62.0%	27.5%	4 mo	7.5 mo
Bernhard et al. JCO 2008	Gem + Capecitabine	26.0%	ND	ND	ND
	Gem	25.0%	ND	ND	ND
Philip et al. JCO 2010	Gem + Cetuximab	49.5%	12.5%	3.4 mo	6.3 mo
	Gem	44.1%	14.0%	3 mo	5.9 mo
Kindler et al JCO 2010	Gem + Bevacizumab	13.0%	13.0%	3.8 mo	5.8 mo
	Gem	10.0%	10.0%	2.9 mo	5.9 mo
Moore et al. JCO 2007	Gem + Erlotinib	57.5%	8.6%	3.75 mo	6.24 mo
	Gem	49.2%	8.0%	3.55 mo	5.91 mo

Table 1. Summary of Results of some important Gemcitabine-based regimen

Oxaliplatin is one of the investigational active agents used in APC. With its synergistic effect, Oxaliplatin shows a higher RR when combined with other drugs. With 5-FU, preclinical data suggested synergistic efficacy which led to investigate the combination in many clinical trials. In a phase II trial in pancreatic cancer patients, this combination was explored and showed encouraging RR which deserve more evaluation *(M. Ducreux, 2004; C. Louvet, R. Labianca, P. Hammel et al. 2005; C. Louvet, T. Andre, G. Liedo et al. 2002).*

Recent publication of the results of a phase II trial performed by our group and assessing the combination of the FOLFOX 6 regimen showed promising results (27.5% partial response and 34.5% stable disease resulting in tumor growth control in 62% of the patients). Grade III or IV toxicities were mild. The median time to progression and the median survival time were 4 and 7.5 months respectively ***(M. Ghosn et al, 2007).***

Results from the randomized phase III study PRODIGE 4/ACCORD 11 trial evaluating the regimen of FOLFORINOX vs. Gemcitabine alone in patients with APC and good performance status showed dramatic improvements in both progression-free survival (6.4 months vs. 3.3 months, $p < 0.001$) and median overall survival (11.1 months vs. 6.8 months, $p < 0.001$) in favor of the group receiving FOLFORINOX. Because of these strong results, NCCN classified FOLFORINOX as a category 1 recommendation for first-line treatment of good performance status patients with either metastatic or locally advanced disease.

There are however some concerns about the toxicity of the FOLFORINOX regimen. The grade ¾ toxicities rates were 12.3% for diarrhea, 15.6% for nausea, 17.2% for vomiting, 24% for fatigue, 47.9% for neutropenia and 5.7% for febrile neutropenia. Despite the high level of toxicity, no toxic deaths have been reported.

The high level of toxicity highlight the need to identify which patients will ultimately benefit from this more aggressive approach.

Summary: Gemcitabine (with or without erlotinib or capecitabine) is still the reference treatment in patients with ECOG performance status 2. **Folfirinox** is a new more toxic and more efficient regimen that may be considered in patients with good performance status. There is a difficulty in improving outcomes in metastatic PC. This continues to be a field of intense interest and regimens that conclusively show benefit in this disease are likely to generate enthusiasm and rapid adoption into clinical practice.

5. References

Agarwal B et al, 2004. Endoscopic ultrasound guided fine needle aspiration and multidetector spiral CT in the diagnosis of pancreatic cancer. Am J gastroenterol; 99: 844 - 850.

Bendell J. C. et al, 2011, Immediate impact of the FOLFIRINOX phase III data reported at the 2010 ASCO Annual Meeting on prescribing plans of American oncology physicians for patients with metastatic pancreas cancer (MPC). J Clin Oncol , 29 (suppl 4): Abstr 286;

Bernhard Jürg et al, 2008. Clinical Benefit and Quality of Life in Patients With Advanced Pancreatic Cancer Receiving Gemcitabine Plus Capecitabine Versus Gemcitabine Alone: A Randomized Multicenter Phase III Clinical Trial. J Clin Oncol, 26 (22): 3695-3701;

Bünger S et al, 2010. biomarkers for improved diagnostic of pancreatic cancer: a current overview. J Cancer Res Clin Oncol. 2011 Mar; 137(3):375-89. .

Burris HA 3rd et al, 1997. Improvements in survival and clinical benefit with gemcitabine as first-line therapy for patients with advanced pancreas cancer: a randomized trial. J Clin Oncol 1997, 15(6): 2403-13.

Colucci Giuseppe et al, 2010. Randomized Phase III Trial of Gemcitabine Plus Cisplatin Compared With Single-Agent Gemcitabine As First-Line Treatment of Patients With Advanced Pancreatic Cancer: The GIP-1 Study. J Clin Oncol, 28: 1645 - 1651.

Conroy T et al, 2011. FOLFIRINOX versus gemcitabine for metastatic pancreatic cancer. N Engl J Med. May 12; 364(19):1817-25.

Ghosn M et al, 2007. FOLFOX-6 combination as the first-line treatment of locally advanced and/or metastatic pancreatic cancer. Am J Clin Oncol, 30 (1): 15-20.

Heinemann V et al. 2007. Increased survival using platinum analog combined with gemcitabine as compared to single-agent gemcitabine in advanced pancreatic cancer: pooled analysis of two randomized trials, the GERCOR/GISCAD intergroup study and a German multicenter study. Ann Oncol, 18 (10): 1652 - 9).

Heinemann V et al., 2008. Capecitabine plus oxaliplatin (CapOx) versus capecitabine plus gemcitabine (CapGem) versus gemcitabine plus oxaliplatin (mGemOx): final results of a multicenter randomized phase II trial in advanced pancreatic cancer. Ann Oncol, 19 (2): 340 - 7.

Jemal A et al. 2001.Global Cancer Statistics, Ca Cancer J Clin 2011, 61: 69 - 90) N Engl J Med. 364(19):1817-25.

Jemal Aet al, 2010. Cancer Statistics 2010, Ca Cancer J Clin, 60: 277 - 300.

Johnson J, de Mejia EG. Dietary factors and pancreatic cancer: The role of food bioactive compounds. Mol. Nutr. Food Res. 2011, 55, 58–73.

Johnson CD. Pancreatic carcinoma: devleoping a protocol for multidetecto row CT. Radiology 2001: 220: 3- 4.

Kindler Hedy Lee et al, 2010. Gemcitabine Plus Bevacizumab Compared With Gemcitabine Plus Placebo in Patients With Advanced Pancreatic Cancer: Phase III Trial of the Cancer and Leukemia Group B (CALGB 80303). J Clin Oncol, 28 (22): 3617-3622.

Li D et al, 2010. Diabetes and risk of pancreatic cancer: a pooled analysis of three large case-control studies. Cancer Causes Control. 2011 Feb; 22(2):189-97.

Lin Y et al, 2011. An Overview of Genetic Polymorphisms and Pancreatic Cancer Risk in Molecular Epidemiologic Studies. J Epidemiol; 21(1):2-12

Low SK et al, 2010. Genome-wide association study of pancreatic cancer in Japanese population. PLoS ONE 2010 Jul 29; 5(7):e11824.

Magruder JT et al. 2011. Diabetes and pancreatic cancer: chicken or egg? Pancreas, 40(3):339-51).

Moore M et al, 2007. Erlotinib plus gemcitabine compared with gemcitabine alone in patients with advanced pancreatic cancer: a phase III trial of the National Cancer Institute of Canada Clinical Trials Group. J Clin Oncol, 25 (15): 1960 - 6

Neoptolemos JP et al, 2010. Adjuvant chemotherapy with fluorouracil plus folinic acid vs gemcitabine following pancreatic cancer resection: a randomized controlled trial. JAMA, 304, 1073–1081.

Oberstein PE, M. Saif. First-Line Treatment for Advanced Pancreatic Cancer. S from the "2011 ASCO Gastrointestinal Cancers Symposium". J Pancreas (Online) 2011, 12(2):96-100.

Philip A. Philip. Phase III Study Comparing Gemcitabine Plus Cetuximab Versus Gemcitabine in Patients With Advanced Pancreatic Adenocarcinoma: Southwest Oncology Group-Directed Intergroup Trial S0205. J Clin Oncol 2010, 28 (22): 3605-3610.

Popli E et al, 2009. Phase III, Randomized Study of Gemcitabine and Oxaliplatin Versus Gemcitabine (fixed-dose rate infusion) Compared With Gemcitabine (30-minute infusion) in Patients With Pancreatic Carcinoma E6201: A Trial of the Eastern Cooperative Oncology Group. J Clin Oncol, 27 (23): 3778-3785.

Song K et al, 2008. A phase II study of capecitabine plus gemcitabine in patients with locally advanced or metastatic pancreatic cancer. Cancer Chemother Pharmacol 2008, 62 (5): 763 - 8.

Stathopoulos S et al, 2006. A multicenter phase III trial comparing irinotecan-gemcitabine (IG) with gemcitabine (G) monotherapy as first-line treatment in patients with locally advanced or metastatic pancreatic cancer. Br J Cancer, 95 (5):587-92.

12

Pancreatic Cancer – Clinical Course and Survival

Birgir Gudjonsson
MACP, FRCP, AGAF
The Medical Clinic, Reykjavik,
Iceland

1. Introduction

The incidence of pancreatic carcinoma varies from 6-20/100.000 in different countries and ethnic groups, but is considered to be on the average 10/100.000 (Gudjonsson 1987) and causes a significant economic burden on health resources (Gudjonsson 1995, Du 2000).

Cancer of the pancreas is the 13th in frequency in the USA but fourth most frequent cause of death from cancer (Jemal 2010) fifth most frequent cause of death in Japan and sixth in China.

Adenocarcinoma constitutes 90% of pancreatic malignancies. Only 50% of patients in tumor registries had histologic confirmation (Gudjonsson 1987).

The cause of pancreatic cancer is unclear but it is more frequent among cigarette smokers. Chronic pancreatitis leads to increased frequency.

2. Genes

Mutations in K-ras genes are found in up to 90% of cases of cancer of the pancreas but are not specific and are also found in patients with chronic pancreatitis. The suppressor genes p16 and p53 are inactivated and DPC4 deleted in 50% of cases of pancreatic cancer. (Cowgill 2003).

3. Clinical features

The disease is slightly more frequent among males than females.

Patients may occasionally be under thirty years of age. Forty percent are between 60-70 years. Thirty percent are between 50-60 years old and twenty percent between 70-80 years old (Gudjonsson 1987).

4. Clinical features

Majority of patients complain of weight loss which is on the average 10 kg. Most complain of pain, which may be deep seated, in a third of patients the pain radiates to the back, a fifth experience relief by bending forward, and 10-15% it is worsened with eating.

Anorexia may be present in half of patients. A third may complain of vomiting. A third complain of acholic stools and dark urine. One in four may report jaundice (Gudjonsson 1987).

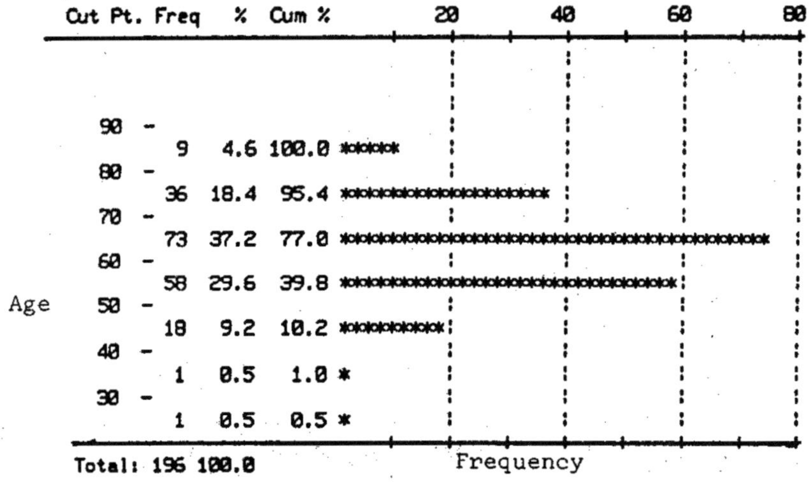

Fig. 1. Age distribution.

Duration of symptoms is variable but 40% have had symptoms less than 1 month, 20% 2 months and 10% 3 months.

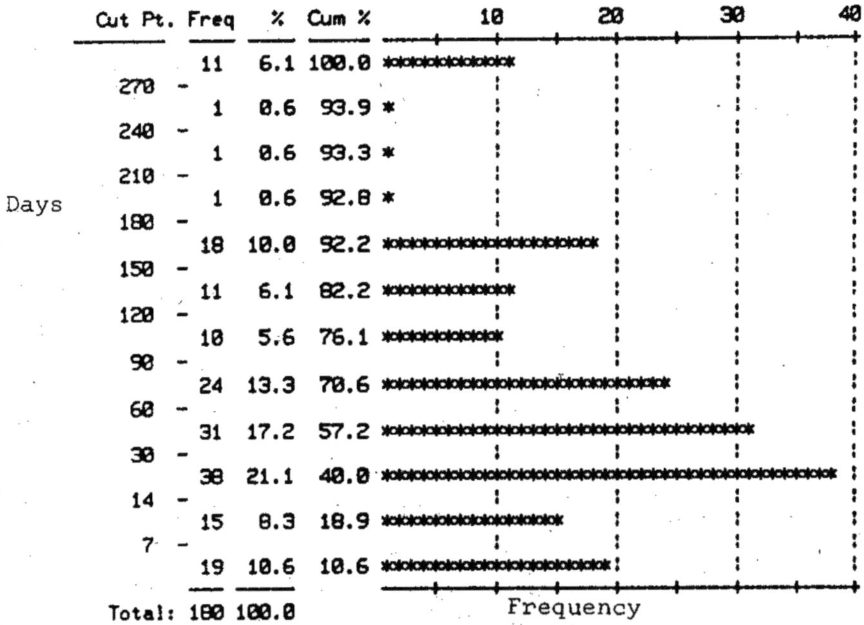

Fig. 2. Duration of symptons.

5. Physical findings

Hepatomegaly may be present in over 50% of patients, 40% may have clinical jaundice, blood in stool may be found in one in four, abdominal mass found in one in five and ascites in more than one in ten.

6. Laboratory values

Elevated alkaline phosfatase and gamma GT are the most frequent abnormalities or in close to 80% of patients, while 60% have elevated SGOT.

Fasting hyperglycemia may be found in close to 60% of patients. Hyperbilirubinemia is initially found in approximately 50%, anemia and elevated lipase in a third.

CA 19-9 may be elevated in 80-90% but is mainly of benefit in monitoring the progress of the disease.

7. Differential diagnosis

The main differential diagnosis are gastric pathology, i.e. cancer or ulcers, gallstones, chronic pancreatitis, or ampullary ca.

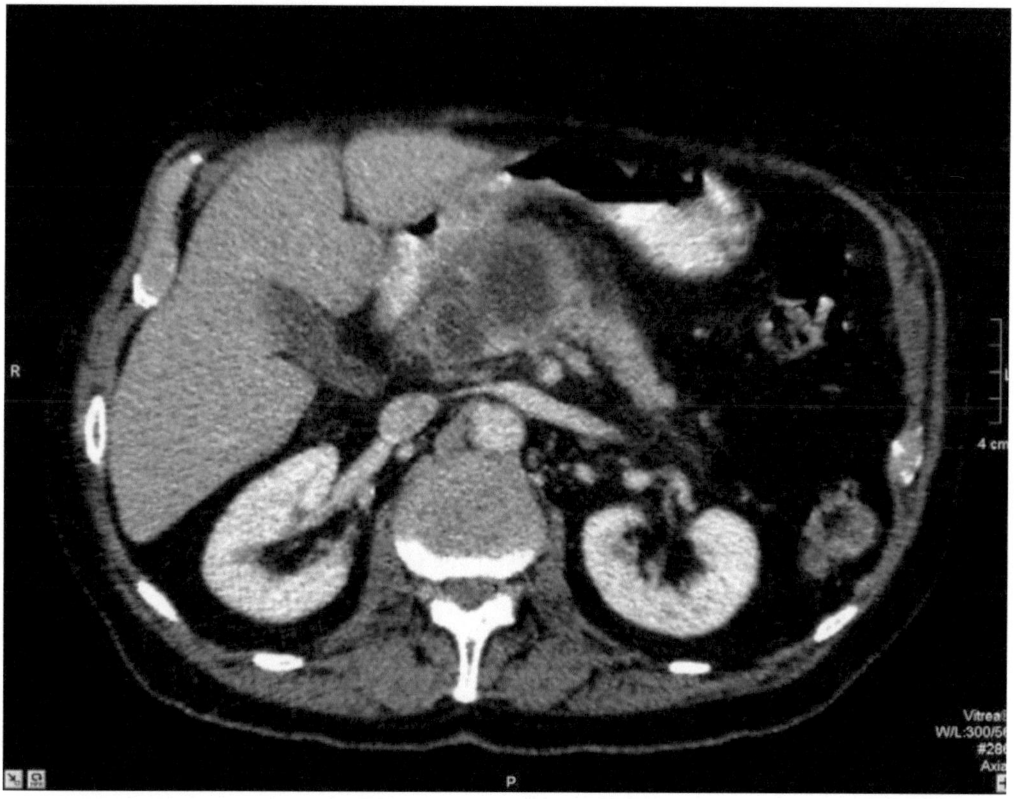

Fig. 3. CT. Pancreatic cancer. Axial view.

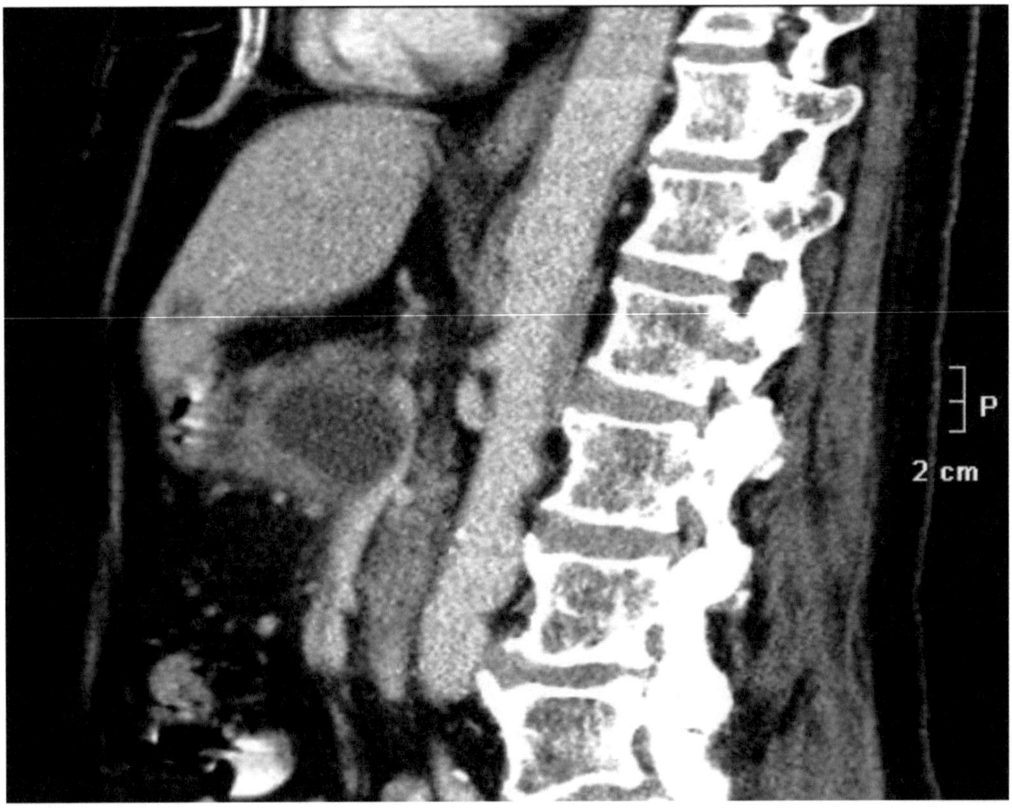

Fig. 4. CT. Pancreatic cancer, Sagital view. Metastases in liver.

8. Diagnostic procedure

In non-jaundice patients it is appropriate to start with upper endoscopy or radiographic upper gastrointestinal studies. In a jaundiced patient ultrasound would establish or rule out gallstones, but also make large tumors and liver metastases obvious. Computerised Tomography, especially the helical form would best confirm the extent of tumor mass and growth beyond the boundaries of the gland. MRI, EUS or ERCP would further delineate the extent of the disease. Angiography and a PET scan are of lesser value (Bipat 2005).

Attempts should be made to obtain tissue diagnosis from the tumour mass or liver by Fine Needle Biopsy guided by CT, US or EUS.

9. Prognosis, statistics

Before doctors embark on attempts at vigorous curative therapy the documented course of this disease and survival statistics so far should be borne in mind (Gudjonsson 1987, 1995).

In 90% of cases it has been found that the disease has progressed beyond the boundaries of the gland to adjacent lymph nodes, liver, omentum, stomach or duodenum.

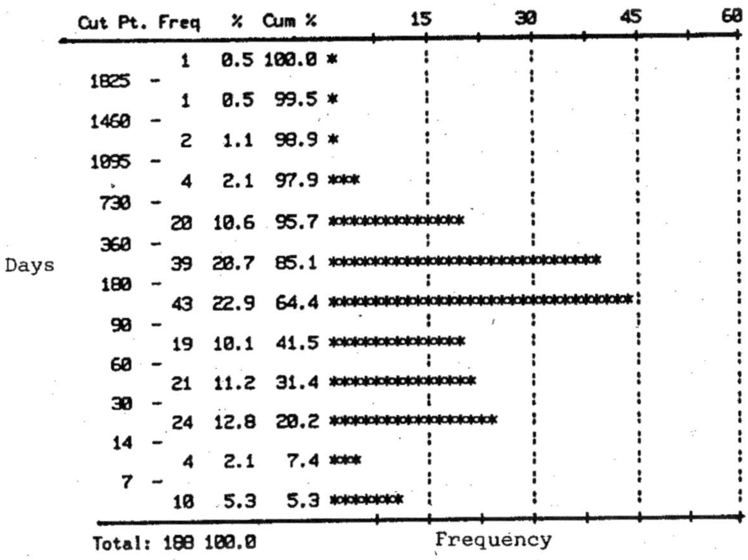

Fig. 5. Survival distribution.

Overall five-year survival is well below 1%. Close to 50% of patients with pancreatic adenocarcinoma will be dead within approximately 3 months, 65-70% within 6 months and 85-90% within 12 months, but an occasional patient may still survive 5 years with or without resection.

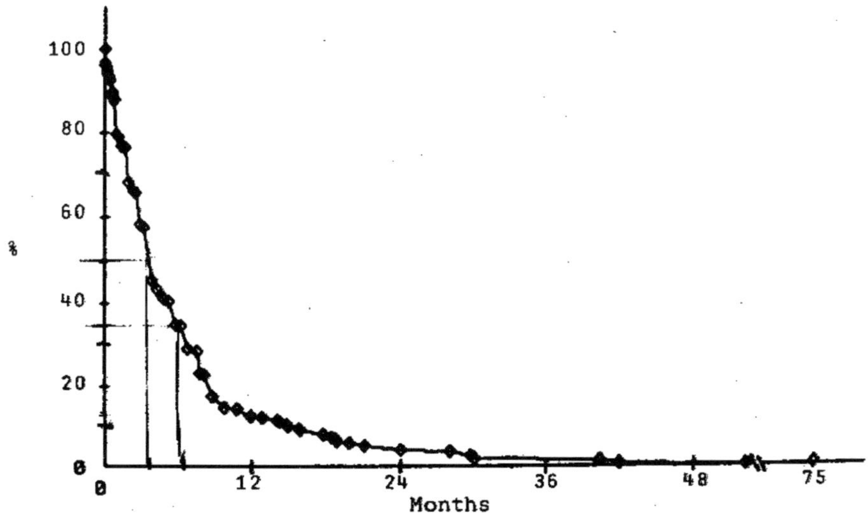

Fig. 6. Survival curve.

The disease will cause pain and obstruction of the biliary and/or gastroduodenal system.

A full 90% of patients will therefore primarily need palliation in the form of relief of pain and relief of the obstruction of the biliary and gastroduodenal system which may occur.

10. Operative findings

Earlier on approximately 80% of patients would have had a surgical laparotomy after imaging studies and in a third of those only a biopsy would have been feasible. Half of those operated on would have had a biliary bypass performed and some of those also a gastric bypass with 5-10% undergoing only a gastric bypass (Brooks 1976).

Now laparoscopy is increasingly used to stage the extent of disease and obtain a biopsy (Nagorney 1999). Either method would reveal that in 2/3 of established cases the tumor would be located in the head of the pancreas and one third in the body and/or tail and have progressed beyond the boundaries of the pancreas. Only about 10% of patients are resectable.

Jaundice will be a significant problem in these patients as the disease progresses. Advances in endoscopic palliative therapy have been significant and stents can now be inserted by skilled hands endoscopically or transhepatically in the biliary system but are associated with complications and primarily have role in those patients who have a short term prognosis (Costamagna 2004).

Many patients will still have laparotomy but are then found to be unresectable. A surgical biliary bypass is then advisable and an operative bypass of the hepatic or common duct is preferred over the gallbladder (Nagorney 1999). If there is no gastric outlet obstruction at that stage the value of a prophylactic gastric bypass is debated but it is well documented that a significant number of those patients who have longer prognosis and initially have only a biliary bypass will later develop gastroduodenal obstruction and will need a second intervention (Gudjonsson 1987).

When a gastroduodenal obstruction occurs later in patients with biliary endoscopic stents, operative gastrojejunostomy may be required, but progress continues in both laparoscopic gastrojejunostomies and also insertion of duodenal stents (Maetani 2004).

Pain is in most cases a major problem. If a laparotomy is performed an intraoperative chemical neurolytic splanchnic block should be done (Lillemoe 1999).

In non-operated patients progress is being made in performing percutaneous, transthoracic (thoracoscopic) splanchnicectomy and endoscopic ultrasonographic splanchnic plexus blocks.

The value of a laparotomy should not be underestimated as by then biopsy, biliary-, gastroduodenalbypass and splanchnic resection can be accomplished (Mann 2009).

Resection is claimed by many to be the only chance of "cure", but is only applicable in 10% of cases. Survival statistics based only on resected patients with actuarial methods and significant censoring are misleading (Yeo 1995, Gudjonssn 2009).

Resections were initially fraught with a high mortality rate but that has certainly decreased at the relatively few centres with high volume, though morbidity is still high.

The poor results of resections is not surprising considering that even in those who are considered resectable, 20-50% of resection margins are positive for cancer (Willet 1993) and nodes are positive in up to 80% of cases and tumor cells can be found in the bone marrow in up to 50% of cases (Z'graggen 2001). Biopsy proof should be mandatory before resections are performed. Radical cancer surgery of 6-10 hours duration for chronic pancreatitis is not justified.

An occasional resected patient may certainly survive 5 years but will then most likely be reported over and over in the literature (Gudjonsson 2009).

Half of those who survive 5 years after resections have recurrence of cancer (Conlon 1996). The post op course of resected patients is not smooth and they may need many readmissions to hospitals (Gudjonsson 1995, Reddy 2009). The value of resections as palliation is unproven.

True cure of pancreatic cancer after resection is exceptional.

11. Chemotherapy

Cancer of the pancreas is a very chemoresistant disease. Gemcitabine and 5 fluoruracil have been used in different forms in numerous trials of resected and nonresected patients and may add to quality of life and prolong life and exceptionally contribute to 5-year survival (Neoptolemos 2004).

Radiation therapy has been used pre- intra- and postoperatively in various forms alone or in conjunction with chemotherapy but has not had any significant effect on survival.

Novel diagnostic and therapeutic approach is needed (Yokoyama 2009).

12. References

Bipat S, Phoa SSKS, Delden OMv, et. al. Ultrasonography, computed tomography and magnetic resonance imaging for diagnosis and determining respectability of pancreatic adenocarcinoma: A meta-analysis. J Comput Assist Tomogr 2005; 29:438-445.

Brooks J, Culebras JM. Cancer of the pancreas. Palliative operation, Whipple procedure, or total pancreatectomy. Am J Surg 1977; 131:516-519.

Conlon K, Klimstra DS, Brennan M. Long-term survival after curative resection for pancreatic ductal adenocarcinoma: Clinicopathologic analysis of 5-year survivors. Ann Surg 1996; 23:273-279.

Costamagna G, Pandolfini M. Endoscopic stenting for biliary and pancreatic malignancies. J Clin Gastroenterol 2004; 38:59-67.

Cowgill SM, Muscarella P. The genetics of pancreatic cancer. Am J Surg 2003; 186:279-286.

Cress RD, Yin D, Clarke L, et al. Survival among patients with adenocarcinoma of the pancreas: a population-based study (United States). Cancer Causes Control 2005; 17:403-409.

Du W, Touchette D, Vaitkevicus VK, et al. Cost analysis of pancreatic carcinoma treatment. Cancer 2000; 89: 1917-24.

Gudjonsson B. Cancer of the pancreas. 50 years of surgery. Cancer 1987; 60:2284-03.

Gudjonsson B. Carcinoma of the pancreas: Critical analysis of costs, results of resections, and the need for standardized reporting. J Am Coll Surg 1995; 181:483-503.

Gudjonsson B. Pancreatic cancer: survival, errors and evidence. Eur J Gastroenterol Hepatol 2009; 21: 1379-1382.

Jemal A, Siegel R, Xu J, et al. Cancer Statistics, 2010. CA: A Cancer J Clin 2010; 60:277-300.

Lillemoe KD. Palliation of pain: Operation. J Gastrointest Surg 1999; 3:345-347.

Lee JK, Kim AY, Kim PN, et al. Prediction of vascular involvement and respectability by multidetector-row CT versus MR imaging with MR angiography in patients who underwent surgery for resection of pancreatic ductal adenocarcinoma. Eur J Radiology 2010; 73: 310-316.

Lockhart AC, Rothenberg ML, Berlin JD. Treatment for pancreatic cancer: Current therapy and continued progress. Gastroenterology 2005; 128:1642-1654.

Maetani I, Tada T, Ukita T, et al. Comparison of duodenal stent placement with surgical gastrojejunostomy for palliation in patients with duodenal obstruction caused by pancreaticobiliary malignancies. Endoscopy 2004; 36:73-78.

Mann CD, Thomasset SC, Johnson NA, et. al. Combined biliary and gastric bypass procedure as effective palliation for unresectable malignant disease. ANZ J Surg 2009; 79: 471-475.

Nagorney DM, et al. Management of unresectable pancreatic duct cancer. The SSAT, AGA, AASLD, ASGE, AHPBA concensus panel. J Gastrointest Surg 1999; 3:331-332.

Neoptolemos JP, Stocken DD, Friess H, et al. A randomised trial of chemotherapy after resection of pancreatic cancer. N Engl J Med 2004; 350: 1200-1210.

Reddy DM, Townsend Jr, Kuo Y-F, et al. Readmission after pancreatectomy for pancreatic cancer in Medicare patients. J Gastrointest Surg 2009; 13: 1963-1975.

Willett CG, Lewandrowski K, Warshaw AL, et al. Resection margins in carcinoma of the head of the pancreas: Implications for radiation therapy. Ann Surg; 1993; 217:144-148.

Yeo CJ, Pitt HA, Cameron JL, et al. Pancreaticoduodenectomy for cancer of the head of the pancreas: 201 patients. Ann Surg 1995; 221:721-733.

Yokoyama Y, Mimura Y, Nagino M. Advances in the treatment of pancreatic cancer: limitations of surgery and evaluation of new therapeutic strategies. Surg Today 2009; 39: 466-475.

Z'graggen K, Centeno BA, Fernandez-del Castillo C. Biological implications of tumor cells in blood and bone marrow of pancreatic cancer patients. Surgery 2001; 129:537-546.

13

Endoscopic Management of Pancreatic Cancer: From Diagnosis to Palliative Therapy

Erika Madrigal and Jennifer Chennat
University of Chicago,
USA

1. Introduction

Pancreatic cancer is the fourth leading cause of cancer death in the U.S. According to the Surveillance Epidemiology and End Results (SEER) program, the median age at diagnosis between 2003-2007 was 72 years of age, and the incidence of new cases diagnosed during this period in all races was 13.3 per 100,000 men and 10.5 per 100,000 women. The median age at death for pancreatic cancer during the same period was 73 years of age, and the mortality rate for all races was 12.3 per 100,000 men and 9.4 per 100,000 women. Pancreatic cancer has a 22.5% 5-year survival rate when localized to the pancreas at diagnosis, and it decreases to 1.9% when metastasized. The lifetime risk to develop pancreatic cancer is 1.41%, and it is the same for men and women. (National Cancer Institute, 2011) Different types of pancreatic cancers originate from different type of pancreatic cells. About 95% of pancreatic cancers originate from exocrine cells. Of these, the most common is pancreatic adenocarcinoma (about 95%). Other less common types of exocrine tumors are: adenosquamous carcinomas, squamous cell carcinomas, giant cell carcinomas, intraductal papillary mucinous neoplasms (IPMN), mucinous cystadenocarcinoma, pancreatoblastoma, cystadenocarcinoma and pseudopapillary tumors. About 5% of pancreatic cancers originate from endocrine cells, and are known as pancreatic neuroendocrine tumors (NETs). Each of these tumors is named according to the hormone they produce: insulinomas, glucagonomas, gastrinomas, somatostatinomas, VIPomas. (American Cancer Society, 2011) Cystic pancreatic lesions are common and have a wide range of malignant potential. These lesions include, but are not limited to, serous cystadenomas (low potential for malignancy), mucinous cystic neoplasms, and IPMN. Based on the degree of dysplasia, these neoplasms are classified into benign (adenomatous), low-grade malignant (borderline) and malignant (carcinoma in situ and invasive cancer). (Brugge et al, 2004)

Pancreatic cancer must be managed with a multidisciplinary approach. Endoscopy has a primary role in the diagnosis and staging of pancreatic cancer. Endoscopic ultrasound (EUS) is the most frequently used modality for this purpose. Treatment with curative intention involves surgery, with adjuvant therapy (chemotherapy and/ or radiation) in some cases. Most cases are diagnosed when curative resection is not possible. Technologic developments have introduced new endoscopic approaches to the palliation of these advanced cases.

This chapter will cover the endoscopic technology currently available for diagnosis, staging and palliation of pancreatic cancer. Promising interventional techniques for the diagnosis and palliation of this neoplasia are currently under development and improvement and will also be discussed here.

2. Diagnosis and staging

The imaging modalities involved in the diagnosis and staging of pancreatic cancer include Computed Tomography (CT), Magnetic Resonance Imaging (MRI), EUS and Endoscopic Retrograde Cholangiopancreatography (ERCP). Only the endoscopic modalities, EUS and ERCP, will be reviewed here.

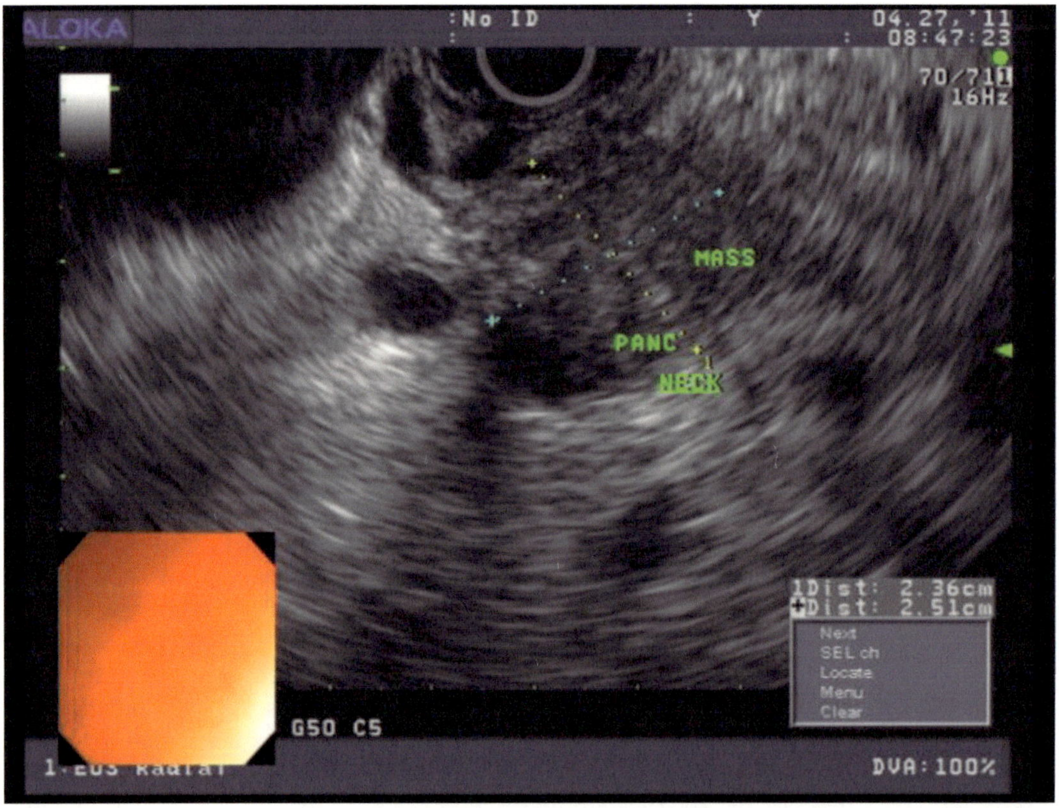

Fig. 1. 55 year-old male with a pancreatic mass found in abdominal CT during work up of abdominal pain and weight loss. EUS revealed a 2.5cm mass located at the neck of the pancreas.

EUS is a combination of endoscopy and intraluminal ultrasound that allows the introduction of high frequency ultrasound waves in the gastrointestinal tract to visualize the wall and adjacent structures. It is considered the procedure of choice for the diagnosis and staging of pancreatic cancer. High resolution endosonographic images can be obtained due to the short distance between the probe and the target lesion. It has become an accepted modality for the diagnosis of pancreato-biliary diseases. (Yamao et al, 2009) EUS has great utility in the diagnosis of pancreatic cancer and other gastrointestinal malignancies, as it allows the etiological diagnosis by tissue acquisition by fine needle aspiration (FNA).

EUS is contraindicated in those circumstances where the lesion cannot be clearly visualized, presence of an interposed vessel in the path between the needle and the target lesion, bleeding diathesis and risk of tumor seeding. (Yamao et al, 2009)

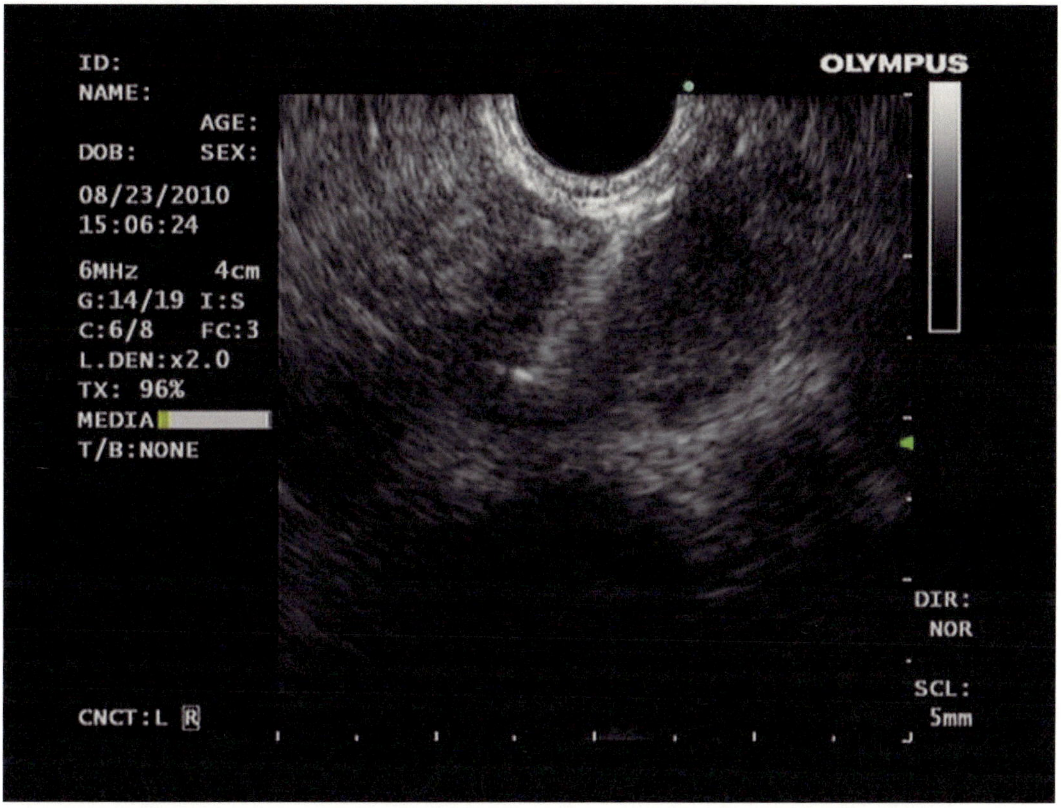

Fig. 2. FNA of a lymph node found during diagnostic EUS in 59 year-old male with metastatic pancreatic adenocarcinoma.

Radial and curve linear array echoendoscopes are available for EUS. Radial echoendoscopes provide a circumferential view at right angle to the shaft of the scope, similar to those provided by CT. The linear array echoendoscope generates longitudinal sector images parallel to the axis of the endoscope giving a 120° to 180° scanning view. The linear echoendoscope also has an instrument channel that ranges in size (2.0 to 3.8mm) and allows not only histological biopsies to be taken by FNA, but also therapeutic interventions that will be discussed later in this chapter. (Yamao et al, 2009; Hawes & Fockens, 2006) EUS-FNA needles can be locked in a fixed position on the echoendoscope and advanced into the lesion by the endoscopist under ultrasonographic guidance. Needle sizes available are 19, 22 and 25 gauge, and allow for a depth of penetration of up to 10cm. A 19 gauge trucut needle is also commercially available and allows for the specimens to be processed for immunohistochemical and gene analysis. (Yamao et al, 2009) The 25 gauge needle has the advantage of being more flexible and passes through the tissue more easily, however is less echogenic and can be more difficult to visualize during FNA. In the other hand, the stiffness of the 22 gauge needle produces less distortion and probably allows for firmer pressure to be applied. (Hawes, 2010a)

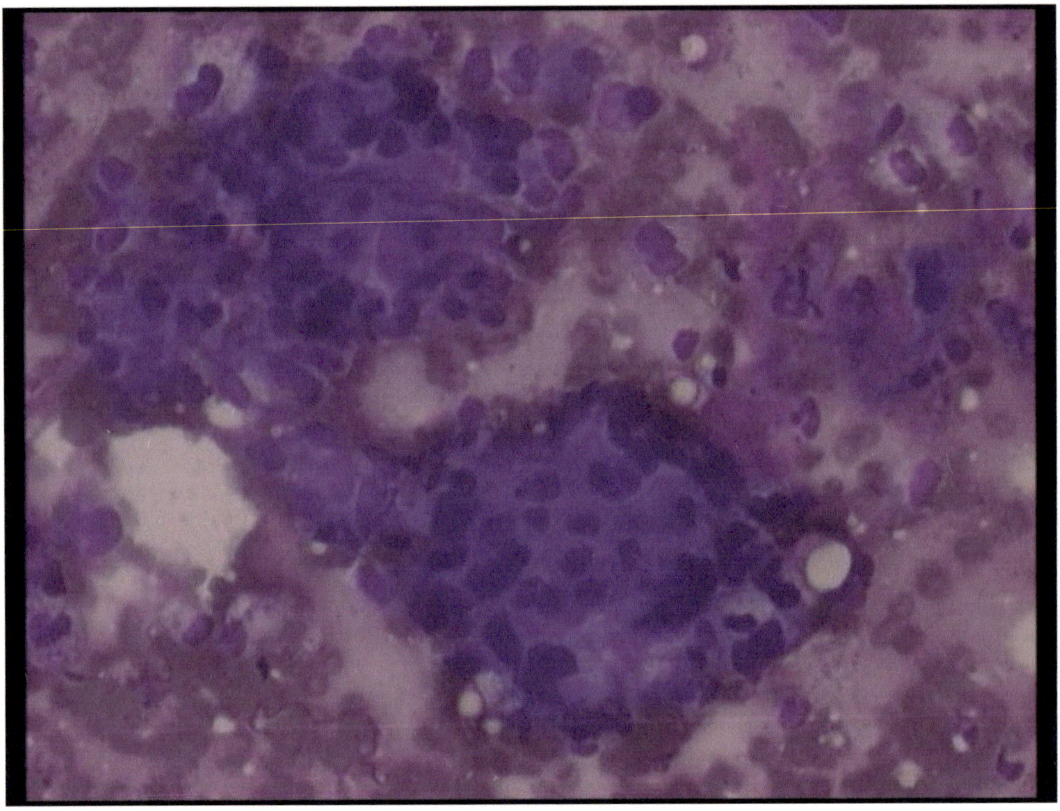

Fig. 3. 55 year-old male with pancreatic neck mass. EUS-FNA was performed and cytology was consistent with adenocarcinoma.

Prior to the development of EUS-FNA, pancreatic FNA or core biopsy were performed either during surgery or percutaneously under US or CT guidance. Intra-operative sampling considerably increases the operating time, and the percutaneous approach has reported sensitivity of about 80%, but at the expense of possible needle-track seeding. (Bret et al, 1986; Ferrucci et al, 1979; Smith et al, 1980; Caturelli et al, 1985) EUS-FNA is associated with high rates of adequate tissue sampling and diagnostic accuracy. A prospective study in 457 patients undergoing EUS-FNA in 554 lesions revealed a sensitivity, specificity, and accuracy of 92%, 93%, and 92% for lymph nodes, 88%, 95%, and 90% for extraluminal masses, and 61%, 79% and 67% for gastrointestinal wall lesions, respectively. (Wiersema et al, 1997) DeWitt summarized the reports of multiple authors on FNA of pancreatic tumors and reported the accuracy, sensitivity and specificity to be 88%, 85% and 98%, respectively in among nearly 1700 patients (DeWitt, 2006, as cited in Hawes & Fockens, 2006). Summarizing the results of 23 studies including 1,096 patients over a 21-year period, the sensitivity of EUS for the detection of a pancreatic mass was in the range of 85-100%. (Al-Haddad & Eloubeidi,

2010; Yasuda et al, 1988; DeWitt et al, 2004; Chhieng et al, 2002; Eloubeidi & Tamhane, 2005) The operating characteristics of EUS-FNA of solid pancreatic masses in 547 patients were: sensitivity 95%, specificity 92%, positive predictive value 98% and negative predictive value 80%, with and overall accuracy of 94.1%. (Eloubeidi et al, 2007) Such accuracy numbers allow for preoperative counseling of patients, minimizing surgeon's operative time in cases of unresectable disease, and avoiding surgical biopsies in those with inoperable disease, also allowing for conservative management of patients with benign pathology results. (Eloubeidi et al, 2007)

To compare the diagnostic yield and complication rates of 22 gauge and 25 gauge needles during EUS-FNA of solid pancreatic masses, a group prospectively randomized 131 patients with suspected pancreatic lesions. (Siddiqui et al, 2009) EUS-FNA with 22 gauge needle was performed in 64 patients and 25 gauge needle was used in 67 patients. Overall, cytology was diagnostic in 120 of 131 patients (91.6%): 87.5% with 22 gauge and 95.5% with 25 gauge. The difference was not statistically different (p=0.18) but there was a trend toward a higher accuracy with the 25 gauge. A similar number of passes was performed in both groups and no complications were reported in either arm.

The 19 gauge Trucut biopsy needle contains an 18mm long specimen tray that acquires larger tissue samples while preserving tissue architecture to allow histologic examination. (Levy, 2007) It was introduced in 2002 and overcomes certain limitations of the FNA needle: certain tumors (stromal tumors, lymphomas and well-differentiated pancreatic tumors) are difficult to diagnose based on cytology alone and the diagnosis accuracy relies on immediate review of the specimen for sampling adequacy by an on-site cytopathologist. When used in conjunction with an echoendoscope, these large caliber needles procure larger specimens for histopathological analysis by means of EUS trucut needle biopsy (EUS-TNB). (Varadarajulu et al 2004) A tissue core sample has several advantages: better distinction between well-differentiated adenocarcinoma and chronic pancreatitis, which accounts for both false-positive and false-negative FNA results; appropriate cellular sub-typing and architectural analysis in the diagnosis of lymphoma, as well as use of special stains, all of which are of limited usefulness with FNA specimens; and elimination of the need for a cytopathologist to assess specimen adequacy, thereby reducing duration and cost of the procedure. (Larghi et al, 2004) A pilot study for the 19 gauge Trucut needle included 18 patients undergoing EUS-FNA and EUS-TNB of different lesions (11 mediastinal masses, 3 pancreatic masses, 3 gastric tumor/ cyst/ lymphoma, and 1 adrenal mass). There was no significant difference in the adequacy of the specimens for evaluation (83% vs. 100% adequate specimens in EUS-TNB and EUS-FNA respectively), or in the diagnostic accuracy of EUS-TNB from EUS-FNA (78% vs. 89% respectively). Two complications were encountered: one patient required surgery for mediastinitis and another patient was managed conservatively for immediate bleeding. (Varadarajulu et al 2004) A group in London prospectively evaluated the safety and accuracy of EUS-FNA alone vs. combined EUS-FNA and EUS-TNB (EUS-FNA/TNB). (Wittmann et al 2006) A total of 159 patients underwent EUS-FNA alone (lesions < 2cm) or the combination of both modalities (lesions of 2cm or more). Adequate samples were obtained in 91%, 88% and 97% by EUS-FNA, EUS-TNB and EUS-FNA/TNB respectively. From the pancreas (n = 83), adequate samples were obtained by FNA in 94% and by TNB in 81%, compared with 87% and 92% from non-pancreatic sites (n = 76) respectively. Overall accuracy for EUS-FNA alone was 77%, for

EUS-TNB alone 73% and for EUS-FNA/TNB 91% (p = 0.008). For pancreatic sampling, the accuracy of FNA alone was 77%, for TNB alone was 56% and for FNA/TNB 83%. For non-pancreatic sampling, the accuracy for EUS-FNA alone was 78%, for EUS-TNB alone 83% and for EUS-FNA/TNB 95% (p = 0.006). The complication rate was 0.6% (one patient with moderate self-limited abdominal pain and another patient with bile leak requiring endoscopic stent replacement). Another group prospectively enrolled 247 patients to determine factors predicting a positive diagnostic yield and the safety of EUS-TBN. (Thomas et al, 2009) The lesions sampled were in the pancreas (113), esophagogastric wall (34), and extrapancreatic areas (100; 52 of those were lymph nodes). The overall accuracy was 75%. The overall complication rate was 2% (bronchopneumonia, minor hemoptysis, minor hematemesis, mucosal tear, retropharyngeal abscess) with no procedure-related deaths. A higher diagnostic yield was found when the lesion was approached through the stomach and when more than two passes were made. With the aim of comparing EUS-FNA using 25 gauge and 22 gauge needles with the EUS guided 19 gauge Trucut needle in solid pancreatic mass, a group in Japan prospectively enrolled 24 patients. (Sakamoto et al, 2009) The 25 gauge EUS-FNA was technically easier and obtained superior overall diagnostic accuracy, especially in lesions of the pancreas head and uncinate process. Overall accuracy for the 25 gauge, 22 gauge and Trucut needle was 91.7%, 79.7% and 54.1%, respectively. Accuracy for cytological diagnosis irrespective the site of lesions with 25 gauge, 22 gauge and Trucut needles was 91.7%, 75% and 45.8%, respectively. For uncinate masses, it was 100%, 33.3%, and 0% respectively.

Most endosonographers consider EUS-FNA the procedure of choice for sampling of pancreatic masses, however, EUS-TNB has a role in selected settings. The most clear advantage of EUS-TNB over EUS-FNA is in the diagnosis of disorders for which histology is necessary and cytology is inadequate, such as autoimmune pancreatitis and chronic 'nonspecific' pancreatitis. For other pancreatic disorders including cystic pancreatic tumors, islet cell tumors, secondary metastatic solid pancreatic tumor, and primary solid pancreatic tumors, EUS-TNB and EUS-FNA have often complementary roles. (Levy, 2007)

Pancreatic masses found in the background of chronic pancreatitis present a particular challenge to endoscopists. Better methods to detect pancreatic tumors in this setting and to better target the fine needle aspiration within a pancreatic mass to optimize sampling are needed. The development of image enhancing techniques and/or the use of contrast agents may fulfill these needs. Elastography is a method for real-time evaluation of tissue stiffness. Elastography uses a hue color map (red-green-blue) to display tissue stiffness: hard or stiff tissue is shown in dark blue, medium hard tissue areas in cyan, intermediate hardness tissue areas in green, medium soft tissue areas in yellow and soft tissue in red. (Hawes, 2010) A group from Spain reported the use of EUS elastography for the characterization of solid pancreatic masses in 130 patients and compared them with 20 normal controls. Four elastographic patterns were described, with high concordance among the 2 blinded investigators. A green-predominant pattern (homogeneous or not) excluded malignancy with high accuracy whereas a blue-predominant pattern (homogeneous or heterogeneous) supported a malignancy diagnosis. Sensitivity, specificity and overall accuracy for the diagnosis of malignancy were 100%, 85.5% and 94% respectively. (Iglesias-Garcia et al, 2009) A Japanese group investigated the usefulness of EUS combined with contrast enhancement in the preoperative localization of pancreatic endocrine tumors (PET) and the differentiation between malignant and benign PETs. (Ishikawa et al, 2010) This group retrospectively studied 62 pathologically confirmed PETs found in 41 patients who had undergone EUS, multiphasic multidetector computed tomography (MDCT) and transabdominal ultrasound (US). Contrast-enhanced EUS had 95% sensitivity in identifying PETs compared with 80% with MDCT and 45% with US. Heterogeneous ultrasonographic texture was the most significant factor for malignancy. It was also noted that when contrast was used with EUS, PETs showed contrast enhancement except in areas of hemorrhage or necrosis. The optimal use of elastography and contrast enhanced EUS would be to define an optimal target area within a pancreatic mass to maximize the cytologic yield. (Hawes, 2010)

Cystic pancreatic lesions are commonly found nowadays given the development and availability of different imaging tests that are often performed for unrelated reasons. Cystic lesions are sometimes difficult to diagnose. Cross-sectional imaging is often non-diagnostic due to the small size of the cystic lesions. EUS has become useful for the diagnosis of these lesions as it provides high resolution images and allows the performance of FNA of the cystic fluid for cytology and tumor marker determinations. A large, prospective multicenter study looking at the imaging, cyst fluid cytology and cyst fluid tumor markers found that

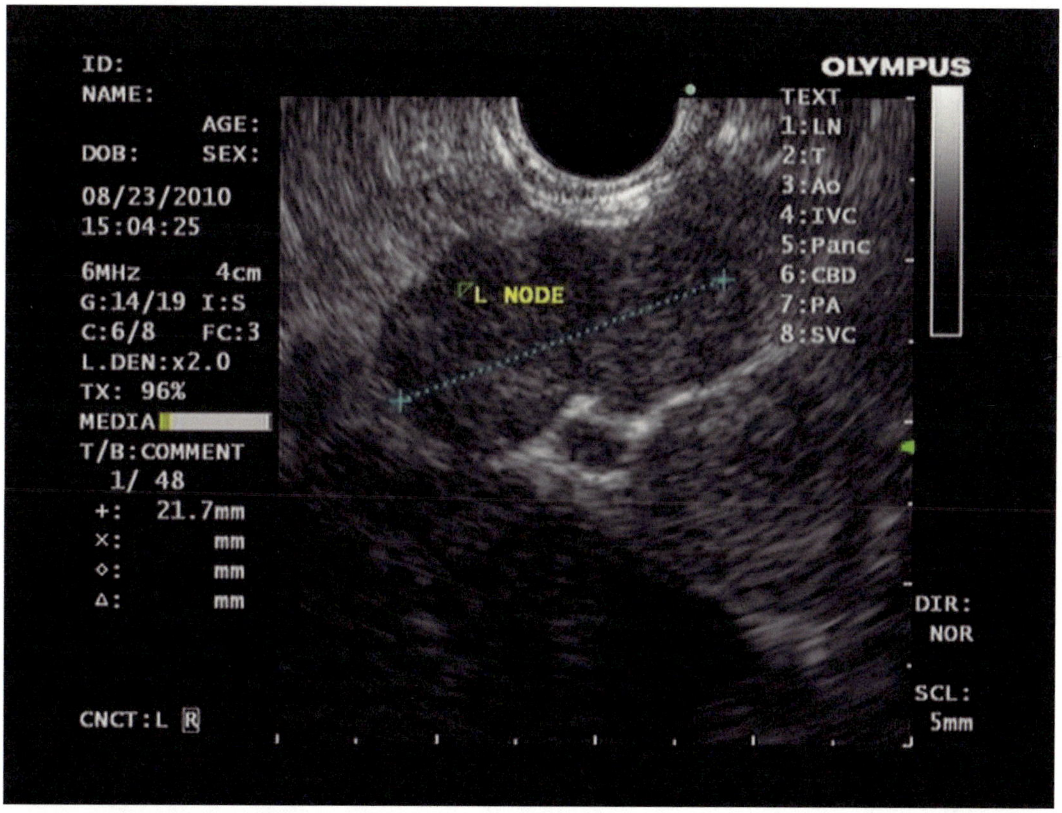

Fig. 4. The picture demonstrates one of the multiple peri-pancreatic lymph nodes found in a patient with metastatic pancreatic adenocarcinoma. The largest measured 25mm. FNA of the lymph node was performed and cytology was consistent with poorly differentiated adenocarcinoma.

the cystic fluid CEA (using a cutoff value of 192 ng/ mL) was able to differentiate mucinous vs. nonmucinous cystic lesions with an accuracy of 79%, which was significantly higher than the accuracy of EUS morphology (51%) or fluid cytology (59%) ($p<0.05$). (Brugge et al, 2004b)

Staging of pancreatic malignancy is done according to the American Joint Committee for Cancer (AJCC) Staging TNM classification. This describes the tumor extension (T), lymph node (N) and distant metastases (M) of tumors, respectively. Accuracy of the T staging by EUS ranges from 63% to 94% and nodal (N) staging ranges from 41% to 86%, (DeWitt et al, 2004; Palazzo et al, 1993; Gress et al, 1999; Rivadeneira et al, 2003) which is superior to CT and trans abdominal ultrasound. (Palazzo et al, 1993; Gress et al, 1999; Rivadeneira et al, 2003; Agarwal et al, 2004) Comparative studies between EUS and cross-sectional imaging have generally shown that EUS is superior for local tumor staging (T and N) in esophageal, pancreatic and rectal cancer, but CT is still necessary for full assessment of metastatic disease. (Hawes, 2010) EUS, however, can be of value when evaluating for metastases. Part of the liver can be visualized by EUS and suspected metastatic lesions can be sampled. Celiac lymph nodes can also be biopsied if appearing suspicious and ascites can be aspirated and sent for cytology to assess for peritoneal metastases. (Al-Haddad & Eloubeidi, 2010)

EUS is associated with a low rate of complications. A study in 322 patients and 345 lesions revealed an overall complication risk of 1.6%. This study involved pancreatic EUS-FNA in 248 cases (134 solid lesions and 114 cystic lesions) and complications were observed in 4 (1.2%) patients with pancreatic cystic lesions (acute pancreatitis in 3, and aspiration pneumonia in 1). No complications resulted from FNA of solid pancreatic lesions. (O'Toole et al, 2001) Despite the low complication risk, life threatening complications have been sporadically reported: fulminant cholangitis after FNA of a liver metastasis and uncontrolled bleeding from a pseudoaneurysm after pancreatic FNA, (Erickson, 2004) massive bleeding from a gastric GIST (Inoue et al, 2006) and acute portal vein thrombosis after FNA of pancreatic cancer. (Matsumoto et al, 2003) A prospective cohort study in 355 patients evaluated the frequency of major complications following EUS-FNA of solid pancreatic masses and found major complications in 2.54% with acute pancreatitis developing in 3 patients (0.85%). (Eloubeidi et al, 2006)

ERCP played a major role in the diagnosis of pancreatic disease since its development in the late 1960s. However, the introduction and advances of imaging studies, especially MRCP, have shifted the ERCP applications toward therapeutic interventions. ERCP is seldom performed for diagnostic purposes, but it provides detailed opacification of the main and branch ducts (pancreatogram). The morphologic changes in the ductal system usually correlate with histologic changes. This is limited in the case of cysts that do not communicate with the pancreatic duct. ERCP also allows collection of pure pancreatic juice for cytology and gene analysis, brush cytology, biopsy of the pancreatic duct, and introduction of baby scopes or ultrasonic probes into the pancreatic duct for pancreatoscopy and intraductal ultrasound (IDUS), respectively. (Fujita et al, 2004)

Pancreatography can suggest the diagnosis of pancreatic cancer. A Japanese study comparing the pancreatographic findings of autoimmune pancreatitis and cancer revealed that an obstructed main pancreatic duct and an upstream duct dilation to a diameter greater than 4mm were significantly more common in cancer cases; meanwhile, autoimmune pancreatitis had a higher prevalence of narrowing of the main pancreatic duct for more than

3cm of its length and a higher prevalence for the presence of side branches in the narrowed portions if the main pancreatic duct. (Nishino et al, 2010) The pancreatographic features suggestive of pancreatic cystic neoplasms include displacement of the pancreatic duct, pancreatic duct strictures, and the degree of pancreatic ductal obstruction. In the case of IPMN, the main pancreatic duct may be dilated diffusely or in a segment fashion depending on the volume of mucus produced, the presence of ductal obstruction and the presence and distribution of intraductal tumors. Enlargement of the main pancreatic duct is a frequent pancreatographic abnormality in IPMN, present in about 77% of patients; side branch ectasia or cystic dilation occurs in about 51% of the cases. (Telford & Carr-Locke, 2002)

Pancreatic juice and mucus can be aspirated directly from the pancreatic duct during ERCP, either by catheter or pancreatoscopy. Stimulation of pancreatic exocrine secretion by administration of secretin may improve the diagnostic yield. The samples are sent for cytology, as well as analysis of mucin, tumor marker levels, and amplification of molecular abnormalities. (Telford & Carr-Locke, 2002) Examination of the pancreatic juice collected during cannulation yielded positive results in 52.3% of pancreatic cancer patients. Higher positive rates were obtained when washing with saline (63.2%) and aspirating after secretin stimulation (51.3%), as well as in cases of pancreatic head cancer (70.6%). (Kameya et al, 1981) For IPMN, the specificity of the cytology of the pancreatic juice is 100%, and the sensitivity is 62.2% when collected by pancreatoscopy and 38.2% when collected by catheter. (Chen 2007; Yamaguchi et al, 2005)

Brush cytology of pancreatic duct strictures or elevated intraductal lesions during ERCP has a sensitivity and specificity to detect malignancy of 48-76% and 100%, respectively, and accuracy of 70-76.4%. (Telford & Carr-Locke, 2002; Chen 2007; Ferrari et al, 1994; Vandervoort et al, 1999; Uchida et al, 2007) Accuracy may be influenced by location of sampling within the pancreas, technical errors and interpretation of the sample. (Chen 2007) Strictures located at the head and body of the pancreas usually yield high rates of positive cytology. The diagnostic yield is overall enhanced by concomitant brushing of pancreatic and bile duct strictures. (McGuire et al, 1996) A retrospective study evaluating the diagnostic yield of combining EUS-FNA with brushing cytology during the work up of pancreatic cancer revealed that the combined use of these two modalities provides a better diagnostic yield in pancreatic adenocarcinoma than either one alone. The sensitivity, specificity and accuracy were 69.2, 93.8, and 77.3% for EUS-FNA alone, 50.8, 100, and 67% for brushing cytology alone, and 84.6, 100, and 89.7% for combination of EUS-FNA with brushing cytology. (Jing et al, 2009) A recent study to determine whether KRAS (proto-oncogene) mutations could be identified in pancreatobiliary stricture brushings and to compare the performance characteristics of KRAS mutation analysis to cytology and fluorescence in situ hybridization (FISH) for detection of carcinoma revealed that combined KRAS mutation and FISH analysis appear to increase the cancer detection rate in patients with pancreatobiliary strictures. The KRAS mutation and polysomic FISH (positive) results were identified in 69% and 63% pancreatic adenocarcinoma specimens, respectively, with a combined sensitivity of 86%. (Kipp et al, 2010) In the case of cysts, a new through the needle cytological brush system (Echo-Brush) seeks to solve the poor cellularity typically obtained by EUS-FNA. This system consists in the introduction of the brush through a 19 gauge EUS needle after aspiration of the cyst fluid. The brush is used to scrub the cystic wall and is processed as standard brushing. Studies have had conflicting results. A group from Spain found that the brush was superior to the aspirated fluid for detecting diagnostic cells but didn't reach statistical significance (73% vs. 36%, p=0.08). In terms of mucinous cells, the yield of the cytobrush was significantly higher (50% vs. 18%, p=0.016). (Sendino et al, 2010) A group from the United Kingdom evaluating the management of cystic pancreatic lesions reported a similar cellularity yield between the FNA group and the brushing group (61.9% and 55.0%, respectively). Greater proportion of patients with malignant cystic lesions diagnosed by EUS sampling were in the brushing group, but this did not reach significance (50% in the brushing group vs. 20% in the FNA group, p=0.524). (Thomas et al, 2010)

Random transpapillary biopsies of the pancreatic duct can be obtained in the presence of a stricture or an elevated lesion. The specificity for the detection of malignancy approaches 100%, but the sensitivity is variable, ranging from 57% to 100%. The accuracy of these biopsies increases when performed during pancreatoscopy. (Telford & Carr-Locke, 2002; Chen, 2007)

Pancreatoscopy is the endoscopy of the pancreatic duct, and it is performed using a mother-baby scope system: a thin endoscope (baby scope) is introduced into the pancreatic duct through the working channel of the duodenoscope (mother scope). This technique has some limitations for small size pancreatic ducts: the wider the scope diameter, the better the quality of images; the tip-bending system, useful for observing the tortuous pancreatic ductal lumen, increases the size of the scope; the use of irrigation and suction system is needed to achieve a good endoscopic view, but also increases the size of the scope. Given these size limitations, the investigation of IPMN is the best indication for the use of pancreatoscopy. (Fujita et al, 2004) The insertion of the pancreatoscope is facilitated by the frequently enlarged papillary orifice present in IPMN. Pancreatoscopy in this condition allows for endoscopic diagnosis in 67% to 83%, (Nguyen et al, 2009) differentiation of a filling defect seen in pancreatography as mucus, tumor or stone, identification of malignant features, endoscopic biopsy, and determination of disease extent. Clusters of papillary projections in IPMN rising <3mm above the ductal surface can represent hyperplasia or adenoma with different degrees of dysplasia. In the other hand, adenocarcinoma is typically polypoid and protrudes >3mm into the ductal lumen. Diffuse hyperemia or distinct vessels may also be observed and are also considered high-risk features. (Telford & Carr-Locke, 2002) The cancer detection rate by pancreatoscopy-guided sampling has a sensitivity of 62.5%, specificity 100%, positive predictive value 100%, and negative predictive value 70.7%. (Iqbal & Stevens, 2009) Despite the usefulness of this diagnostic tool, pancreatoscopy requires expensive, very fragile equipment and two experience endoscopists to operate it. Hence, it is not performed often. (Telford & Carr-Locke, 2002)

IDUS uses a thin caliber (approximately 2mm in diameter) ultrasound probe with high-frequency ultrasound (12-30 MHz). For pancreatic IDUS, the ultrasonic probe is advanced into the pancreatic duct over a guidewire during an ERCP. However, in some situations it is not possible for even a thin caliber prove to pass a stenotic site caused by a mass in the pancreatic duct. (Fujita et al, 2004) A study comparing the detection rates of different imaging technologies in patients with mucin-producing tumors revealed a detection rate of 21% for CT, 29% for ultrasound, 83% for pancreatoscopy, 86% with EUS, and 100% for IDUS. (Chen, 2007) IDUS is useful in assessing the indications for surgery by revealing mural nodules in mucin-producing tumors, evaluating the feasibility of partial resection of the tumor, locating multiple lesions in pancreatic islet-cell cancer, and differentiating benign from malignant cases of localized stenosis of the main pancreatic duct. (Furukawa et al, 1997)

Cancer detection rate can be improved by techniques that allow better visualization, such as narrow-band imaging (NBI) or by developing techniques that image the lesion at microscopic level, such as confocal laser microscopy. NBI during pancreatoscopy has been shown to provide better visualization of vascular pattern and tumor vessels than conventional white light. (Iqbal & Stevens, 2009) Some authors have reported the ability of NBI to identify both the surface structure and mucosal vessels as good as, or even better than, conventional white light, regardless of benign or malignant etiology. (Itoi et al, 2009)

The use of a confocal microscope enables subsurface in vivo histological assessment during ongoing endoscopy. This technology also requires the application of a flourophore for mucosal fluorescence imaging. Endomicroscopic images can be acquired after intravenous application of fluorescein, which also makes the blood vessels clearly visible. The use of this technology in the investigation of biliary pathologies has escalated since the introduction of a flexible probe-based confocal laser endomicroscopy (pCLE) system. Certain hallmarks and patterns have been identified to differentiate benign from malignant epithelium. (Meining, 2009) The experience in pancreatic pathologies is more limited and developing. A group was able to use pCLE to detect and further differentiate pancreatic strictures such as IPMN. (Meining et al, 2009) The use of this technology may be helpful to clarify location and types of IPMN for a targeted surgical resection. Confocal endomicroscopy is being developed further and a new miniprobe small enough to be introduced through a 22 gauge puncture needle was developed. Feasibility studies to evaluate the ability of this needle-based confocal laser endomicroscopy (nCLE) for in vivo histology of various organs, including pancreas, have been carried in animal models with good results. (Becker et al, 2010; Mennone & Nathanson, 2011) A multicenter trial assessing the use of nCLE in humans is currently being carried.

3. Therapeutic Interventions

Endoscopy has no role in the treatment of pancreatic cancer, as the only definite treatment is surgical resection when the disease is diagnosed in early stages. For advanced cases, palliation is indicated and endoscopy plays an important role. The procedures currently performed for palliation of pancreatic cancer involve stent placement for the drainage of biliary or pancreatic duct obstruction by ERCP or under EUS guidance, celiac plexus neurolysis (CPN), injection of anti-tumor agents, and implantation of fiducial markers to guide radiation therapy. Other experimental procedures are being developed to evaluate the role of EUS in the application of radiofrequency ablation (RFA) and photodynamic therapy (PDT).

ERCP for drainage of biliary obstruction is the most commonly performed endoscopic procedure for palliation of pancreatic cancer. Endoscopic treatment of these malignant biliary obstructions is often successful in alleviating symptoms such as jaundice and pruritus, reducing the incidence of cholangitis, and increasing biliary drainage so that hepatically metabolized chemotherapeutic agents can be offered. (Rogart, 2010) The first biliary stents available were made of polyethylene (plastic), and had the drawback of occlusion with sludge in about 30% of cases, resulting in recurrence of symptoms and development of cholangitis. Self-expanding metal stents (SEMS) had previously been used for vascular and urethral indications, and were later developed for biliary applications. Initial non-comparative studies reported an occlusion rate of SEMS of 10-18%. In 1992, the

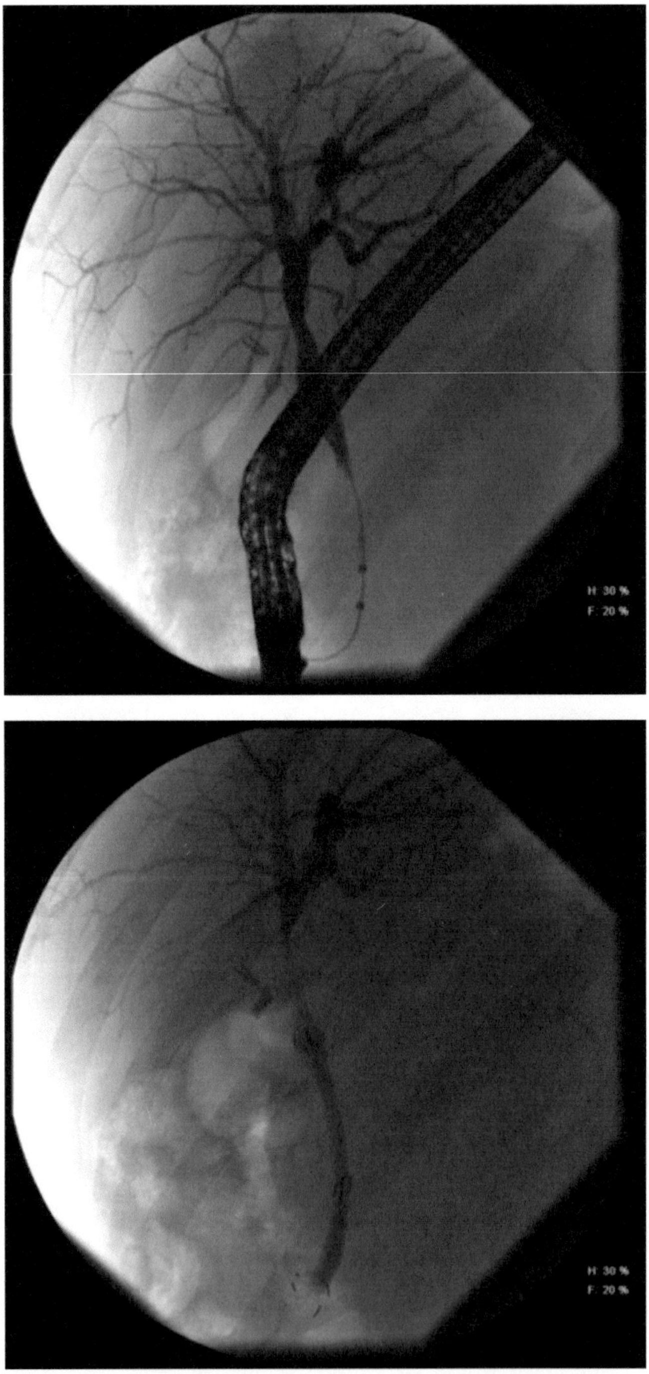

Fig. 5. 59 year-old male with biliary obstruction secondary to pancreatic head mass (adenocarcinoma). An ERCP was performed and a distal common bile duct stricture can be appreciated in the left image. The patient had metastatic disease, and a SEMS was placed for palliation of jaundice and pruritus.

first prospective randomized clinical trial reporting the patency and cost-effectiveness of SEMS vs. plastic stents was published: the median patency of the stent was significantly prolonged in patients with metal stent compared with those with a polyethylene stent (273 days vs. 126 days, p=0.006), and the incremental cost-effectiveness analysis showed that initial placement of a SEMS results in a 28% decrease of endoscopic procedures. (Davids et al, 1992) Since the introduction of biliary SEMS, several groups have concluded that their placement represent a cost-saving strategy, as plastic stents are associated with higher risk of recurrent biliary obstruction, which translates into additional procedures, hospitalizations, etc. (Arguedas et al, 2002; Kaassis et al, 2003; Moss et al, 2006) There was initial concern on the possibility of interfering with subsequent pancreaticoduodenectomy after biliary metal stent placement in patients with uncertain surgical status or with resectable masses, but this has not been well substantiated. There are actually some reports on the cost-benefit that these stents offer to these patients, as well as the longer patency rate, need for fewer procedures and fewer episodes of cholangitis. (Rogart, 2010; Wasan et al, 2005; Chen et al, 2005; Boulay et al, 2010) In addition, insertion of SEMS is advised as the treatment of biliary SEMS occlusion, as it provides longer patency and survival, decreases the number of subsequent procedures by 50% (compared to plastic stents) and is cost-effective. (Rogart et al, 2008)

However, technical failure during ERCP is encountered in up to 10% of cases due to various factors including duodenal obstruction, anatomical variations, periampullary diverticulum and tightness of the stricture. In these cases, percutaneous transhepatic biliary drainage (PTBD) and surgical drainage are options available. The technical success rate for PTBD placement is 90% if the intrahepatic system is dilated and 70% in a non-dilated system. The morbidity is 7% and the mortality is 5%, and it is contraindicated in the presence of ascites and coagulopathy. Surgical drainage, although a possibility, is associated with high morbidity and mortality rates (66% and 32%, respectively), as the patients in need for this procedure are usually very deconditioned. Hence, the drainage of the biliary system using a transgastric or transduodenal approach under EUS guidance has been introduced with a reported technical success rate of 92%. Once the common bile duct (CBD) is localized from the duodenal bulb or the intrahepatic system is visualized from the stomach, the biliary system is accessed under EUS guidance and a stent is deployed under fluoroscopic guidance to form a choledochoduodenostomy or a hepaticogastrostomy, respectively. The reported technical success rate for hepaticogastrostomy is 90-100% and the clinical success rate is 75-100%. The complication rate associated with EUS-guided biliary drainage is 19%, with 8% being due to focal biliary peritonitis. Other complications include bleeding, pneumoperitoneum, infection caused by stent occlusion/migration, and death. (Ramesh & Varadarajulu, 2008; Irisawa et al 2009) Plastic stents are the most commonly used during this approach; however, transduodenal and transgastric placement of self-expandable metal stents (SEMS) for palliation of malignant biliary obstruction has been reported and some authors report antegrade placement achieving transpapillary or, in case of post-surgical anatomy, transanastomotic placement. (Siddiqui et al, 2011; Nguyen et al, 2010; Artifon et al, 2010)

EUS-guided pancreatic duct drainage can also be accomplished. There are two techniques: 1) transmural drainage of the main pancreatic duct; and 2) rendezvous approaches for ERCP assistance of transpapillary drainage. (Irisawa et al, 2009) The main indication for the pancreatic duct drainage is to alleviate pain caused by pancreatic ductal obstruction associated with chronic pancreatitis and other inflammatory processes. For this reason, this will not be discussed further in this chapter.

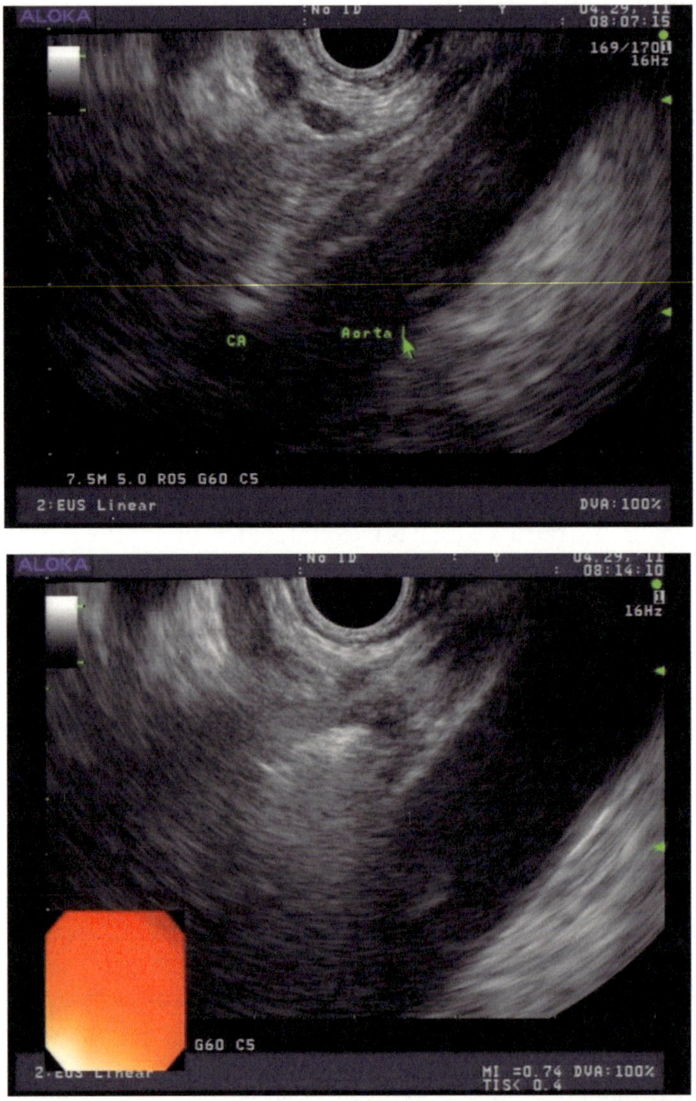

Fig. 6. 40 year-old female with locally advanced pancreatic cancer and severe abdominal pain with poor response to narcotics. Patient had EUS guided CPN. Celiac axis is localized under EUS (left image) and absolute alcohol was then injected to both sides of the celiac axis (seen as a white cloud surrounding the aorta in the right image) .

Pain is reported in the majority of patients with advanced pancreatic cancer (90%), and effective pain control can be achieved in 70-90% of these patients with CPN. (Ramesh & Varadarajulu, 2008; Puli et al, 2009; Kaufman et al, 2010) This procedure entails the injection of absolute alcohol under EUS guidance to destroy the sympathetic plexus near the celiac axis. A similar technique involving the injection of triamcinolone is performed in patients with chronic pancreatitis for pain control. (Ramesh & Varadarajulu, 2008) Significant reduction of pain scores 12 weeks after CPN was observed in 30 patients with advanced intra-abdominal malignancy, while 91% of these patients required same or less pain medication and 88% of patients had persistent improvement in their pain score. (Wiersema et al, 1996) Similarly, in another study of 58 patients with unresectable pancreatic cancer, EUS-guided CPN lowered pain scores in 78% at 2 weeks and a sustained response was noted until 24 weeks. (Naresh et al, 2001) The most commonly reported complications after CPN are orthostatic hypotension in 10-15% and transient diarrhea in 9%. (Gunaratnam et al, 2001) Recently, a retrospective analysis to determine predictors of response to CPN in a cohort of 64 patients with pancreatic cancer revealed that visualization o the celiac ganglia was the best predictor of response: patients with visible ganglia were >15 times more likely to respond ($p < 0.001$). (Ascunce et al, 2011)

Percutaneous ethanol injection is an effective treatment for cystic and solid lesions in the liver. Successful ethanol ablation of cysts in the thyroid, parathyroid, kidneys, and spleen have been reported with minimal side effects. EUS offers minimally invasive access to perform ablation of pancreatic lesions. This EUS-guided ablative therapy may have important clinical applications in the treatment of solid (adenocarcinomas, neuroendocrine tumors) and cystic pancreatic lesions (mucinous cystic neoplasm, IPMN), especially in nonoperative candidates. A pilot study in porcine models showed that ethanol injection into normal porcine pancreas results in focal inflammation, necrosis and fibrosis at the injection site. (Aslanian et al, 2005) Another pilot study reported the safety and feasibility in humans, after 25 patients underwent ethanol lavage of different cystic pancreatic lesions (mucinous cystic neoplasms, IPMNs, serous cystadenomas, and pseudocysts) with no side effects or complications reported in short and long-term follow up. (Gan et al, 2005) The approach to this technique involves aspirating the cyst content with a 22 gauge needle until collapse is achieved. Ethanol is then injected into the cyst, and the cyst is lavaged for 3 to 5 min. The cystic lesion is finally drained of fluid at the conclusion of the lavage. (Trevino & Varadarajulu, 2011) Studies in animals have revealed that EUS-guided injection of ethanol into the pig pancreas results in a localized concentration-depended tissue necrosis without complications, with a visible necrotic area of 20.8mm (+/- 4.3mm) after injection of 40% to 100% ethanol. (Matthes et al, 2007) A small study demonstrated no cyst recurrence by CT after a median follow up of 26 months (including suspected mucinous cysts). However, longer follow up is still needed before considered these patients cured. (DeWitt et al, 2010) The main potential problem of EUS-guided ethanol ablation is the risk of acute pancreatitis due to diffusion of alcohol outside the lesion into the main pancreatic duct and/or the pancreatic parenchyma. (Giovannini, 2007)

EUS-guided fine needle injection (FNI) has been proposed as a new technique for delivery of anti-tumor agents for patients with locally advanced malignancy. Few small size studies (8-37 patients) have been published, reporting the safety and feasibility of direct injection of different agents, such as allogenic mixed lymphocyte culture or cytoimplant (cytokine production within a tumor may lead to regression by host immune mechanisms, and cytoimplants produce such a cytokine response), ONYX-015 (adenovirus that selectively replicates and kills malignant cells) and TNFerade [replication-deficient adenovector containing the human tumor necrosis factor (TNF)-α gene, regulated by radiation-inducible promoter Egr-1]. The commonly reported side effects are low grade fever without leukocytosis, nausea, abdominal pain and elevated liver enzymes and bilirrubin. No pancreatitis has been reported, but few cases of sepsis and two cases of duodenal perforation occurred prior to the institution of prophylactic antibiotic and due to the rigid endoscope tip during transduodenal approach, respectively. These studies revealed partial response or at least tumor stabilization. Perhaps combination of systemic chemotherapy and/or radiation with EUS-FNI would improve outcomes. This field will continue to expand with the refinement of echoendoscopes, delivery systems and novel local antitumor agents. (Trevino and Varadarajulu, 2010; Klapman & Chang, 2005; Verna & Dhar, 2008; Chang, 2006)

Implantation of fiducial markers to facilitate stereotactic radiotherapy and radioactive seeds for brachytherapy can be performed under EUS guidance. Fiducials can be placed into tumors to enable higher doses of targeted radiotherapy while sparing adjacent healthy tissue with low risk of complications. This technique has a reported technical success rate of 84-94%, and its direct impact on patient management is promising but still under clinical investigation. A total of 3-6 gold fiducials are placed within the tumor in different planes under EUS guidance. Immediate complications are uncommon and involve needle malfunction and minor bleeds with no significant drop in hemoglobin. Although fiducials can spontaneously migrate from the initial injection site, the reported rate of migration is low (7%), and no migration-related complications have been documented. (Ramesh & Varadarajulu, 2008; Park et al, 2010; Sanders et al, 2010) The EUS-guided placement of fiducials has traditionally involved the use of 19 gauge needles. However, a recently published case series reported the feasibility of using a 22 gauge needle, which may permit greater access when compared to a 19 gauge needle technique. (Ammar et al, 2010) Brachytherapy is a useful method for local control of malignant tumors, including pancreas. After the placement of the radioactive seeds, the tissue is exposed to steady radiation, leading to localized ablation and avoiding the radiation of normal tissues surrounding the malignant lesion. EUS-guided brachytherapy has been performed to place radioactive iodine seeds into the locally advanced pancreatic tumor mass, with significant improvement in pain scores and also improvement in performance status scores. When assessing the tumor response, an 80% rate of positive response (decrease in tumor size) or stable disease has been reported. Hematologic toxicity is usually mild, but includes neutropenia, thrombocytopenia, and anemia. Other reported complications reported less frequently are pancreatitis and pseudocyst formation. (Sun et al, 2006) Small size studies have demonstrated the technical feasibility of EUS-guided implantation of radioactive seeds in pancreatic tumors, and the technique appears to be well tolerated. (Ramesh & Varadarajulu, 2008; Sun et al, 2006) However, larger studies evaluating this technique and its role in a multimodality approach in combination with chemotherapy and/ or external beam radiation are needed.

Radiofrequency ablation (RFA) is a well-established procedure that provides palliation for various malignant diseases. RFA causes a relatively predictable zone of coagulation necrosis by intense tissue heating. Accurate and precise targeting of the tumor is important to maximize the yield and minimize the morbidity. (Klapman & Chang, 2005) This technique is emerging as one of the safest and most predictable for thermal tumor ablation and is traditionally administered with percutaneous or surgical approaches. (Verma & Dhar, 2008) The feasibility and effectiveness of EUS-guided RFA has been evaluated in animal models and the probe is deployed by a 19 gauge needle inducing coagulative necrosis. (Ramesh &

Varadarajulu, 2008) Further application of this technique has been impeded because of the lack of a retractable needle electrode array to ablate large areas. This was overcome by the development of a retractable umbrella-shaped electrode array that has delivered effective coagulation necrosis of large areas in the porcine model. (Varadarajulu et al, 2009)

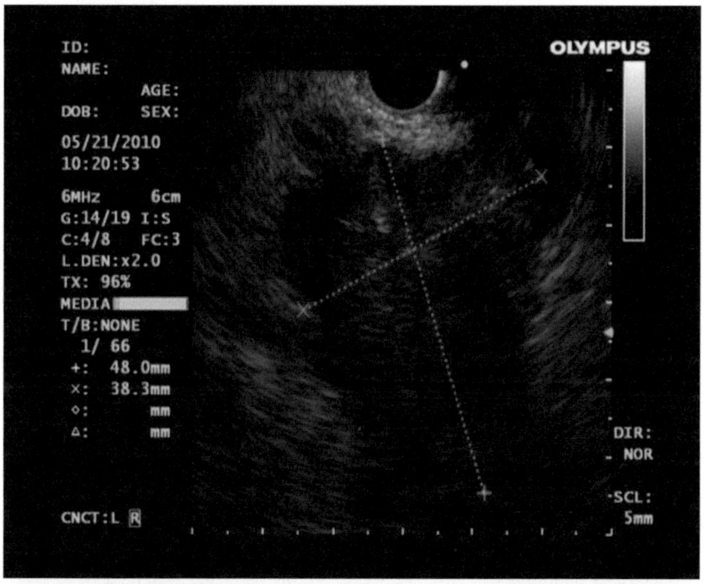

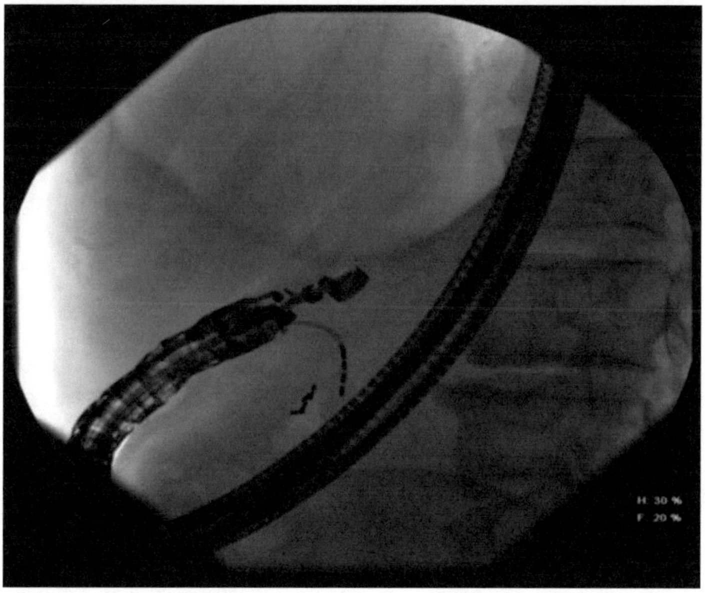

Fig. 7. 66 year-old male with locally advanced, non resectable, pancreatic cancer that underwent EUS-guided of fiducials in the pancreatic head for stereotactic radiotherapy. A 5cm pancreatic head mass was identified by EUS (left image), followed by placement of a total of 9 gold fiducials into the inferior and superior aspects of the tumor under fluoroscopy (right image)

Another experimental technique is photodynamic therapy (PDT), which involves the systemic administration of a photosensitizing agent, followed by placement of light-diffusing photodynamic fibers into the target malignant tissue. This is usually accomplished percutaneously, but it has recently been placed endoscopically with EUS guidance in the pancreas of porcine models. (Verma & Dhar, 2008) In animal models, the EUS-guided PDT of pancreas and other organs has proved to be safe and effective. (Chan et al, 2004)

These two EUS-guided ablative techniques, RFA and PDT, have only been performed in animal models and further studies in the safety and efficacy in humans are needed before considering their use in the palliation of advanced pancreatic cancer.

4. Conclusion

Endoscopy is a constantly evolving field with a major role in the diagnosis of pancreatic cancer as well as palliation of advanced cases. Pancreatic cancer must be managed with a multidisciplinary approach. EUS is the most frequently used modality for the diagnosis and staging of pancreatic cancer. Treatment with curative intention involves surgery, with the use of adjuvant therapy (chemotherapy and/ or radiation) in some cases. Most cases are diagnosed when curative resection is not possible and different endoscopic approaches can be used in a palliative attempt for symptomatic relieve of pain, jaundice or obstruction.

5. References

Agarwal B, Abu-Hamda E, Molke KL, Correa AM, Ho L. Endoscopic ultrasound-guided fine needle aspiration and multidetector spiral CT in the diagnosis of pancreatic cancer. Am J Gastroenterol 2004;99:844-50.

Al-Haddad M, Eloubeidi MA. Interventional EUS for the diagnosis and treatment of locally advanced pancreatic cancer. JOP 2010;11:1-7.

Ammar T, Cote GA, Creach KM, Kohlmeier C, Parikh PJ, Azar RR. Fiducial placement for stereotactic radiation by using EUS: feasibility when using a marker compatible with a standard 22-gauge needle. Gastrointest Endosc 2010;71:630-3.

Arguedas MR, Heudebert GH, Stinnett AA, Wilcox CM. Biliary stents in malignant obstructive jaundice due to pancreatic carcinoma: a cost-effectiveness analysis. Am J Gastroenterol 2002;97:898-904.

Artifon EL, Takada J, Okawa L, Moura EG, Sakai P. EUS-guided choledochoduodenostomy for biliary drainage in unresectable pancreatic cancer: a case series. JOP 2010;11:597-600.

Ascunce G, Ribeiro A, Reis I, Rocha-Lima C, Sleeman D, Merchan J, Levi J. EUS visualization and direct celiac ganglia neurolysis predicts better pain relief in patients with pancreatic malignancy (with video). Gastrointest Endosc 2011;73:267-74.

Aslanian H, Salem RR, Marginean C, Robert M, Lee JH, Topazian M. EUS-guided ethanol injection of normal porcine pancreas: a pilot study. Gastrointest Endosc 2005;62:723-7.

Becker V, Wallace MB, Fockens P, von Delius S, Woodward TA, Raimondo M, Voermans RP, Meining A. Needle-based confocal endomicroscopy for in vivo histology of intra-abdominal organs: first results in a porcine model (with videos). Gastrointest Endosc 2010;71:1260-6.

Boulay BR, Gardner TB, Gordon SR. Occlusion rate and complications of plastic biliary stent placement in patients undergoing neoadjuvant chemoradiotherapy for pancreatic cancer with malignant biliary obstruction. J Clin Gastroenterol 2010;44:452-5.

Bret PM, Nicolet V, Labadie M. Percutaneous fine-needle aspiration biopsy of the pancreas. Diagn Cytopathol 1986;2:221-7.

Brugge WR, Lauwers GY, Sahani D, Fernandez-del Castillo C, Warshaw AL. Cystic neoplasms of the pancreas. N Engl J Med 2004;351:1218-26.

Brugge WR, Lewandrowski K, Lee-Lewandrowski E, Centeno BA, Szydlo T, Regan S, del Castillo CF, Warshaw AL. Diagnosis of pancreatic cystic neoplasms: a report of the cooperative pancreatic cyst study. Gastroenterology 2004;126:1330-6.

Caturelli E, Rapaccini GL, Anti M, Fabiano A, Fedeli G. Malignant seeding after fine-needle aspiration biopsy of the pancreas. Diagn Imaging Clin Med 1985;54:88-91.

Chan HH, Nishioka NS, Mino M, Lauwers GY, Puricelli WP, Collier KN, Brugge WR. EUS-guided photodynamic therapy of the pancreas: a pilot study. Gastrointest Endosc 2004;59:95-9.

Chang KJ. EUS-guided fine needle injection (FNI) and anti-tumor therapy. Endoscopy 2006;38 Suppl 1:S88-93.

Chen VK, Arguedas MR, Baron TH. Expandable metal biliary stents before pancreaticoduodenectomy for pancreatic cancer: a Monte-Carlo decision analysis. Clin Gastroenterol Hepatol 2005;3:1229-37.

Chen YK. Pancreatoscopy: present and future role. Curr Gastroenterol Rep 2007;9:136-43.

Chhieng DC, Jhala D, Jhala N, Eltoum I, Chen VK, Vickers S, Heslin MJ, Wilcox CM, Eloubeidi MA. Endoscopic ultrasound-guided fine-needle aspiration biopsy: a study of 103 cases. Cancer 2002;96:232-9.

Davids PH, Groen AK, Rauws EA, Tytgat GN, Huibregtse K. Randomised trial of self-expanding metal stents versus polyethylene stents for distal malignant biliary obstruction. Lancet 1992;340:1488-92.

DeWitt J, Devereaux B, Chriswell M, McGreevy K, Howard T, Imperiale TF, Ciaccia D, Lane KA, Maglinte D, Kopecky K, LeBlanc J, McHenry L, Madura J, Aisen A, Cramer H, Cummings O, Sherman S. Comparison of endoscopic ultrasonography and multidetector computed tomography for detecting and staging pancreatic cancer. Ann Intern Med 2004;141:753-63.

DeWitt J, DiMaio CJ, Brugge WR. Long-term follow-up of pancreatic cysts that resolve radiologically after EUS-guided ethanol ablation. Gastrointest Endosc 2010;72:862-6.

Eloubeidi MA, Tamhane A. EUS-guided FNA of solid pancreatic masses: a learning curve with 300 consecutive procedures. Gastrointest Endosc 2005;61:700-8.

Eloubeidi MA, Tamhane A, Varadarajulu S, Wilcox CM. Frequency of major complications after EUS-guided FNA of solid pancreatic masses: a prospective evaluation. Gastrointest Endosc 2006;63:622-9.

Eloubeidi MA, Varadarajulu S, Desai S, Shirley R, Heslin MJ, Mehra M, Arnoletti JP, Eltoum I, Wilcox CM, Vickers SM. A prospective evaluation of an algorithm incorporating routine preoperative endoscopic ultrasound-guided fine needle aspiration in suspected pancreatic cancer. J Gastrointest Surg 2007;11:813-9.

Erickson RA. EUS-guided FNA. Gastrointest Endosc 2004;60:267-79.

Ferrari Junior AP, Lichtenstein DR, Slivka A, Chang C, Carr-Locke DL. Brush cytology during ERCP for the diagnosis of biliary and pancreatic malignancies. Gastrointest Endosc 1994;40:140-5.

Ferrucci JT, Wittenberg J, Margolies MN, Carey RW. Malignant seeding of the tract after thin-needle aspiration biopsy. Radiology 1979;130:345-6.

Fujita N, Noda Y, Kobayashi G, Kimura K, Ito K. Endoscopic approach to early diagnosis of pancreatic cancer. Pancreas 2004;28:279-81.

Furukawa T, Oohashi K, Yamao K, Naitoh Y, Hirooka Y, Taki T, Itoh A, Hayakawa S, Watanabe Y, Goto H, Hayakawa T. Intraductal ultrasonography of the pancreas: development and clinical potential. Endoscopy 1997;29:561-9.

Gan SI, Thompson CC, Lauwers GY, Bounds BC, Brugge WR. Ethanol lavage of pancreatic cystic lesions: initial pilot study. Gastrointest Endosc 2005;61:746-52.

Giovannini M. Concentration-dependent ablation of pancreatic tissue by EUS-guided ethanol injection. Gastrointest Endosc 2007;65:278-80.

Gress FG, Hawes RH, Savides TJ, Ikenberry SO, Cummings O, Kopecky K, Sherman S, Wiersema M, Lehman GA. Role of EUS in the preoperative staging of pancreatic cancer: a large single-center experience. Gastrointest Endosc 1999;50:786-91.

Gunaratnam NT, Sarma AV, Norton ID, Wiersema MJ. A prospective study of EUS-guided celiac plexus neurolysis for pancreatic cancer pain. Gastrointest Endosc 2001;54:316-24.

Hawes RF, P. Endosonography. Elsevier, 2006.

Hawes RH. The evolution of endoscopic ultrasound: improved imaging, higher accuracy for fine needle aspiration and the reality of endoscopic ultrasound-guided interventions. Curr Opin Gastroenterol 2010;26:436-44.

Iglesias-Garcia J, Larino-Noia J, Abdulkader I, Forteza J, Dominguez-Munoz JE. EUS elastography for the characterization of solid pancreatic masses. Gastrointest Endosc 2009;70:1101-8.

Inoue H, Mizuno N, Sawaki A, Takahashi K, Aoki M, Bhatia V, Matuura K, Tabata T, Yamao K. Life-threatening delayed-onset bleeding after endoscopic ultrasound-guided 19-gauge Trucut needle biopsy of a gastric stromal tumor. Endoscopy 2006;38 Suppl 2:E38.

Institute NC. Surveillance Epidemiology and End Results. http://seer.cancer.gov/statfacts/html/pancreas.html, 2011.

Iqbal S, Stevens PD. Cholangiopancreatoscopy for targeted biopsies of the bile and pancreatic ducts. Gastrointest Endosc Clin N Am 2009;19:567-77.

Irisawa A, Hikichi T, Shibukawa G, Takagi T, Wakatsuki T, Takahashi Y, Imamura H, Sato A, Sato M, Ikeda T, Suzuki R, Obara K, Ohira H. Pancreatobiliary drainage using the EUS-FNA technique: EUS-BD and EUS-PD. J Hepatobiliary Pancreat Surg 2009;16:598-604.

Ishikawa T, Itoh A, Kawashima H, Ohno E, Matsubara H, Itoh Y, Nakamura Y, Nakamura M, Miyahara R, Hayashi K, Ishigami M, Katano Y, Ohmiya N, Goto H, Hirooka Y. Usefulness of EUS combined with contrast-enhancement in the differential diagnosis of malignant versus benign and preoperative localization of pancreatic endocrine tumors. Gastrointest Endosc 2010;71:951-9.

Itoi T, Neuhaus H, Chen YK. Diagnostic value of image-enhanced video cholangiopancreatoscopy. Gastrointest Endosc Clin N Am 2009;19:557-66.

Jing X, Wamsteker EJ, Li H, Pu RT. Combining fine needle aspiration with brushing cytology has improved yields in diagnosing pancreatic ductal adenocarcinoma. Diagn Cytopathol 2009;37:574-8.

Kaassis M, Boyer J, Dumas R, Ponchon T, Coumaros D, Delcenserie R, Canard JM, Fritsch J, Rey JF, Burtin P. Plastic or metal stents for malignant stricture of the common bile duct? Results of a randomized prospective study. Gastrointest Endosc 2003;57:178-82.

Kameya S, Kuno N, Kasugai T. The diagnosis of pancreatic cancer by pancreatic juice cytology. Acta Cytol 1981;25:354-60.

Kaufman M, Singh G, Das S, Concha-Parra R, Erber J, Micames C, Gress F. Efficacy of endoscopic ultrasound-guided celiac plexus block and celiac plexus neurolysis for managing abdominal pain associated with chronic pancreatitis and pancreatic cancer. J Clin Gastroenterol 2010;44:127-34.

Kipp BR, Fritcher EG, Clayton AC, Gores GJ, Roberts LR, Zhang J, Levy MJ, Halling KC. Comparison of KRAS mutation analysis and FISH for detecting pancreatobiliary tract cancer in cytology specimens collected during endoscopic retrograde cholangiopancreatography. J Mol Diagn 2010;12:780-6.

Klapman JB, Chang KJ. Endoscopic ultrasound-guided fine-needle injection. Gastrointest Endosc Clin N Am 2005;15:169-77, x.

Larghi A, Verna EC, Stavropoulos SN, Rotterdam H, Lightdale CJ, Stevens PD. EUS-guided trucut needle biopsies in patients with solid pancreatic masses: a prospective study. Gastrointest Endosc 2004;59:185-90.

Levy MJ. Endoscopic ultrasound-guided trucut biopsy of the pancreas: prospects and problems. Pancreatology 2007;7:163-6.

Matsumoto K, Yamao K, Ohashi K, Watanabe Y, Sawaki A, Nakamura T, Matsuura A, Suzuki T, Fukutomi A, Baba T, Okubo K, Tanaka K, Moriyama I, Shimizu Y. Acute portal vein thrombosis after EUS-guided FNA of pancreatic cancer: case report. Gastrointest Endosc 2003;57:269-71.

Matthes K, Mino-Kenudson M, Sahani DV, Holalkere N, Brugge WR. Concentration-dependent ablation of pancreatic tissue by EUS-guided ethanol injection. Gastrointest Endosc 2007;65:272-7.

McGuire DE, Venu RP, Brown RD, Etzkorn KP, Glaws WR, Abu-Hammour A. Brush cytology for pancreatic carcinoma: an analysis of factors influencing results. Gastrointest Endosc 1996;44:300-4.

Meining A. Confocal endomicroscopy. Gastrointest Endosc Clin N Am 2009;19:629-35.

Meining A, Phillip V, Gaa J, Prinz C, Schmid RM. Pancreaticoscopy with miniprobe-based confocal laser-scanning microscopy of an intraductal papillary mucinous neoplasm (with video). Gastrointest Endosc 2009;69:1178-80.

Mennone A, Nathanson MH. Needle-based confocal laser endomicroscopy to assess liver histology in vivo. Gastrointest Endosc 2011;73:338-44.

Moss AC, Morris E, Mac Mathuna P. Palliative biliary stents for obstructing pancreatic carcinoma. Cochrane Database Syst Rev 2006:CD004200.

Nguyen NQ, Binmoeller KF, Shah JN. Cholangioscopy and pancreatoscopy (with videos). Gastrointest Endosc 2009;70:1200-10.

Nguyen-Tang T, Binmoeller KF, Sanchez-Yague A, Shah JN. Endoscopic ultrasound (EUS)-guided transhepatic anterograde self-expandable metal stent (SEMS) placement across malignant biliary obstruction. Endoscopy 2010;42:232-6.

Nishino T, Oyama H, Toki F, Shiratori K. Differentiation between autoimmune pancreatitis and pancreatic carcinoma based on endoscopic retrograde cholangiopancreatography findings. J Gastroenterol 2010;45:988-96.

O'Toole D, Palazzo L, Arotcarena R, Dancour A, Aubert A, Hammel P, Amaris J, Ruszniewski P. Assessment of complications of EUS-guided fine-needle aspiration. Gastrointest Endosc 2001;53:470-4.

Palazzo L, Roseau G, Gayet B, Vilgrain V, Belghiti J, Fekete F, Paolaggi JA. Endoscopic ultrasonography in the diagnosis and staging of pancreatic adenocarcinoma. Results of a prospective study with comparison to ultrasonography and CT scan. Endoscopy 1993;25:143-50.

Park WG, Yan BM, Schellenberg D, Kim J, Chang DT, Koong A, Patalano C, Van Dam J. EUS-guided gold fiducial insertion for image-guided radiation therapy of pancreatic cancer: 50 successful cases without fluoroscopy. Gastrointest Endosc 2010;71:513-8.

Puli SR, Reddy JB, Bechtold ML, Antillon MR, Brugge WR. EUS-guided celiac plexus neurolysis for pain due to chronic pancreatitis or pancreatic cancer pain: a meta-analysis and systematic review. Dig Dis Sci 2009;54:2330-7.

Ramesh J, Varadarajulu S. Interventional endoscopic ultrasound. Dig Dis 2008;26:347-55.

Rivadeneira DE, Pochapin M, Grobmyer SR, Lieberman MD, Christos PJ, Jacobson I, Daly JM. Comparison of linear array endoscopic ultrasound and helical computed tomography for the staging of periampullary malignancies. Ann Surg Oncol 2003;10:890-7.

Rogart JN. The plastic biliary stent: an obsolete device for managing pancreatic cancer? J Clin Gastroenterol 2010;44:389-90.

Rogart JN, Boghos A, Rossi F, Al-Hashem H, Siddiqui UD, Jamidar P, Aslanian H. Analysis of endoscopic management of occluded metal biliary stents at a single tertiary care center. Gastrointest Endosc 2008;68:676-82.

Sakamoto H, Kitano M, Komaki T, Noda K, Chikugo T, Dote K, Takeyama Y, Das K, Yamao K, Kudo M. Prospective comparative study of the EUS guided 25-gauge FNA needle with the 19-gauge Trucut needle and 22-gauge FNA needle in patients with solid pancreatic masses. J Gastroenterol Hepatol 2009;24:384-90.

Sanders MK, Moser AJ, Khalid A, Fasanella KE, Zeh HJ, Burton S, McGrath K. EUS-guided fiducial placement for stereotactic body radiotherapy in locally advanced and recurrent pancreatic cancer. Gastrointest Endosc 2010;71:1178-84.

Sendino O, Fernandez-Esparrach G, Sole M, Colomo L, Pellise M, Llach J, Navarro S, Bordas JM, Gines A. Endoscopic ultrasonography-guided brushing increases cellular diagnosis of pancreatic cysts: A prospective study. Dig Liver Dis 2010;42:877-81.

Siddiqui AA, Sreenarasimhaiah J, Lara LF, Harford W, Lee C, Eloubeidi MA. Endoscopic ultrasound-guided transduodenal placement of a fully covered metal stent for palliative biliary drainage in patients with malignant biliary obstruction. Surg Endosc 2011;25:549-55.

Siddiqui UD, Rossi F, Rosenthal LS, Padda MS, Murali-Dharan V, Aslanian HR. EUS-guided FNA of solid pancreatic masses: a prospective, randomized trial comparing 22-gauge and 25-gauge needles. Gastrointest Endosc 2009;70:1093-7.

Smith FP, Macdonald JS, Schein PS, Ornitz RD. Cutaneous seeding of pancreatic cancer by skinny-needle aspiration biopsy. Arch Intern Med 1980;140:855.

Society AC. Learn About Cancer. Pancreatic Cancer. http://www.cancer.org/Cancer/PancreaticCancer/DetailedGuide/pancreatic-cancer-what-is-pancreatic-cancer, 2011.

Sun S, Xu H, Xin J, Liu J, Guo Q, Li S. Endoscopic ultrasound-guided interstitial brachytherapy of unresectable pancreatic cancer: results of a pilot trial. Endoscopy 2006;38:399-403.

Telford JJ, Carr-Locke DL. The role of ERCP and pancreatoscopy in cystic and intraductal tumors. Gastrointest Endosc Clin N Am 2002;12:747-57.

Thomas T, Bebb J, Mannath J, Ragunath K, Kaye PV, Aithal GP. EUS-guided pancreatic cyst brushing: a comparative study in a tertiary referral centre. JOP 2010;11:163-9.

Thomas T, Kaye PV, Ragunath K, Aithal G. Efficacy, safety, and predictive factors for a positive yield of EUS-guided Trucut biopsy: a large tertiary referral center experience. Am J Gastroenterol 2009;104:584-91.

Trevino JM, Varadarajulu S. Endoscopic ultrasonography-guided ablation therapy. J Hepatobiliary Pancreat Sci 2011;18:304-10.

Uchida N, Kamada H, Tsutsui K, Ono M, Aritomo Y, Masaki T, Kushida Y, Haba R, Nakatsu T, Kuriyama S. Utility of pancreatic duct brushing for diagnosis of pancreatic carcinoma. J Gastroenterol 2007;42:657-62.

Vandervoort J, Soetikno RM, Montes H, Lichtenstein DR, Van Dam J, Ruymann FW, Cibas ES, Carr-Locke DL. Accuracy and complication rate of brush cytology from bile duct versus pancreatic duct. Gastrointest Endosc 1999;49:322-7.

Varadarajulu S, Fraig M, Schmulewitz N, Roberts S, Wildi S, Hawes RH, Hoffman BJ, Wallace MB. Comparison of EUS-guided 19-gauge Trucut needle biopsy with EUS-guided fine-needle aspiration. Endoscopy 2004;36:397-401.

Varadarajulu S, Jhala NC, Drelichman ER. EUS-guided radiofrequency ablation with a prototype electrode array system in an animal model (with video). Gastrointest Endosc 2009;70:372-6.

Verna EC, Dhar V. Endoscopic ultrasound-guided fine needle injection for cancer therapy: the evolving role of therapeutic endoscopic ultrasound. Therap Adv Gastroenterol 2008;1:103-9.

Wasan SM, Ross WA, Staerkel GA, Lee JH. Use of expandable metallic biliary stents in resectable pancreatic cancer. Am J Gastroenterol 2005;100:2056-61.

Wiersema MJ, Vilmann P, Giovannini M, Chang KJ, Wiersema LM. Endosonography-guided fine-needle aspiration biopsy: diagnostic accuracy and complication assessment. Gastroenterology 1997;112:1087-95.

Wiersema MJ, Wiersema LM. Endosonography-guided celiac plexus neurolysis. Gastrointest Endosc 1996;44:656-62.

Wittmann J, Kocjan G, Sgouros SN, Deheragoda M, Pereira SP. Endoscopic ultrasound-guided tissue sampling by combined fine needle aspiration and trucut needle biopsy: a prospective study. Cytopathology 2006;17:27-33.

Yamaguchi T, Shirai Y, Ishihara T, Sudo K, Nakagawa A, Ito H, Miyazaki M, Nomura F, Saisho H. Pancreatic juice cytology in the diagnosis of intraductal papillary mucinous neoplasm of the pancreas: significance of sampling by peroral pancreatoscopy. Cancer 2005;104:2830-6.

Yamao K, Bhatia V, Mizuno N, Sawaki A, Shimizu Y, Irisawa A. Interventional endoscopic ultrasonography. J Gastroenterol Hepatol 2009;24:509-19.

Yasuda K, Mukai H, Fujimoto S, Nakajima M, Kawai K. The diagnosis of pancreatic cancer by endoscopic ultrasonography. Gastrointest Endosc 1988;34:1-8.

14

Role of Guided - Fine Needle Biopsy of the Pancreatic Lesion

Luigi Cavanna, Roberto Di Cicilia, Elisabetta Nobili,
Elisa Stroppa, Adriano Zangrandi and Carlo Paties
Oncology – Hematology and Pathology Departments,
Hospital of Piacenza,
Italy

1. Introduction

Pancreatic cancer (PC) is the fifth leading cause of cancer death in the United States, with 28,000 to 30,000 number of deaths annually (American Cancer Society,2002).

Survival in patients with untreated pc is very poor, the one year survival rate is 19% and the 5- year survival rate is 4% for all stages combined (American Cancer Society,2002).

It must be emphasized that the majority of patients with pancreatic cancer are diagnosed in the metastatic phase; however when complete surgical resection with margin negative and node negative is possible, it offers the best opportunity for long survival or even cure, with 5-year survival approaching 40% when performed at specialized center. (Sohn et al, 2000).

Epithelial neoplasia of pancreas can be divided into those with predominantly exocrine differentiation and those with endocrine differentiation.

Neoplasia of exocrine differentiation can be further subdivided into solid and cystic tumors; the majority of malignancies of the pancreas are solid infiltrating ductal adenocarcinomas.

2. Histology

About 80% of pancreatic malignancies are ductal adenocarcinomas, of which approximately 70% occur in the head of the pancreas.

A variety of uncommon types of pancreatic carcinoma have been described, including acinar, adenosquamous, anaplastic, papillary, mucinous and microadenocarcinomas, each of which composes less than 5% of the total. All of these have similarly poor prognoses and are treated in a similar fashion. Also uncommon are mucinous cystic neoplasms (cystadenoma/cystadenocarcinoma) of the pancreas, which occur most frequently in the middle-aged women, and these are tipically located in the tail of the pancreas.

Clinical behavior can be difficult to predict pathologically, leading some to conclude that all mucinous cystic neoplasms of pancreas have malignant potential.

Other rare neoplasms include pancreatoblastomas, most of which occur in children, primary lymphoma of the pancreas and metastasis.

3. Diagnosis of pancreatic neoplasia

Currently, imaging modalities for detection of pancreatic masses include ultrasonography (US), computed tomography (CT) scan, magnetic resonance imaging (MRI)/ magnetic resonance cholangiopancreatography, endoscopic ultrasonography (EUS).

In clinical practice differential diagnosis of pancreatic masses is frequently a clinical challenge; often therapeutic decision in this context is mainly based on the ability to perform a diagnosis of malignancy or to exclude malignancy (Tamm & Charnsangavej, 2001).

It is well known that ductal adenocarcinoma is the most frequent cause of pancreatic mass, however other neoplasms such as lymphoma, metastasis, cystic tumors or benign conditions as chronic pancreatitis with different prognosis and treatment options can arise within the pancreas (Iglesias et al., 2010).

A pathologic diagnosis becomes therefore relevant for an adequate therapeutic strategy (Cohen et al., 2000).

At least 80% of the patients with suspected pancreatic cancer, have unresectable disease at diagnosis because of locoregional involvement or distant metastases , and it as been reported that only 7% of the patients have a tumour that is confined within the pancreas (National Cancer Institute, 2007).

Patients with suspected pancreatic cancer and imaging studies suggesting resectable tumour should undergo directly to surgery since no histologic diagnosis confirmation is required prior to surgical exploration unless neoadjuvant therapy is indicated (Zamboni et al., 2010).

As a matter of fact preoperative cytohistological diagnosis may risk dissemination of cancer cells, or developing complications (bleeding, pancreatitis, pancreatic leak) that can delay surgery and increase costs.

On the other hand a negative biopsy results in a patient with a high suspicion of cancer neoplasm that is not of help, due to a high possibility of a false negative result (Tillou et al., 1996).

Patients with metastatic or locally advanced but unresectable disease at imaging studies should undergo biopsy prior chemotherapy or radiation since a cytohistological diagnosis is recommended before initiating a cytostatic therapy coherently with the National Comprehensive Cancer Network (NCCN) guidelines for suspected pancreatic cancer. (Hartwig et al, 2009; Itani et al., 1997) Biopsies allow a cytohistological diagnosis and can differentiate pancreatic cancer between primary pancreatic lymphoma (Arcari et al., 2005), metastasis or benign focal lesion such as focal pancreatitis.

3.1 Primary pancreatic lymphoma and pancreatic metastasis

Primary pancreatic lymphoma (PPL) is a very rare disease, representing fewer than 2% of extra-nodal malignant lymphoma and 0,5% of all pancreatic masses (Arcari et al., 2005).

Fewer than 150 cases of PPL have been reported in the literature in English. Imaging techniques such as Us and CT scan can suggest a diagnosis of PPL but a cyto-hystological examination is mandatory for diagnosis and treatment planning of patients with suspicious PPL. Our group reported five cases of PPL and reviewing the literature it was concluded that 1) imaging techniques can suggest the suspicion of PPL, however are unable to distinguish PPL from pancreatic adenocarcinoma, 2) histological diagnosis can be easily obtained by percutaneous Us-guided tissue core biopsy 3)surgery can be avoided both for diagnosis and therapy, but the treatment of choice of PPL may only be evaluated on a larger series of patients (Arcari et al., 2005).

Metastases to the pancreas are rare; in a survey of 4,955 autopsies (Adsay et al., 2004) a rate of metastasis to the pancreas of 3,83% was described and a significantly different distribution of metastatic neoplasms, with lung and gastrointestinal tumors comprising by far the largest proportion.

In a retrospective review of 1,172 pancreatic endoscopic ultrasound-guided fine-needle aspiration biopsy , 25 cases (2,1%) had a confirmed diagnosis of pancreatic metastasis.

This included 12 cases of renal cell carcinoma, 3 (12%) melanomas, 3 (12%) small cell carcinomas and 7 (28%) other malignancies.

In these metastatic tumors involving the pancreas 20 (80%) of the lesions were solitary.

Four cases (16%) had no prior history of malignancy; the average time of diagnosis of pancreatic metastasis was 5.3 years.

Immunohistochemistry and special stains were performed in 22 (88%) and 9 (36%) cases respectively (Gilbert et al., 2011).

4. Staging of pancreatic cancer (table 1)

Staging procedures include US, CT scanning, MRI, and EUS. A diagnostic laparoscopy may also be performed to detect peritoneal disease that is not visible radiologically. Regardless of these studies, an accurate histologic diagnosis is necessary to distinguish benign disease from carcinoma, islet cell tumors, and retroperitoneal lymphomas, because of the major therapeutic and prognostic differences among these disease entities. Criteria for surgical resection include absence of metastatic disease and absence of invasion of prominent local blood vessels.

5. Guide for pancreatic biopsy

Intraoperative needle biopsy of the pancreas has been performed with the fine-needle aspiration biopsy (FNAB) technique since the 1960's (Moossa & Altorki, 1983) and with the core tissue biopsy technique since 1970's (Ingram et al., 1978) subsequently ultrasound , computed tomography and endoscopic ultrasound became available to evaluate and characterize pancreatic masses and above all to guide a needle for the biopsy, avoiding the costs, morbidity and mortality of a major surgical procedure performed only to obtain a tissue sample for a cytohistological diagnosis (Civardi et al.,1986; Turner et a.l, 2010).

For many years percutaneous US and /or CT guided biopsy was routinely performed in situations in which a pancreatic biopsy was necessary, in 2002 the American Joint Committee on cancer has selected endoscopic ultrasound guided FNAB as "the procedure of choice" if available (Greene et al., 2002).

However, as recently reported, local expertise in and the availability of EUS and interventional radiology may determine the first procedure selected for a cytohistological diagnosis for a pancreatic mass (Zamboni et al., 2010).

Prymary Tumor (T)			
TX	Primary tumor cannot be assessed		
T0	No evidence of primary tumor		
Tis	In situ carcinoma		
T1	Tumor limited to the pancreas 2 cm or less in greatest dimension		
T2	Tumor limited to the pancreas more than 2 cm in greatest dimension		
T3	Tumor extends beyond the pancreas but without involvement of celiac axis or the superior mesenteric artery		
T4	Tumor involves the celiac axis or the superior mesenteric artery (unresectable primary tumor)		
Regional Lymph Nodes (N)			
NX	Regional lymph nodes cannot be assessed		
N0	No regional lymph node metastasis		
N1	Regional lymph node metastasis		
Distant Metastasis (M)			
MX	Distant metastasis cannot be assessed		
M0	No distant metastasis		
M1	Distant metastasis		
Stage grouping			
Stage 0	Tis	N0	M0
Stage IA	T1	N0	M0
Stage IB	T2	N0	M0
Stage IIA	T3	N0	M0
Stage IIB	T1-3	N1	M0
Stage III	T4	Any N	M0
Stage IV	Any T	Any N	M1

Table 1. Staging of pancreatic carcinoma

5.1 Methods of percutaneous guided biopsy

Patient preparation before any type of invasive procedure includes ruling out coagulation disorders with laboratory tests and obtaining written informed consent for the biopsy. Local anesthesia (lidocaine) is not routinely performed. (Zamboni et al., 2010; Civardi et al., 1986).

5.2 Percutaneous ultrasound

In the past for performing abdominal US-guided FNAB the "free-hand" technique was utilized (Civardi et al., 1986; Bret et al., 1982; Livraghi, 1984) subsequently puncturing probe became available and two types of probes are commonly used for interventional procedures: probes with lateral support and probes with noncontinuous crystals and central support; the former allow only oblique needle tracks, whereas the latter allow both vertical and oblique tracks.

Prior to perform the biopsy, a pancreatic lesion can be studied with conventional US, Doppler US, and CT, to evaluate the content of the lesion and to select the best route for biopsy, avoiding vessels and pleura.

In clinical practice when liver metastases are present in patients with suspected pancreatic cancer, the biopsy can be done in the liver metastasis, if safer for the patient and easier for the psysician.

5.3 Computed tomography

Computed tomography allows optimal visualization of the lesion and is superior to US in large fat patients , however radiation dose and the procedure length are the major limits of CT -guided pancreatic biopsy.

CT fluoroscopy can reduce procedure length because it allows a fast reconstruction of images, with a continuous update and the possibility of controlling acquisition and visualizing images in the room while performing the examination.

In addiction CT fluoroscopy allows visualizing the needle track from the entry point to the target, allowing faster and more efficient procedure (Zamboni et al., 2010).

5.4 Endoscopic ultrasound

Over the past decade, EUS has proven to be one of the most significant advantages in gastrointestinal endoscopy (Turner et al., 2010; Erickson, 2004) Since its introduction, EUS has offered improved accessibility to small pancreatic lesions, and its usefulness as a diagnostic tool has greately changed the therapeutic approach to pancreatic masses.

Since it was first reported in (Chang et al, 1994), EUS-guided FNAB of the pancreas has become a popular technique for the diagnosis and staging of cystic and solid lesions of the pancreas because it is relatively safe and accurate (Carrara et al., 2010;).

Thus, this diagnostic modality has become important in the management of patients with symptomatic or incidentally discovered pancreatic masses.

5.4.1 US, CT, or EUS for guide pancreatic FNAB

The relative diagnostic accuracy, safety and cost of US and CT-guided FNAB favor their use over EUS-FNAB for the diagnosis of unresectable pancreatic tumors. (Zamboni et al., 2010 ; Levy, 2006).

A randomized controlled trial EUS-FNAB and US/CT-FNAB failed to observe any statistically significant difference between the endoscopic and percutaneous approach in the diagnosis of pancreatic malignancy (Horwhat et al.,2006).

Several authors support the use of EUS-FNAB over percutaneuos approach because of the lower risk of seeding (Gilbert et al, 2001; Turner et al, 2010). In a review of 1406 cases with advanced pancreatic cancer who underwent nonsurgical biopsy (percutaneous-guided or EUS-guided sampling) were compared with cases who did not undergo biopsy, without observing any difference in overall median survival, so it was concluded that the risk of seeding is remote. (Hernandez et al., 2009). It was reported that the risk of seeding can be related to the number of needle passes: more number of needle passes more risk of seeding (Civardi et al., 1986; Fornari et al., 1989).

It must be emphasized that one-site cytopathological evaluation can improve the diagnostic yield of guided FNAB and can reduce the number of needle passes (Garcia et al., 2011).

A review of 182 patients undergoing EUS-guided FNAB of solid pancreatic lesions over a 2 years study period was reported (Garcia et al., 2011). Sample were either evaluated on site by a cytopathologist or processed by the endoscopist and sent to the pathology department for evaluation.

Diagnostic accuracy for malignancy, number of needle passes, adequate - specimen collection rate, cytological diagnosis , and final diagnosis and complications rate according to the presence or absence of on-site cytopathologist were evaluated.

A significantly higher number of needle passes was performed when an on-site cytopathologist was not available (3.5+- 1.0 vs 2.0+-0.7; p< 0.001). The presence of an on-site cytopathologist was associated with a significant lower number of inadequate samples (1.0 vs 12.6%; p=0.002) and a significantly higher diagnostic sensivity (96.2 vs 78.2%; p=0.002), and overall accuracy (96.8 vs 86.2%; p=0.013) for malignancy (Garcia et al., 2011).

Already, in 1988 our group reported the value of rapid staining and assessment of percutaneous ultrasound-guided fine needle aspiration biopsy in a series of 160 patients. (Civardi et al., 1988) The total series of FNAB had a sensitivity of 95.6%, a specificity of 100% and an overall accuracy of 97.3%.

The cumulative accuracy after each pass was calculated: a significant increase in diagnostic accuracy was found only after the second pass, the third and the fourth passes gave little further improvement. These results indicate that a rapid evaluation of the aspirated material during US-guided FNAB can reduce the number of punctures needed per case resulting in less disconfort and, probably a reduced likelihood of complications for the patient.

It must be emphasized that in this study the same physicians that performed the US-FNAB performed also the rapid staining evaluation for the adequacy avoiding the cytopathologist, minimizing the costs and improving the educational benefit of physicians. (Civardi et al., 1988).

5.4.2 Type of needle and results of guided biopsy

Biopsies of the pancreas can be performed with needle ranging in size from 18 to 25 gauge (G). Aspiration biopsies for cytological evaluation are performed with fine-needle (< 1mm in external diameter : from 20 to 25 G), cutting needle are used to obtain tissue cores, which allow hystopathological evaluation , these needle ranging in size from 18 to 23 G.

In table 2 are reported the results of sensitivity, specificity, overall accuracy, method of guidance, needle size of percutaneous pancreatic fine-needle aspiration biopsy.

Our group (Di Stasi et al., 1998) in a multicenter study reviewed 510 patients who had a final diagnosis available and who had undergone ultrasound-guided fine needle biopsy of the

N° of patients	sensitivity (%)	specificity (%)	accuracy (%)	guidance	needle size	authors
510	87	100	95	US	21-22	Di Stasi et al (1998)
267	81	-	-	US	22	Bhatia et al (2008)
222	89	98	91	US	22 (20,25)	Garre Sanchez et al (2007)
104	77.9	100	81.7	US	-	Volmar et al; Zamboni (2005)
70	80	100	81	CT/US	-	Mallery et al (2002)
59	93	100	93	US	22	Matsubara et al (2008)
50	78.6	100	82	CT	-	Volmar et al (2005)
36	62	100	72	CT/US	20-22	Horwhat et al (2006)
545	99.4	-	99.4	US	21-22	Zamboni et al (2010)

Table 2. Sensitivity, specificity, accuracy method of guidance and needle size (gauge) of percutaneous fine needle aspiration biopsy of pancreatic masses

pancreas. Retrieval rate, sensitivity, specificity, and overall diagnostic accuracy of the whole series, by three different bioptic procedures (cytology, histology and cytology plus histology) were evaluated. The reliability of ultrasound-guided fine needle biopsy to allow a correct diagnosis in the different pancreatic pathologies was calculated for cytology, histology, and cytology plus histology, retrieval rate values were: 94%, 96%, and 97%; sensitivity was: 87%, 94%, and 94%, specificity:100%; and diagnostic accuracy: 91%, 90% and 95%, respectively.

In a series of 545 US-guided FNAB, 93,4% procedures were diagnostic, with an overall 99,4% sensitivity and 99.4% accuracy (Zamboni et al., 2010).

The largest series reporting in the literature percutaneous FNAB of pancreatic masses show sensitivities ranging between 62% and 93%, accuracies between 72% and 94%. The majority of percutaneous FNAB are ultrasound guided, and the needle size range from 21 to 22 G (Tab 2).

FNAB cytology of pancreatic cancer are reported in figure 1 a , b, 2 a, b, 3 a, b;

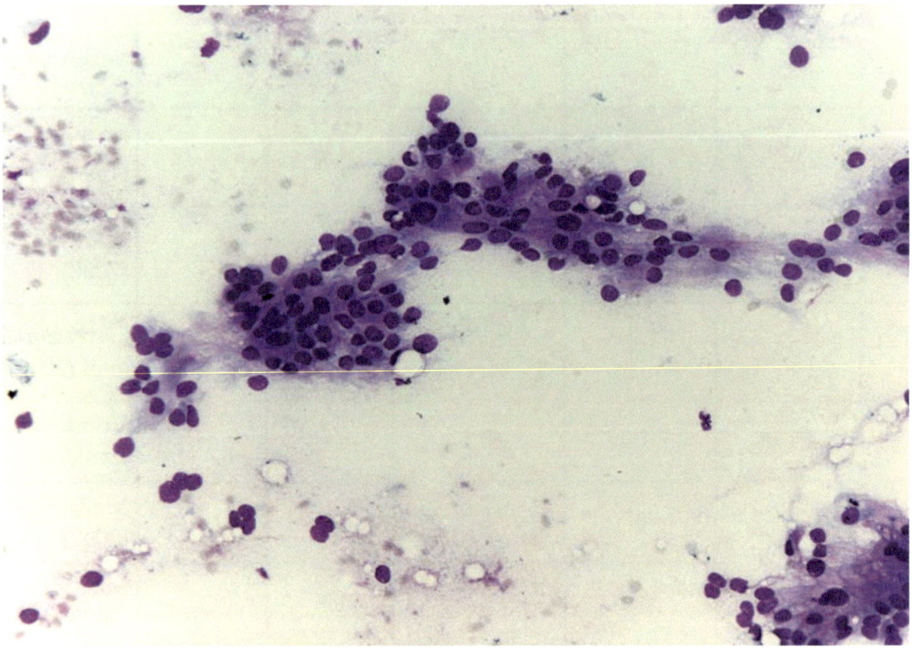

Fig. 1. a. FNAB of pancreatic well-differentiated adenocarcinoma, (a) relatively mild nuclear atypia, but nuclear crowding. MGG x 200

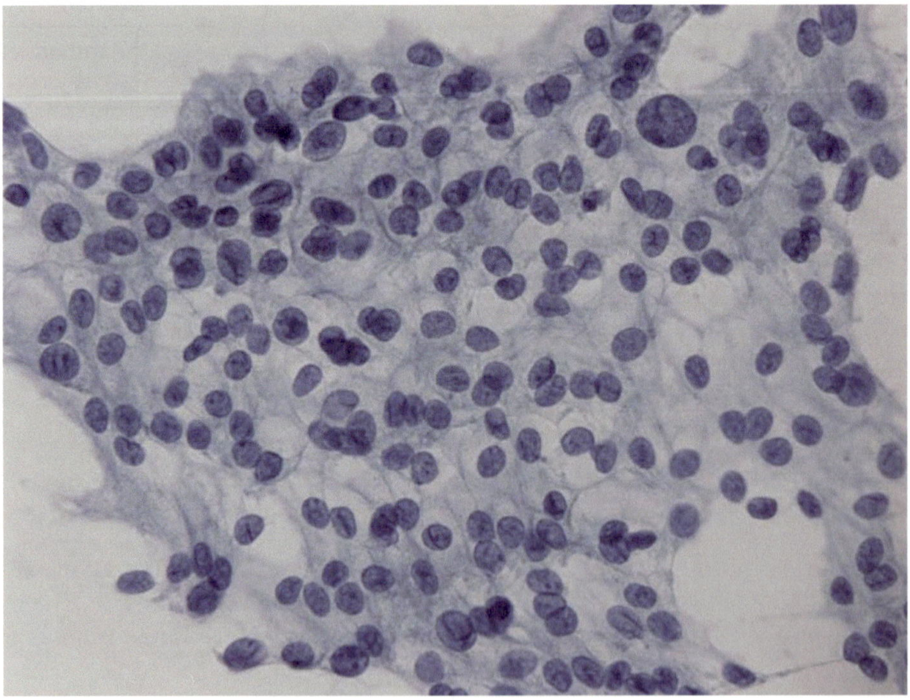

Fig. 1. b. Well evident microglandular arrangement. PAP x 400

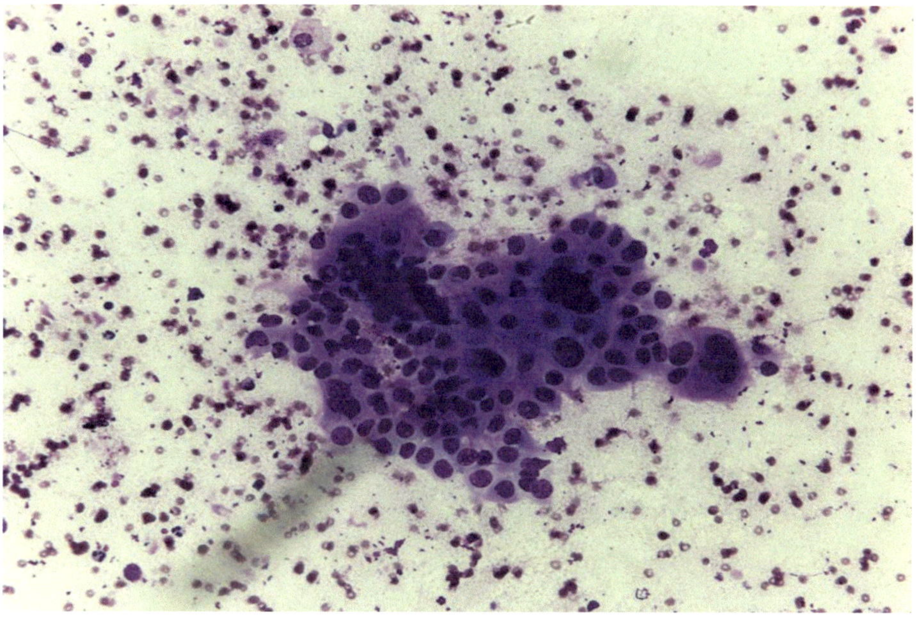

Fig. 2. a. FNAB of pancreatic moderately differentiated pancreatic adenocarcinoma. MMG x 200

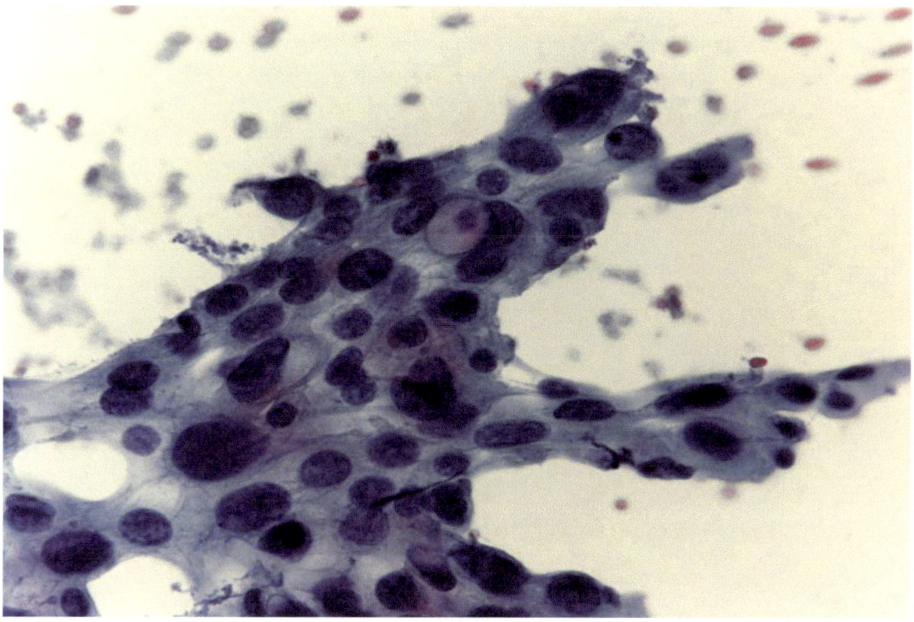

Fig. 2. b. Clusters of cells with some acinar arrangement. PAP x 400

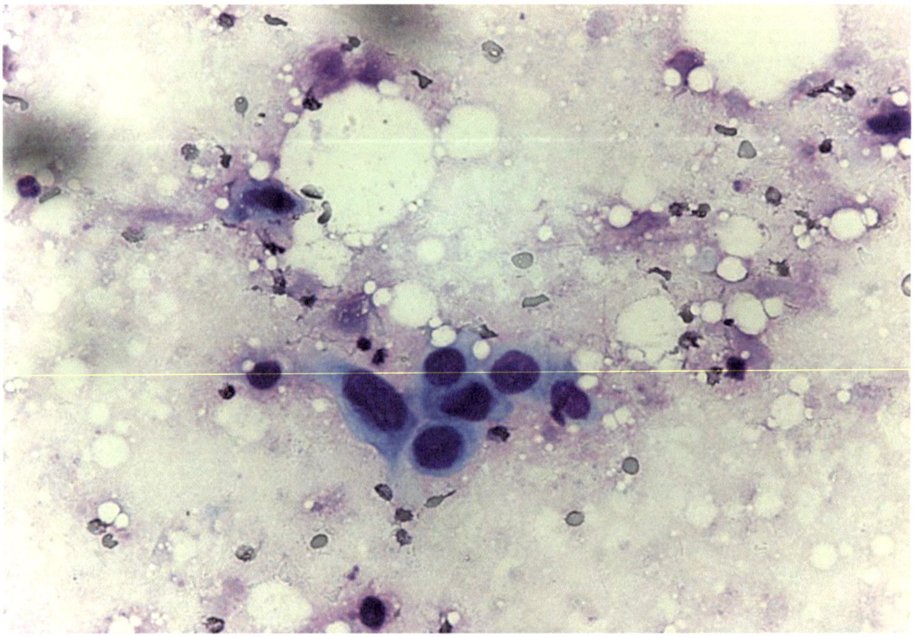

Fig. 3. a. FNAB of pancreatic poorly differentiated pancreatic adenocarcinoma, a cluster of cancer cells. MGG x 400

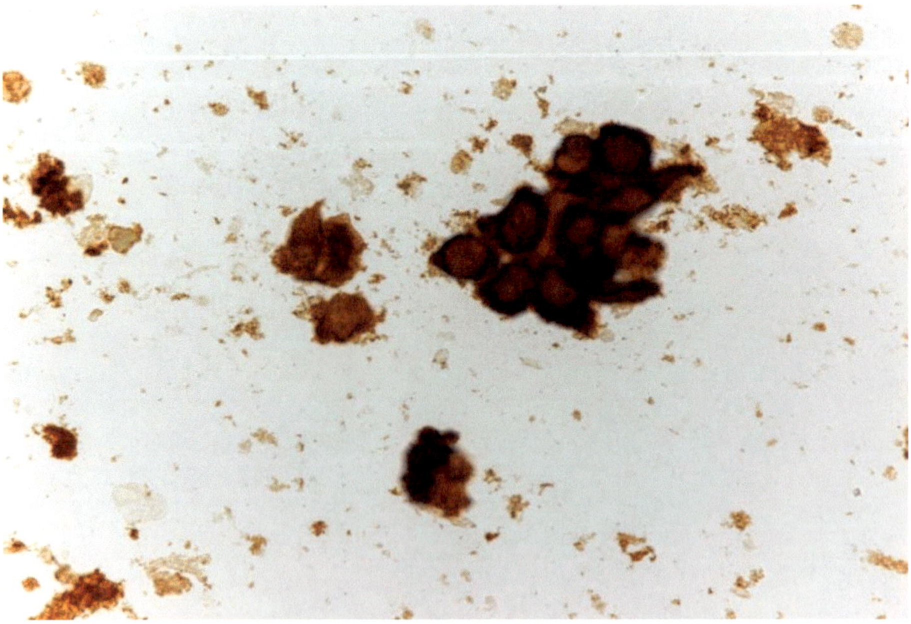

Fig. 3. b. Cancer cells with strong reactivity to CK 7 antiboby. X 400

and FNAB cytology of pancreatic metastasis is reported in figure 4 a, b.

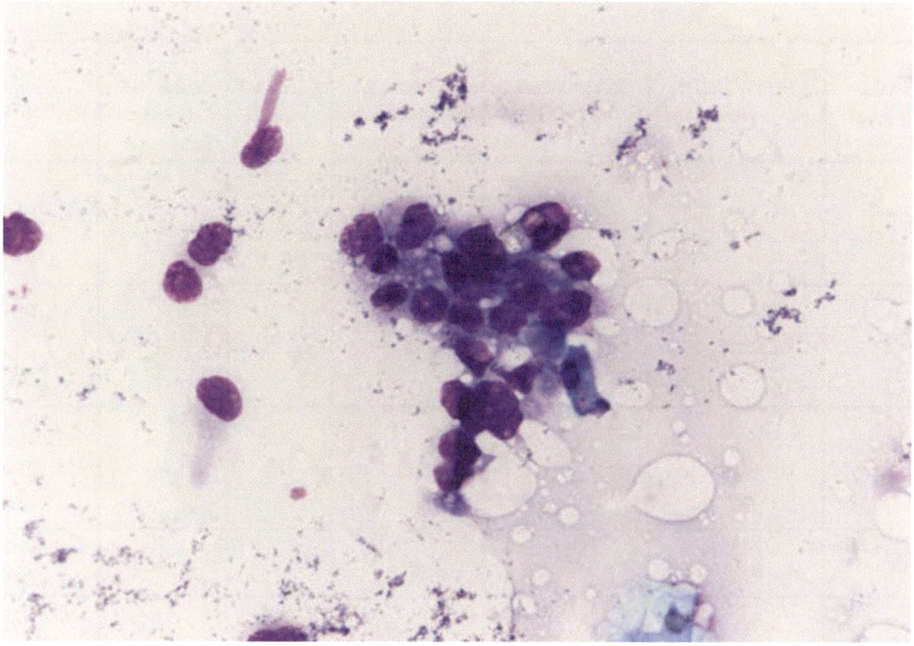

Fig. 4. a. FNAB of pancreatic mass showing metastatic melanoma large cells. MGG x 400

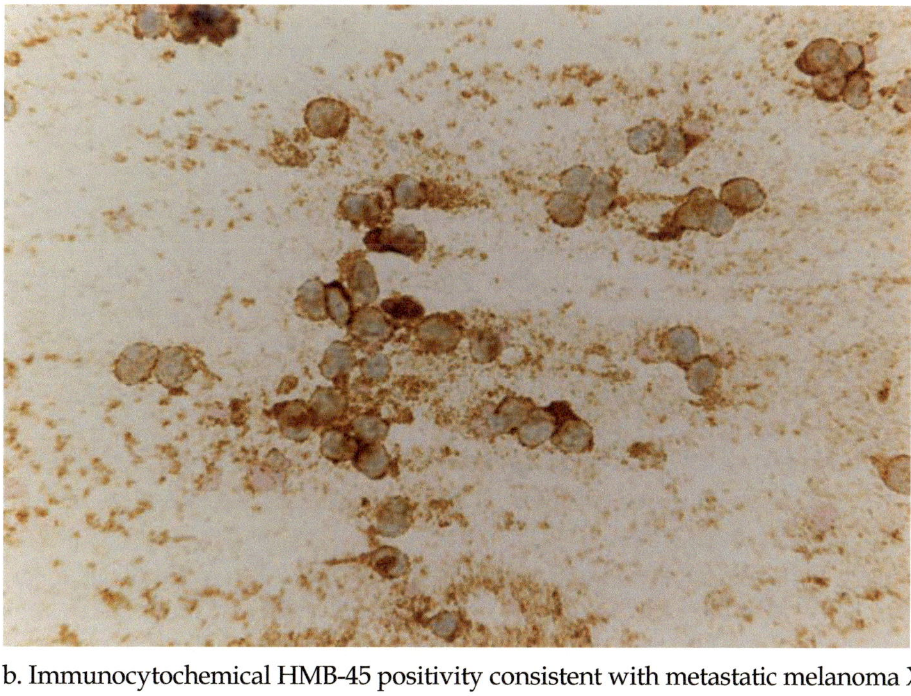

Fig. 4. b. Immunocytochemical HMB-45 positivity consistent with metastatic melanoma X 400

Sensitivity, specificity, accuracy method of guidance and needle size of percutaneous tissue core biopsy of pancreatic masses are reported in table 3.

N° of patients	sensitivity (%)	specificity (%)	accuracy (%)	guidance	needle size	authors
372	90	-	90	CT	18	Amin et al (2006)
212	86	100	86	US	21	Matsubara et al (2008)
142	90.9	-	92.6	US	-	Jennings et al (1989)
100	90	-	-	US	-	Karlson et al (1996)
92	92.5	100	93.3	US	18	Paulsen et al (2006)
50	90.4	-	92	US	-	Elvin et all (1990)
18	100	1	100	CT	18	Paulsen et al (2006)

Table 3. Sensitivity, specificity, accuracy method of guidance and needle size (gauge) of percutaneous tissue core biopsy of pancreatic masses

372 CT-guided pancreatic biopsies with a 18 G cutting needle showed 90% sensitivity and accuracy (Karlson et al., 1996); similar results were reported in a series of 212 US guided percutaneous tissue core pancreatic biopsies, with 86% sensitivity and accuracy (Paulsen et al., 2006).

The largest series in the literature on percutaneous tissue core biopsy of pancreatic lesions report sensitivities and accuracies between 86% and 100% (Tab 3). Tissue core biopsy of primary pancreatic lymphoma and metastatic adenocarcinoma are reported in fig 5 a b and 6 a b c. Percutaneous core biopsy of pancreatic lesions is considered sensitive, safe and accurate (Zanaboni et al., 2010) however this procedure may have a higher complication rate than percutaneous FNAB (Fornari et al., 1989).

At our institution we routinely use FNAB with 22G needles when a pathologic diagnosis of pancreatic mass is required while tissue core biopsy with 20G or 21G needles is reserved when cytological diagnosis is inadequate or when lymphoma is suspected on cytological evaluation (Arcari et al., 2005) Fig 5 a, b.

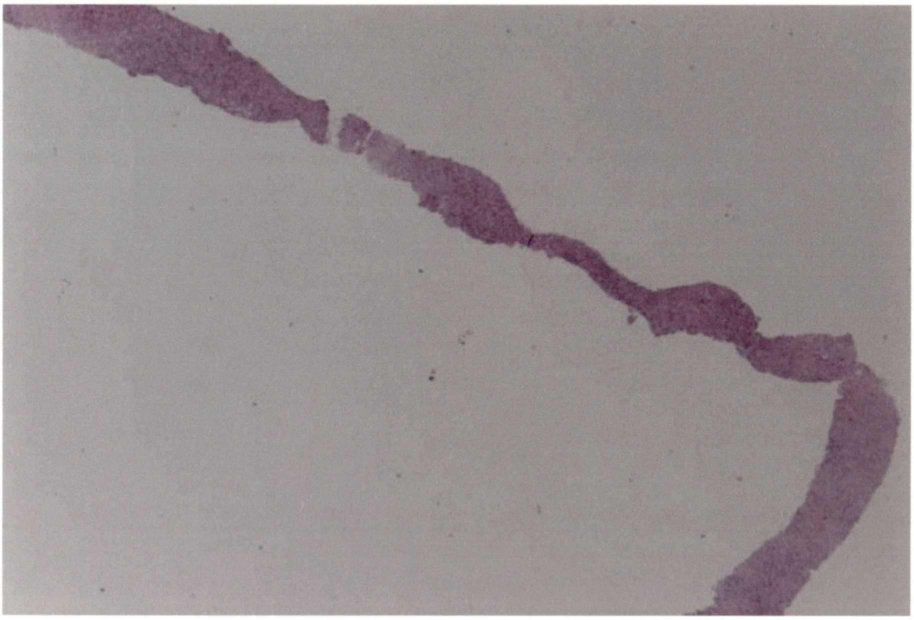

Fig. 5. a. Tissue core biopsy of a pancreatic mass. H&E X 20

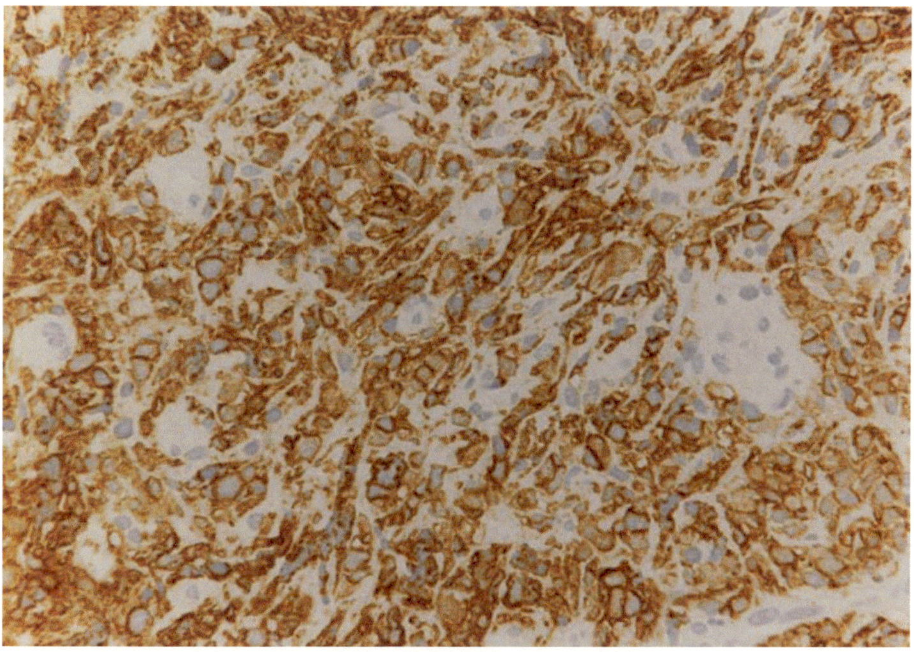

Fig. 5. b. Diffuse large B-cell Lymphoma CD20 positive. X 400

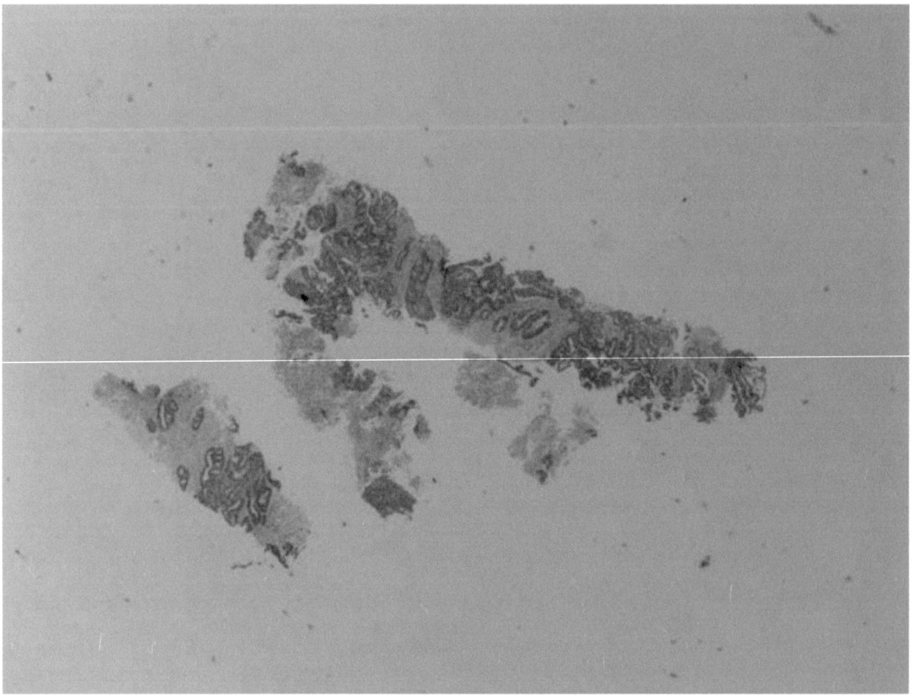

Fig. 6. a. Tissue core biopsy of a pancreatic mass. H&E x 20

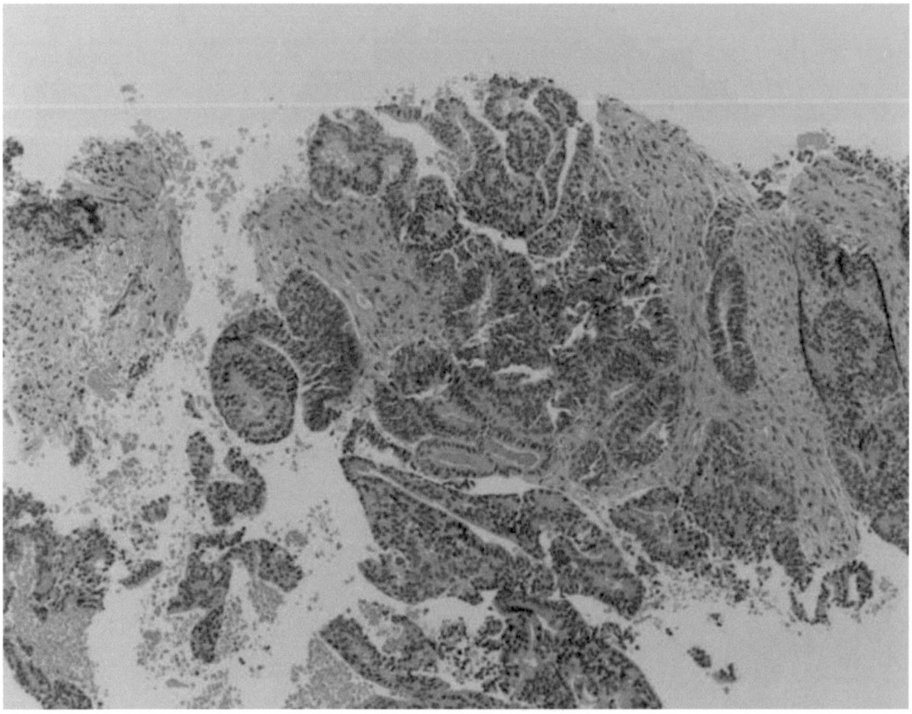

Fig. 6. b. Histology shows metastasis from endometrial adenocarcinoma. H&E X 100

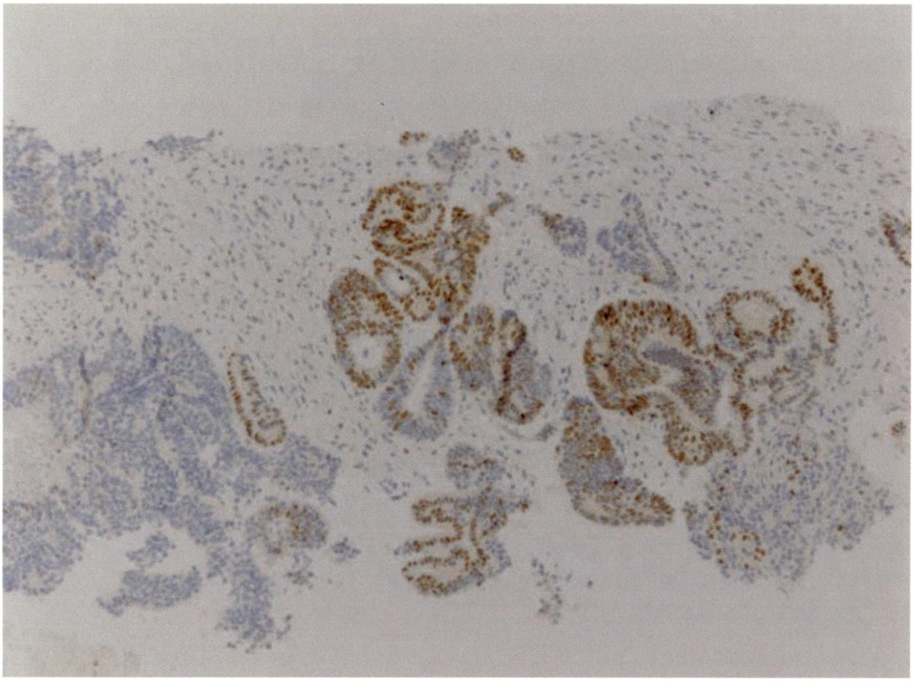

Fig. 6. c. Estrogen receptor positive neoplastic cells. X100

Since it was developed endoscopic ultrasound-guided fine needle aspiration biopsy has been widely used and has been adapted for gastrointestinal and perigastrointestinal lesions.

A medical literature review to evaluate the role of EUS-FNAB for diagnosis of pancreatic masses showed a 78-95% sensitivity, 75-100% specificity, 98-100% positive predictive value and a 78-95% accuracy (Yoshinaga et al, 2011) (Tab 4).

N of patients	Sensitivity %	Specificity %	Accuracy%	Needle size	Authors
583	84	86	84	22-26	Siddiqui et al (2011)
100	78	75	78	22	Touchefeu et al (2009)
182*	78.2-96.2*	98.4	86.2-96.8*	22	Garcia et al (2011)
737	77	99	80	22-25	Turner et al (2010)
207	92.6	88.6	91.8	22	Klimet et al(2010)

* The presence of an on site-cytopathologist was associated with a significantly higher diagnostic sensitivity and overall accuracy for malignancy.

Table 4. Sensitivity, specificity, accuracy needle size of endoscopic-guide pancreatic biopsy

6. Complications of pancreatic biopsy

US, EUS or CT guided fine-needle biopsy are considered to be a low risk procedure.

Interventions with needle with a larger diameter seem cause more complications.

The major complication of pancreatic biopsy can be hemorrhage, needle track seeding and pancreatitis.

Our group (29) reported the complications following 10.766 US-guided fine-needle abdominal biopsies. The mortality was 0.018%: the two reported deaths were due to hemoperitoneum and occurred in patients with hepatocellular carcinoma arizing in cirrotic liver.

The biopsy of pancreatic carcinoma was more dangerous for needle –track seeding (five of eight reported cases), however, it has been reported that peritoneal carcinomatosis may occur more frequently in patients who undergo percutaneous FNAB compared with those who have FUS-FNAB for the diagnosis of pancreatic cancer (Micames et al, 2003).

6.1 Conclusions

There is consensus in the literature of the appropriateness of obtaining a cytohystological diagnosis in patients with unresectable pancreatic neoplastic lesion, prior to initiate chemotherapy and/or radiation.

Although the American Joint Committeee on Cancer has selected EUS-guided FNAB as the procedure of choice, if available, we recall that there is wide variability in the world on the modalities for guide biopsy (US ; CT ; EUS) and for needle biopsy choice (FNAB or tissue core biopsy).

There is a consensus that local expertise, the availability of EUS and interventional percutaneous procedures may determine the choice for pancreatic biopsy.

In agreement with other authors (Zamboni et al., 2010) at our institution , in the appropriate setting, percutaneous US-guided FNAB is considered the first invasive approach of obtaining tissue diagnosis confirmation in patients with unresectable lesions.

However, guided FNAB or guided tissue core biopses remain invasive procedures and must be performed when informations so obtained benefits the patient.

7. Acknowledgments

Authors thanks Michela Monfredo, Gabriele Cremona and MariaRosa Cordani for the important support.

8. References

Adsay NV, Adea A, Basturk O, Kilnc N, Nassar H, Cheng JD. Secondary tumours of the pancreas: An analisys of a surgical and autopsy database and review of the literature. Virchows Arch 2004; 444:527-35.

American Cancer Society. (2002) Facts and figures. Atlanta, GA: American Cancer Society.

Amin Z, Theis B, Russel RC, et al (2006) Diagnosing pancreatic cancer: the role of percutaneous biopsy and Ct. Clin Radiol 61:996-1002

Arcari A, Anselmi E, Bernuzzi P, et al (2005). Primary pancreatic lymphoma. Report of five cases. Haematologica; 90: (3) e23-e26.

Bhatia P, Srinivasan R, Rajwanshi A, et al (2008) 5 Year review and reappraisal of ultrasound-guided percutaneous transabdominal fine needle aspiration of pancreatic lesions. Acta Cytol 52:523-529

Bret PM, Fond A, Bretagnolle M, et al. (1982) Une technique simple de guidage des Ponctions Percutanees Par l'echographie en temps reel. J Radiol ; 63 : 363-365.

Carrara S, Arcidiacono PG, Mezzi G,et al, (2010). Pancreatic Endoscopic Ultrasound-guided Fine Needle Apiration: Complication rate and clinical course in a single centre. Dig Liver Dis; 42:520-3

Chang KJ, Albers CG, Erickson RA, et al (1994). Endoscopic ultrasound-guided fine needle aspiration of pancreatic carcinoma. Am J Gastroenterol ; 89:263-6.

Civardi G, Fornari F, Cavanna L et al. (1988) Value of rapid Staining and Assessment of Ultrasound-guided Fine Needle Aspiration Biopsies. Acta Cytologica 32;4.

Civardi G, Fornari F, Cavanna L, et al (1986). Ultrasonically guided fine needle aspiration biopsy (UG-FNAB): a useful technique for the diagnosis of abdominal malignancies. European Journal of Cancer & Clinical Oncology; 2: 225-227.

Clin Ultrasound 1984; 12: 60-62.

Cohen SJ, Pinover WH, Watson JC et al. (200) Pancreatic cancer. Curr TRat Options Oncol; 1:375-86.

Di Stasi M, Lencioni R, Solmi L, et al (1998) Ultrasound-guided fine needle biopsy of pancreatic masses: results of a multi center study. Am J Gastroenterol 93:1329-1333

Elvin A, Andersson T, Scheibenpflug L, et al (1990) Biopsy of the pancreas with a biopsy gun. Radiology 176.677-679

Erickson RA, EUS-guided FNA. Gastrointest Endosc 2004; 60:267-79.

Fornari F, Civardi G, Cavanna L et al. (1989) Complications of ultrasonically guided fine-needle abdominal biopsy. Results of a multicenter Italian study and review of the literature. The Cooperative Study Group. Scand J Gastroenterol 24(8):949-55

Garcia JI, Larino-Noia J, Abdulkader I et al. Quantitative endoscopic ultrasound elastography: an accurate method for the differentiation of solid pancreatic masses. Gastroenterology 2010; 139:1172-80.

Garcia JI, Dominguez-Munoz E, Abdulkader I et al. (2011) Influence of On-Site Cytopathology Evaluation on the Diagnostic Accuracy of Endoscopic Ultrasound-Guided Fine Needle Aspiration (EUS-FNA) of Solid Pancreatic Masses. Am J Gastroenterol.

Garre Sanchez MC, Rendon Unceta P, Lopez Cano A, et al (2007) Ultrasound-guided biopsy of the pancreas: a multicenter study. Rev Esp Enferm Dig 99:520-524

Gilbert CM, Monaco SE, Cooper ST, Khalbuss WE. (2011) Endoscopic ultrasound-guided fine-needle aspiration of metastases to the pancreas: a sudy of 25 cases. Cyjournal 2011; 8:1

Greene F, Fritz A, Balch C et al. (2002) Exocrine pancreas. Cancer Staging Handbook. American Joint Committee on Cancer. New York: Springer.

Hartwig W, Schneider L, Diener MK, et al (2009) Preoperative tissue diagnosis for tumours of the pancreas. Br J Surg (96(1): 5-20.

Hernandez LV, Bhutani MS, Eisner M et al. (2009) Non-surgical tissue biopsy among patients with advanced pancreatic cancer: effect on survival. Pancreas 38(3):289-292

Horwhat JD, Paulson EK, McGrath K, et al. (2006)A randomized comparison of EUS-guided FNA versus CT or US-guided FNA for the evaluation of pancreatic mass lesions. Gastrointest Endosc; 63: 966-975.

Ingram DM, Sheiner HJ, Shilkin KB. (1978) Operative biopsy of the pancreas using the Trucut needle. Aust N Z J Surg; 48: 203-206

Itani KM, Taylor TV, Green LK. Needle biopsyfor suspicious lesions of the head of the pancreas: pitfalls and implications for therapy. J Gastrointest Surg 1997; 1: 337-341

Jennings PE, Donald JJ, Coral A, et al (1989) Ultrasound -guided core biopsy. Lancet 1:1369-1371

Karlson BM, Forsman CA, Wilander E, et al (1996) Efficiency of percutaneous core biopsy in pancreatic tumor diagnosis. Surgery 120: 75-79

Klimet M, Urban O, CEgan M et al, (2010) Endoscopic ultrasound-guided fine-needle aspiration of pancreatic masses: the utility and impact of management of patients. Scandinavian Journal of Gatroenter; 45: 1372-1379

Levy MJ. (2006)Know when to biopsy 'em, know when to walk away. Gastrointest Endosc; 63: 630-634.

Livraghi T. (1984) A simple no-cost technique for real-time biopsy. J Clin Utrasound; 12 (1): 60 - 62.

Mallery JS, Centeno BA, Hahn PF, et al (2002) Pancreatic tissue sampling guided by EUS, CT/US, and surgery: a comparison of sensitivity and specificity. Gastrointest Endosc 56: 218-224

Matsubara J, Okusaka T, Morizane C, et al (2008) Ultrasound-guided percutaneous pancreatic tumor biopsy in pancreatic cancer: a comparison with metastatic liver tumor biopsy, including sensitivity, specificity, and comlications. J Gastroenterol 43: 225-232

Micames C, Jowell PS, White R, et al (2003) Lower frequency of peritoneal carcinomatosis in patients with pancreatic cancer diagnosed by EUS-guided FNA vs percutaneous FNA. Gastrointest Endosc 58: 5

Moossa AR, Altorki N. (1983) Pancreatic biopsy. Surg Clin North Am; 63: 1205-1214.

Paulsen SD, Nghiem HV, Negussie E, et al (2006) Evaluation of imaging-guided core bipsy of pancreatic masses. AJR Am J Roentgenol 187:769-772

Siddiqui AA, Brown JL, Hong SSK, et al (2011) Relashionship of pancreatic mass size and diagnostic yield of endoscopic ultrasound-guided fine needle aspiration. Dig Dis Sci; DOI 10. 1007s 10620-011-1782-z

Sohn TA, Yeo CJ, Cameron JL, et al. (2000) Resected adenocarcinoma of the pancreas -616 patients: results, outcomes, and prognostic indicators. J Gastrointest Surg; 4: 576.

Surveillance, Epidemiology, and End Results (SEER)Program (www.seer.cancer.gov) , National Cancer Institute, DCCPS, Surveillance Research Program, Cancer Statistics Branch, released April 2008, based on the November 2007 submission

Tamm E, Charnsangavej C. (2001) Pancreatic cancer: current concepts in imaging for diagnosis and staging. CancerJ; 7: 298-311.

Tillou A, Schwartz MR, Jordan PH Jr. (1996) Percutaneous needle biopsy of the pancreas: when should it be performed? World J Surg; 20: 283-286, discussion 287

Touchefeu Y, Le Rhun M, Coron E, et al (2009) Endoscopic ultrasound-guided fine-needle aspiration for the diagnosis of solid pancreatic masses: the impact of patient-management strategy. Alimentary Pharmacology and Therapeutics 30: 1070-1077

Turner BG, Cizginer S, Agarwal D, (2010) Diagnosis of pancreatic neoplasia with EUS and FNA: a report of accuracy. Gastrointestinal endoscopy; 71: 1.

Varadarajulu S, Wallace MB. (2004) Applications of endoscopic ultrasonography in pancreatic cancer. Cancer Control; 11:15-22.

Volmar K, Vollmer R, Jowell P; et al (2005) Pancreatic FNA in 1000 cases: a comparison of imaging madalities. Gastrointest Endosc 61:854-861

Yeo TP, Hruban RH, Leach SD et al (2002) Pancreatic Cancer. Curr Probl Cancer; 26: 176

Yoshinaga S, Suzuki H, Oda I, et al (2011) Role of endoscopic ultrasound-guided fine needle aspiration (EUS-FNA) for diagnosis of solid pancreatic masses. Dig Endosc 1:29-33

Zamboni GA, D'Onofrio M, Principe F, et al. (2010) Focal pancreatic lesions: accuracy and compliactions of US-guided fine-needle aspiration cytology. Abdom Imaging; 35: 362-366

15

Coagulation Disorders in Pancreatic Cancer

A. Albu, D. Gheban, C. Grad and D.L. Dumitrascu
University of Medicine and Pharmacy "Iuliu Hatieganu", Cluj-Napoca, Romania

1. Introduction

The association between cancers and thrombosis is well known for a long period of time. In 1865 Armand Trousseau noted for the first time that unexpected or migratory thrombophlebitis could be a sign of an undiagnosed visceral malignancy (Trousseau, 1865). Some years later it is said that he observed this complication on himself in the context of an occult gastric cancer that cased his death (Khorana, 2003).

The risk of developing thrombosis in cancer patients is considered to be increased 2- 7 fold compared with persons without cancer (Bloom et al, 2005; Heit et al, 2004). This risk is dependent on many factors. According to the type of tumor, the risk is thought to be the highest in tumors of the ovary, pancreas and central nervous system. Also the extent of the tumor, the presence of metastasis, age, immobility and the type of therapy increase this risk. Surgery for cancers (Rahr & Sørensen, 1992) and chemotherapy (Levine, 1997) are both associated with an important risk of venous thrombosis and embolism. In a large case-control study that included 3220 patients with cancer, it was reported an overall 7 times increased risk for venous thrombosis that depend on type of cancer and time since the cancer diagnosis. A very high relative risk was found for gastrointestinal, lung and hematological malignancies. Advanced stage of disease was associated with a further increase in risk (Blom et al, 2005).

Patients with cancer who develop venous thromboembolism have a poor prognosis than those without this vascular complication. The risk of recurrent thromboembolism and death from any cause is greater than three fold in patients with cancer compared to those without malignancy (Levitan et al, 1999).

Epidemiological studies looking for the incidence of cancer in patients with thromboembolic events found out that in 15-20% of patients, thromboses were associated with malignancy (Er & Zacharsky, 2006).

The association of cancer and thrombosis raises two distinct problems. On one hand, the diagnosis of thrombosis in one patient may represent, in some situations, a sign of an occult malignancy. On the other hand, a patient with cancer may develop some time, in the evolution of his malignant disease, a thromboembolic event, which may worsen his prognostic. That is why, for the clinical practice, the diagnosis of these associated diseases is very important.

2. Epidemiology of thrombosis in pancreatic cancer

Pancreatic cancer (PC) is known to be associated with a higher incidence of venous thromboembolism than other cancers. The first publication that noted the high incidence of thrombosis in PC was a postmortem study done in 1938 (Sproul, 1938). Since that, several other studies have been conducted and the incidence found ranges from 5% to 60% (Sack et al, 1977; Khorana & Fine, 2005).

In a cohort study of 202 patients with a first diagnosis of pancreas carcinoma the authors found that the risk of venous thrombosis is 6-fold increased compared with the general population, at a cumulative risk of 10% (Blom et al, 2006). In this study, tumors of the corpus and cauda of the pancreas had a 2-3-fold increase risk of venous thrombosis than tumors of the caput of the pancreas (Blom et al, 2006). Similar results showing a higher incidence of thrombotic events for tumors located in the corpus and cauda of the pancreas were reported by other authors (Sproul, 1938; Sack et al, 1977; Bick, 1992; Pinzon et al, 1986).

In a retrospective single institute study 6,870 patients with pancreatic cancer were evaluated for venous and arterial thrombosis. The incidence of all thrombotic events was 19%with venous thrombosis accounting for 17%, arterial thrombotic events for 2% and associated venous and arterial events in 0.9% of cases. Pulmonary embolism was found in 25% of patients with venous thrombosis (Epstein et al, 2010)

The risk of venous thrombosis increases in the presence of metastases. Blom and colab. found a 2-fold increase risk of venous thrombosis in patients with distant metastases, after adjusting for age, sex, surgery and chemo- or radiotherapy (Blom et al, 2006).

The risk of developing thrombosis is further increased with chemotherapy (Heit, 2002; Wall, 1989) and also with surgical treatment. Patients with PC treated with chemotherapy had a 4.8-fold increased risk of thrombosis compared to those without chemotherapy. The same study showed no significant increase in thrombotic risk patients treated with radiotherapy (Blom et al, 2006).

Patients with malignancies submitted to surgery have at least twice the risk of postoperative venous thrombosis and more than 3 times the risk of fatal PE compared with non-cancer patients undergoing a similar procedure (Geerts et al, 2004).

In patients with PC submitted to surgery there was a 4.5-folf increase in the risk of venous thrombosis during the postoperative period of 30 days (Blom et al, 2006).

The incidence of fatal pulmonary embolism was also evaluated. In one study 4 out of 541 (0.7%) died from pulmonary embolism (Neoptolemos et al, 2001). Concordant results were reported in another study that found 2 of 202 patients (1%) with fatal pulmonary embolism (Blom et al, 2006).

3. Pathogenesis of thrombosis in pancreatic cancer

The mechanisms underlying the association of venous thromboembolism with pancreatic cancer are not completely understood. Large and relevant data suggest an implication of coagulation systems and increased angiogenesis. It is considered that activation of hemostasis in pancreatic cancer causes thrombosis but also tumor angiogenesis (Browder et al, 2000).

The key molecule in this process seems to be ***tissue factor*** (TF), the main physiologic initiator of the extrinsic pathway of coagulation (Gouaulthelimann & Josso, 1979; Nemerson, 1988). TF plays also an important role in angiogenesis (Mechtcheriakova et al, 1999; Zhang et al, 1994).

TF, also called platelet tissue factor, factor III, or CD142 is a protein present in subendothelial tissue, platelets, and leukocytes. TF consists of three domains: extracellular that binds factor VIIa, transmembrane and intracellular involved in the signaling function (Nemerson, 1988). In healthy individuals there are little circulating amounts of active TF. In response to specific stimuli such as inflammation, malignant processes, its expression increases (Ruf et al, 2000; Wada et al, 1995).

As an initiator of coagulation, TF binds and activates factor VIIa, resulting in TF-VIIa complex which activates factor X leading to the synthesis of thrombin essential in clot formation (Gilbert & Arena, 1995). The activity of TF is regulated by several factors. The most important is TF pathway inhibitor which is composed of three different domains: the first inhibits FVII, the second inhibits FX and the function of the last one is still unknown (Broze, 1995; Girard et al, 1989; Echrish et al, 2011). TF pathway inhibitor is secreted by endothelial cells.

The expression of TF can be controlled by epidermal growth factor receptor (Milsom et al, 2008) and by FX activated. Increased concentrations of FX activated inhibit the synthesis of TF (Ettelaie et al, 2007).

In cancers, TF is present on malignant cells and also on endothelial cells (Rickles et al, 2003). Some previous data indicate that TF is expressed in pancreatic malignant cells. It correlated with advanced histological stages and with a poor prognosis (Kakkar et al, 1995; Nitori et al, 2005). In a retrospective study, Khorana and colab. investigated the expression of TF in non invasive and invasive pancreatic cancers. They found an increased expression of TF in 77% of patients with pancreatic intraepithelial neoplasia and in 91% of patients with intraductal papillary mucinous neoplasms, two non invasive precursors of invasive pancreatic cancer. They concluded that TF expression is an early event in pancreatic cancer. In patients with pancreas resection, TF expression correlated with expression of vascular endothelial growth factor (VEGF) and increased neovascularization, suggesting an implication of TF in angiogenesis. They found an incidence of thromboembolism of 26.3% in patients with high TF expression levels compared to 4.5% in those with low expression of TF, suggesting an important role of TF in cancer associated thrombotic complications. (Khorana et al, 2007).

Angiogenesis has been documented in pancreatic cancer and it was associated with a rapid tumor growth and a poor prognosis (Lomberk, 2010).

The process of angiogenesis represents the formation of new blood vessels from the pre-existing vascular bed. In cancers angiogenesis contributes to tumor growth (Folkman, 1995).

Pancreatic cancer seems to be accompanied by an important increase in angiogenesis that is linked to the activation of coagulation. Proteins of coagulation are involved in angiogenesis in two different ways, one clotting dependent and the other one clotting independent (Echrish et al, 2011). The clotting dependent mechanism is initiated by the activation of TF receptors. TF activates then the coagulation cascade that leading to fibrin formation and platelet activation (Falanga & Rickles, 1999). Activated platelets release mediators that promote angiogenesis such as VEGF, beta fibroblast growth factor (β-FGF) and platelet grows factor (PGF) (Palumbo et al, 2000; Echrish et al, 2011). In clotting independent mechanism thrombin plays a very important role by inducing the proteolytic cleavage of protease-activated receptors (PAR) (Traynelis & Trejo, 2007). The activation of PAR stimulates the synthesis of factors implicated in angiogenesis such as VEGF (Liu & Mueller, 2006).

Another mediator that involved in thrombosis and angiogenesis of pancreatic cancer is epithelial growth factor receptor (EGFR). An increased expression EGFR was noted in pancreatic cancer and correlated with enhanced angiogenesis, tumor growth and unfavorable evolution (Yamanaka et al, 1993).

Microparticles have also been studied in relation with thromboembolism in cancer. Microparticles are membrane vesicles released from stimulated or apoptotic cells in normal persons but they are also implicated in the activation of coagulation (Diamant et al, 2004).

Many recent data support the role of microparticles (MP) and of TF-MP complex in thrombotic complications of patients with malignancies (Tilley et al, 2008).

The level of TF activity associated with TF/MP seems to be higher in PC compared with other types of cancer. From the group of patients with cancer and thrombosis those with pancreatic malignancies have the highest TF activity (Tesselaar et al, 2009).

The role of ***P-selectin*** in thrombosis in these patients was also studied during the last two decades. P-selectin is released from platelets and endothelial cells and contributes to the adhesion of leucocytes on activated platelets and thrombus formation and to adhesion of cancer cells to stimulated endothelial cells. Experimental studies that have been done on primates suggest that P-selectin inhibition is as effective as low molecular weight heparin in promoting thrombus resolution and in preventing re-occlusion (Chen & Geng, 2006). In humans elevated levels of P-selectin may be predictive of thromboembolism in patients with cancers (Ay et al, 2008).

A large case-control study of venous thrombosis in patients with cancer found that the presence of factor V Leiden or prothrombin 20210A mutation increases by 12 to 17-fold the risk of developing thrombosis compared to those with out these modifications (Blom et al,2005).

Activation of endothelium by tumor-derived inflammatory cytokines, which could induce expression of various adhesive molecules such as V-CAM and E-selectin may promote the thrombotic process in cancer patients (Varki, 2007).

Thromboembolic events in PC patients are also influenced by particular conditions that generally increase the risk of thrombosis such as immobilization, advanced age, comorbidities (infections, cardiac or respiratory failure, obesity, etc.), history of venous thrombosis (Offord et al, 2004; Echrish et al, 2011). Also, the local effects of a great tumour, such as venous compression, that can predispose to an increased risk of thromboembolism (Dumitrascu et al, 2010) .

Central vein catheterization used for the administration of cancer therapy represents a risk factor for thrombosis in these patients. Patients with distant metastases have more increased risk for thrombosis in absence of antithrombotic prophylaxis. The incidence of clinically overt venous thrombosis in cancer patients with central venous catheter ranges from 0.3% to 28%, and rises to 27% - 66% when the diagnosis was assessed by venography (Verso & Agnelli, 2003; Verso et al, 2008).

Chemotherapy has been shown to be an independent risk factor for thrombosis in cancer patients. In a large population based study, the risk of thrombosis was increased 6.5 fold in patients receiving chemotherapy and 4,1 fold in patients with cancer not receiving this kind of therapy, compared to patients without malignancies (Heit et al, 2000, Kirwan et al, 2011). The risk is additionally increased if chemotherapy is combined with steroids (Shen et al, 2011) or erythropoietin (Bennet et al, 2008). The inhibitors of angiogenesis (thalidomide, lenalidomide, bevacizumab, sunitinib, sorafenib, and sirolimus) used as novel antineoplasic therapy are associated with an increase in arterial and venous thromboembolism and hemorrhage (Zangari et al, 2009). Gemcitabine is a deoxycytidine analogue related to cytarabine, that has been shown to improve evolution in patients with advanced PC. Deep venous thrombosis was found in one study in 3.2% of patients treated with gemcitabine (Kaye,1994).

4. Clinical outcome in pancreatic cancer patients with thrombosis

Patients with PC may present with signs of venous or arterial thrombosis. Venous thrombosis is more frequent and it can affect peripheral or visceral veins (Blom et al, 2006). Migratory superficial thrombophlebitis is highly suggestive for a malignancy (Fig. 1). Of the visceral vein thrombosis portal thrombosis has a very high incidence. In one study portal vein thrombosis was found in 32 of 108 patients (30%) and it was associated with a poor prognosis (Price et al, 2010). Perpancreatic veins may also be involved (Fig.2).

The diagnosis is suggested by clinical signs and is usually confirmed ultrasonographically (Fig. 3 and 4).

Disseminated intravascular coagulation is another coagulation disturbance described in PC. It was associated with an increase in circulating TF (Ueda, 2001). This complication was also observed in patients suffering from metastatic pancreatic cancer treated with a recombinant adenoviral vector containing the cloned human wild type p53 suppressor gene (Haag, 2000).

It is generally reported that patients with cancer and thrombotic complications have a poor prognosis (Levitan et al, 1999; Sorensen et al, 2000). In the retrospective study by Epstein and colab., 24% of patients with PC and thromboembolism, experienced pulmonary embolism. The authors found a reduced overall survival for patients with a thromboembolic event (12.9 month) if compared to those without (13.4 month). Treatment consisted of low molecular weight heparin, in 95% of patients and inferior vena cava filter was necessary in 19%. Patients with occult thrombotic events or with thrombosis diagnosed at the time of cancer diagnosis, had a poorer survival (6.2 month) compared with those with secondary thrombotic events (13.7 month) (Epstein et al, 2010; Shah& Saif, 2010).

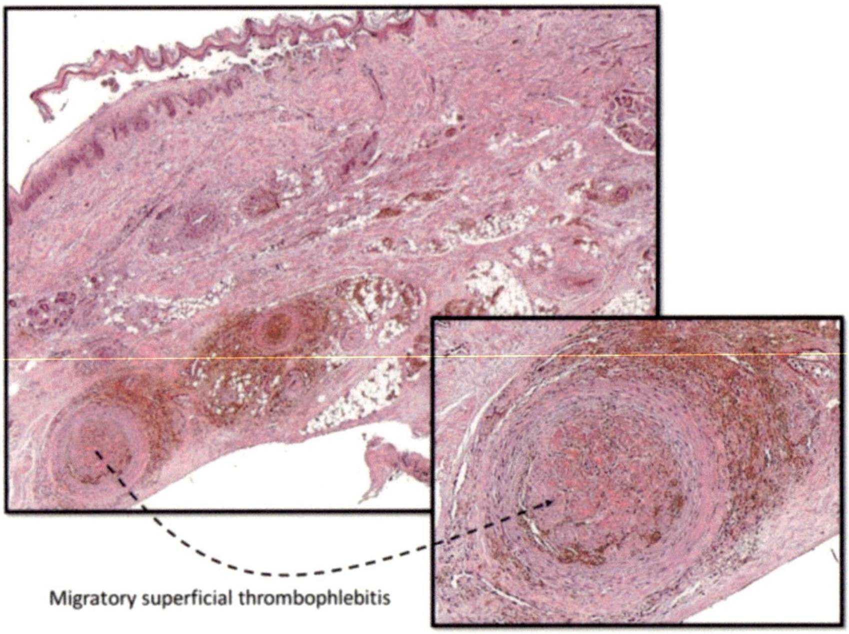

Fig. 1. Migratory superficial thrombophlebitis in a case of PC (hematoxylin-eosin staining of superficial veins)

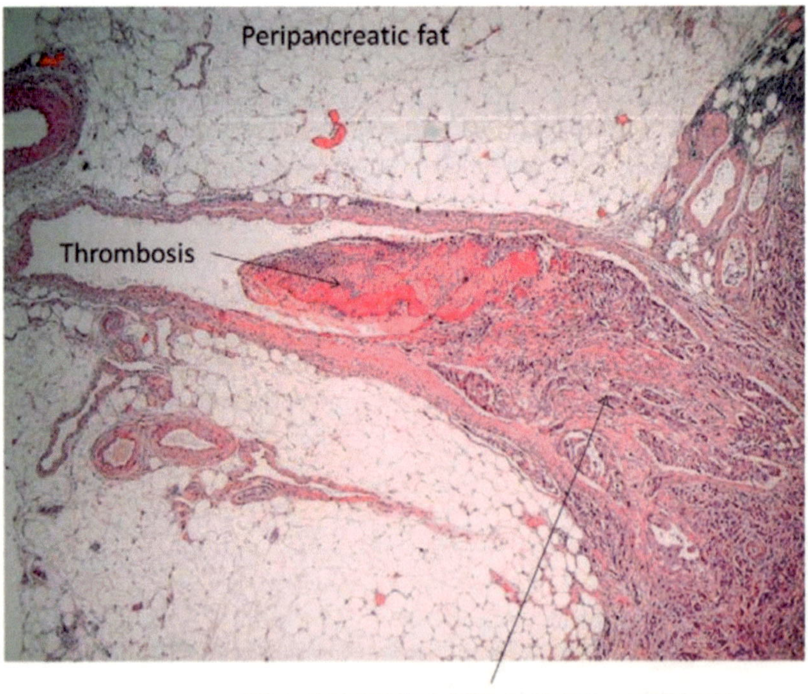

Fig. 2. Vascular invasion of PC with local vein thrombosis (hematoxylin-eosin staining)

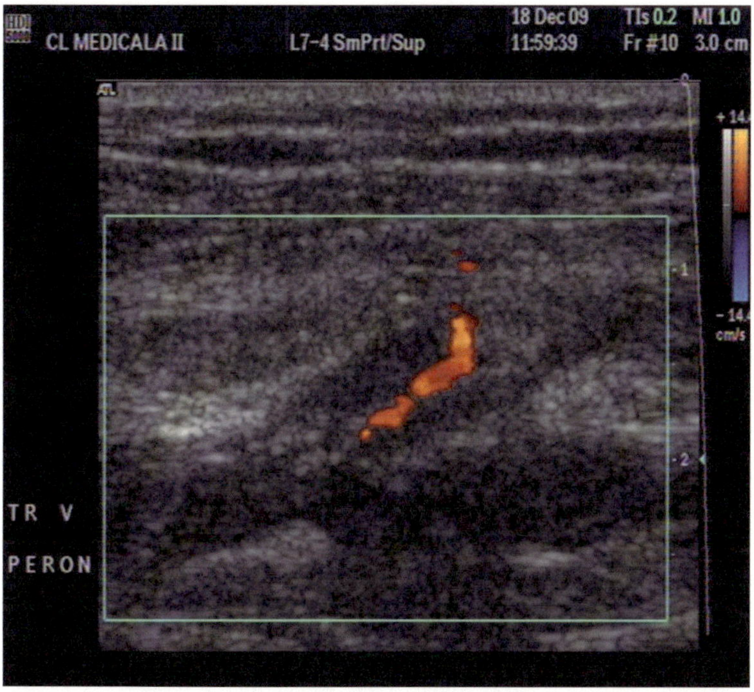

Fig. 3. Thrombosis of peroneal vein in a patient with PC (2D and colour Doppler echographic examination)

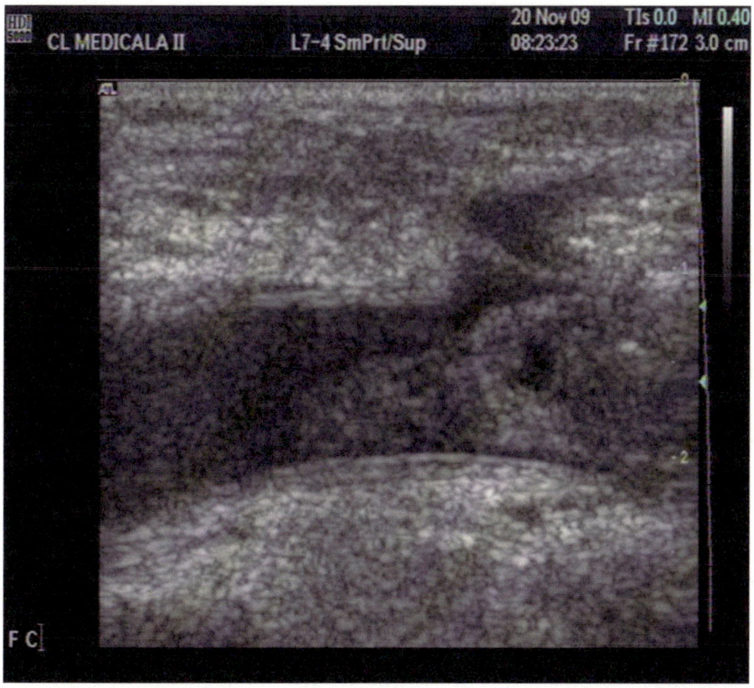

Fig. 4. Thombosis of femoral vein in a patient with PC (2D echographic examination)

Looking for possible predictors of thromboembolism in pancreatic cancer, one previous study showed that higher levels of TF expression in tumor cells were associated with nearly 4 fold increase in venous thrombosis (Khorana et al, 2007). In a recent retrospective study that included patients diagnosed with pancreaticobiliary cancers between January 2005 and December 2008, looked for the association of TF with thromboembolism and survival. This study included 117 patients with a median age of 65 years of which 68% had pancreatic cancer and 29% biliary cancers. Thrombotic complications were found in 52 (44.4%) patients. Elevated levels of TF (greater than 2.5pg/ml) were associated with thromboembolic events (odds ratio=1.22;p=0.04). Also, TF levels were predictive for a worse overall survival (hazard ratio=1.05; p=0.01) (Barthuar et al, 2010). These results if confirmed in prospective studies suggest that TF expressed by neoplastic cells or plasma levels of TF could be used as independent predictive biomarkers for thromboembolic events in PC patients and also in other cancers (Khorana et al,2007; Barthuar et al, 2010).

5. Prevention and treatment of thromboembolism in PC

5.1 Prophylaxis of venous trombosis

Epidemiologic and pathogenic data clearly indicate that patients with malignancy had an important risk of thormboembolic events. In practice, risk stratification can be used to classify patients according to their thrombotic risk. The ACCP guidelines consider the patient with cancer in the very high risk category particularly when surgery is recommended. Other factors that may increase patient's risk are age, immobilization, prior history of venous thrombosis, obesity and central venous catheter (Geerts et al, 2004; Caprini et al, 2001).

Prophylaxis in cancer is indicated mainly in two distinct situations: in patients undergoing surgery and in medical patients receiving chemotherapy.

Patients undergoing abdominal surgery are a particularly high-risk population who may benefit for extended thromboprophylaxis. Low molecular weight heparins are preferred as they showed to be as effective and safe as unfractionated heparin. Several studies showed a reduction in thromboembolic complications in patients receiving prolonged prophylaxis for 3 or 4 weeks compared to those with 1 week of treatment in postoperative period. This beneficial effect was not accompaneied by an increase in hemorrhagic complications (Bergqvist et al, 2002; Rasmussen et al, 2003).

In patients treated with chemotherapy antithrombotic prophylaxis showed also a reduction in thromboembolic risk. There are 2 trials in patients with PC treated with gemcitabine and a low molecular weight heparin and another one in wich a low molecular weight heparin was associated to a combined chemotherapy gemcitabine and cisplatinum.

The results of the Charité Onkologie (CONKO)-004 trial were recently published. The principal objective of this trail was the evaluation of the reduction in symptomatic thromboembolic events in patients with advanced PC. The second end point was the overall survival. Between April 2004 and January 2009, 312 patients with histological confirmed advanced PC were randomized into two groups as follows: 160 patients received treatment with enoxaparin 1 mg/kg once a day for 3 month, followed by 40 mg daily and 152 did not receive antithrombotic prophylaxis. The results indicated a significant reduction of symptomatic thromboembolism in treated patients after 3 month (1.25% compared to 9.87% in non treated patients). This significant difference was also found after 12 months with an incidence of 5% in treated patients compared to 15.13% in non treated arm of the trial. There were no significant major hemorrhagic complications in both groups. The median overall survival was not different between the two groups (9.92 month in treated patients versus 8.15 month in no treatment group; p=0.054), for a median follow up period of 45.44 months (Reiss et al, 2010).

In the FRAGEM (Chemotherapy With or Without Dalteparin) trial, 123 patients were randomised to receive dalteparin. This study showed also a significant reduction in thromboembolic events in patients receiving prophylaxis (Maraveyas et al, 2007).

The third trial aimed to assess the effects of the addition of low molecular weight heparin (nadoparin) to gemcitabine plus cisplatinum combination in 42 patients with advanced PC. The results showed a better mean time to progression in the group receiving prophylaxis (6.0+/-0.9 months) when compared to control group (3.0+/-1.5 months) (p=0.0001). Also median overall survival time for the nadoparin group was 9.0+/-1.9 months compared to 4.0+/-0.4 months (p=0.0034) in the control group (Icli et al, 2007).

The results of these trials showed that the association of a low molecular weight heparin to chemotherapy in advanced pancreatic cancer patients reduces the risk of thromboembolic events. However, the CONKO-004 did not found any improvement in the overall survival and time to progression. This needs to be verified in future prospective trials.

In patients with central vein catheter used commonly for the administration of chemotherapeutic agents and parenteral nutrition, anticoagulation is not recommended for routine prophylaxis of catheter related thrombosis in cancer patients (Geerts et al, 2004). Even if early studies showed risk of venous thrombosis related to central vein catheters (Montreal et al, 1996), a large multinational trial that investigated the efficacy of dalteparin in preventing catheter related thrombosis, found that the risk of thrombosis was not significantly different in the group treated with dalteparin compared to placebo-treated patients (Karthaus et al, 2006). Prophylaxis in patients with central vein catheters may be imposed sometimes when additional risk factors are detected.

5.2 Treatment of venous thrombosis

Treatment of venous thombotic complications in patients with cancer is usually difficult due to the risk of recurrences and at the same time of bleeding with severe consequences. The aims of treatment are reduction of clinical manifestations of thrombosis and of the risks pulmonary embolism and postthrombotic syndrome.

The treatment of choice is the administration of a low molecular weight heparin for one week followed by an oral anticoagulant (vitamin K antagonist). Low molecular weight heparins have been shown to be as effective and save as unfractionated heparin. They are preferred like first line treatment because usually no laboratory monitoring is necessary, and the risks of developing heparin induced thrombocytopenia and osteoporosis is reduced. Also the administration of this type of heparin is convenient using once or twice daily doses as subcutaneous injection (Dolovich et al, 2000; van den Belt et al, 2000, Er &Zacharski, 2006).

Recurrent thrombosis needs long-term management. In cancer patients prolonged anti thrombotic, particularly with oral antivitamin K medication, is associated with increased risk of hemorrhagic complications that may be linked to malnutrition, liver dysfunction and metastases, reduced alimentary intake or vomiting. The risk of bleeding appears to correlate with the extent of the disease. In a study that investigated the risk of bleeding in patients with different extent of the disease, patients with moderately extensive cancer had a 2-3-fold increase in risk of major bleeding; patients with extensive cancer had a 5-fold increase in this risk (Prandoni et al, 2002).

Low molecular weight heparins are now preferred as long term secondary prevention treatment in these patients. This indication is based on the results of several randomized trials that showed a superior efficacy and safety of low molecular weight heparins compared with oral anticoagulants in long term administration. In a multicenter randomized trial patients were treated for 3 month with enoxaparin or with warfarin. Of the group receiving warfarin 15 (21%) of 71 patients had a major bleeding or a thrombotic recurrence, compared to 7 (10.5%) of 67 patients treated with enoxaparin (Meyer et al, 2002). A large multicenter trail, „The Randomized Comparison of Low-Molecular-Weight Heparin versus Oral Anticoagulant Therapy for the Prevention of Recurrent Venous Thromboembolism in Patients with Cancer (CLOT) compared treatment with dalteparin with oral anticoagulant therapy. After 6 months of treatment the probability of recurrent venous thrombosis was 17% in patients receiving oral anticoagulation compared to 9% in those treated with dalteparin. There were no significant differences between groups for the hemorrhagic complications (Lee et al, 2003).

5.3 Antineoplastic effects of anticoagulants

There are evidences that anticoagulant therapy may have also anticancer effects. Heparins in addition to activation of antithrombin, may promote the release of the tissue factor pathway inhibitor from the endothelium that blocks tissue factor expressed by tumor cells (Alban, 2001; Sandset et al, 2001). Heparin is also able to bind to and to inhibit some inflammatory cytokines that can activate endothelial cells and increase expression of adhesion molecules (Elsayed & Becker, 2003; Varki ,2007). Heparin may interfere with formation of the platelet "cloak" around tumor cells suggesting a possible effect in metastasis prevention (Borsig et al, 2001).

Several clinical studies support the efficacy of heparins in improuving tumor response and survival. The administration of nadroparin in patients with advanced solid cancers increased median survival to 8 month compared to 6.6 months in patients receiving placebo, after 6 weeks of treatment (Klerk et al, 2005). Dalteparin associated in the treatemnt of patients with small cell lung cancer, for 18 weeks improved tumor response and median overall survival from 8 to 13 months (Altinbas et al, 2004).

Beneficial effects have also been reported for warfarin in cancer patients. A prospective randomized trial showed that survival of patients with small-cell lung carcinoma had a significant prolonged survival if warfarin was added to standard therapy. The median survival and the time to first evidence of disease progression were increased in patients receiving warfarin (Zacharski et al, 1981).

Data suggesting the participation of coagulation mechanisms in tumour growth are important arguments for researchers to explore this novel therapeutic strategy in cancer patients.

6. Conclusions

Pancreatic cancer is associated with a very increased risk of thromboembolic events. The mechanisms underlying this association are complex and multifactorial but are not yet clearly understood. Thromboembolic complications in patients with PC indicate a poor prognosis and a reduction of life expectancy. Antithrombotic prophylaxis in advanced PC treated with chemotherapy reduces the risk of embolic complications and it may also improve survival and time to progression of cancer in these patients. The medication of choice in preventing and treating thrombosis are low molecular weight heparins. Anticoagulant therapy may help cancer patients due also to a possible antitumor effect.

7. Acknowledgements

This work was partly funded by the research grant INFORAD of the Romanian Ministry of Education and Research.

8. References

Alban, S. (2001). Molecular weight-dependent influence of heparin on the form of tissue factor pathway inhibitor circulating in plasma. *Semin Thromb Hemost*. Vol.27, pp. 503-511. ISSN 0094-6176.

Altinbas, M.; Coskun, H.S.; Er, O.; Ozkan, M.; Eser, B.; Unal, A., et al. (2004). A randomized clinical trial of combination chemotherapy with and without low-molecular-weight heparin in small cell lung cancer. *J Thromb Haemost,* vol.2, pp. 1266-1271, ISSN 1538-7933.

Ay, C.; Simonek, R.; Vormittag, R., et al. (2008). High plasma levels of soluble P-selectin are predictive of venous thromboembolism in cancer patients. Results from the Vienna cancer and thrombosis study. *Blood,* vol. 112, no.7, pp. 2703-2708, ISSN 0268-960X.

Barthuar, A.; Khorana, A.A.; Hutson, A., et al (2010). Association of elevated tissue factor (TF) with survival and thromboembolism (TE) in pancreaticobiliary cancers (PBC). *J Clin Oncol,* vol. 28 (15 suppl),pp. 4062, ISSN 2218-4333.

Bennett, C.L.; Silver, S.M.; Djulbegovic, B. et al. (2008) . Venous thromboembolism and mortality associated with recombinant erythropoietin and darbepoetin administration for the treatment of cancer-associated anemia. *JAMA,* vol. *299,* pp. 914-924, ISSN 00987484.

Bergqvist, D.; Agneli, G.; Cohen A., et al. (2002). Duration of prophylaxis against venous thromboembolism with enoxaparin after surgery for cancer. *N Engl J Med* vol. 346, pp. 975-980, ISSN 0028-4793.

Bick, R.L. (1992). Coagulation abnormalities in malignancy; a review. *Semin Thromb Hemost,* vol.18, no.4, pp.353-372, ISSN 0094-6176.

Blom, J.W.; Doggen, C.J.M.; Osanto, S. & Rosendaal, F.R. (2005) Malignancies, prothrombotic mutations, and the risk of venous thrombosis. *JAMA,* vol. *293,* pp. 715-722, ISSN 00987484.

Blom, J.W.; Osanto, S. & Rosendaal, F.R. (2006). High risk of venous thrombosis in patients with pancreatic cancer: A cohort study of 202 patients. *Eur J Cancer,* vol.42, pp. 410-414, ISSN 1359-6349.

Borsig, L.; Wong, R.; Feramisco, J.; Nadeau, D.R.; Varki, N.M. & Varki, A. (2001). Heparin and cancer revisited: mechanistic connections involving platelets, P-selectin, carcinoma mucins, and tumor metastasis. *Proc Natl Acad Sci USA*, vol. 98, pp. 3352-3357, ISSN 0027-8424.

Browder, T.; Folkmen, J. & Pirie-Shepherd, S. (2000). The hemostatic system as a regulator of angiogenesis. *J Biol Chem*; vol. 275, pp.1521-1524, ISSN 0021-9258.

Broze, G.J.(1995). Tissue factor pathway inhibitor and the revised theory of coagulation. *Annu. Rev.Med.*, vol. *46*, pp. 103-112, ISSN 0066-4219.

Caprini, J.A.; Arcelus, J.I. & Reyna, J.J. (2001). Effective risk stratification of surgical and nonsurgical patients for venous thromboembolic disease. *Semin Hematol*, vol. 38(2Suppl 5), pp. 12-19, ISSN 0037-1963.

Chen, M. & Geng, J.G. (2006). P-selectin mediates adhesion of leukocytes, platelets, and cancer cells in inflammation, thrombosis, and cancer growth and metastasis. *Arch Immunol Ther Exp* (Warsz). Vol. 54, pp. 75-84, ISSN 0004-069X.

Diamant, M.; Tushuizen, M.E.; Sturk, A. & Nieuwland R. (2004). Cellular microparticles: new players in the field of vascular disease? *Eur J Clin Invest*, vol. 34, pp. 392–401, ISSN 0014-2972.

Dolovich, L.R.; Ginsberg, J.S.; Douketis, J.D., et al. (2000). A meta-analysiscomparing low-molecular-weight heparins with unfractionated heparin in the treatment of venous thromboembolism:examining some unanswered questions regarding location of treatment, product type, and dosing frequency. *Arch Intern Med*,vol. 160, pp.181-188, ISSN 0003-9926.

Dumitrascu, D.L.; Suciu, O.; Grad, C. & Gheban, D. (2010). Thrombotic complications of pancreatic cancer: classical knowledge revised. Dig Dis, vol. 28, pp. 350-354.

Echrish, H.; Madden, L.A.; Greenman, J. & Maraveyas, A. (2011). The hemostasis apparatus in pancreatic cancer and its importance beyond thrombosis. *Cancers*, vol. *3*, pp. 267-284, ISSN 2072-6694.

Elsayed, E. & Becker, R.C. (2003). The impact of heparin compounds on cellular inflammatory responses: a construct for future investigation and pharmaceutical development. *J Thromb Thrombolysis*, vol. 15, pp. 11-18, ISSN 0929-5305.

Epstein, A.S.; Crosbie, C.; Gardos, S. at al. (2010). A single institution, (MSKCC) analysis of incidence and clinical outcomes in patients with thromboembolic events and exocrine pancreas cancer. *J Clin Oncol*, vol. 28(15 suppl), pp.4126, ISSN 2218-4333.

Er, O. & Zacharsky, L. (2006). Management of cancer associated venous thrombosis. *Vasc Health Risk Manag*, vol. 2, pp. 351-356, ISSN 1176-6344.

Ettelaie, C.; Li, C.; Collier, M.E.W.; Pradier, A.; Frentzou, G.A.; Wood, C.G.; Chetter, I.C.; McCollum, P.T.; Bruckdorfer, K.R. & James, N.J. (2007). Differential functions of tissue factor in the trans-activation of Cell Signall pathways. *Atherosclerosis*, vol. *194*, pp. 88-101, ISSN: 0021-9150.

Falanga, A. & Rickles, F.R. (1999). Pathophysiology of the thrombophilic state in the cancer patient. *Sem Throm Hemost*, vol. *25*, pp. 173-182, ISSN 0094-6176.

Folkman, J. (1995). Angiogenesis inhibitors generated by tumors. *Mol Med*, vol.*1*, pp. 120-122, ISSN 1226-3613.

Geerts, W.H.; Pineo, G.F.; Heit, J.A.; Bergqvist, D.; Lassen, M.R.; Colwell, C.W., et al. (2004). Prevention of venous thromboembolism: the Seventh ACCP Conference on

Antithrombotic and Thrombolytic Therapy. *Chest*, vol. 126, pp. 338-400S, ISSN 0012-3692.

Gilbert, G.E. & Arena, A.A. (1995). Phosphatidylethanolamine induces high-affinity binding sites for factor-VIII on membranes containing phosphatidyl-L-serin. *J Biol Chem*, vol. *270*, pp. 18500-18505, ISSN 0021-9258.

Girard, T.J.; Warren, L.A.; Novotny, W.F.; Likert, K.M.; Brown, S.G.; Miletich, J.P.& Broze, G.J. (1989). Functional significance of the kunitz-type inhibitory domains of lipoprotein-associated coagulation inhibitor. *Nature*, vol.*338*, pp. 518-520, ISSN 0028-0836.

Gouaulthelimann, M. & Josso, F. (1979). Initiation invivo of blood coagulation-role of white blood-cells and tissue factor. *Nouv Presse Med*, vol. *8*, pp. 3249-3253, ISSN 0755-4982.

Haag, C.; Thiede C.; Hanig V. & Ehninger G. (2000). Disseminated Intravascular Coagulation (DIC) After Intraarterial Injection of Adenoviral Vector Containing P53 in Patients with Pancreatic Cancer in a Phase I/II Study. Proc Am Soc Clin Oncol vol. 19, (abstr 1813). 2000 ASCO Annual Meeting, New Orleans, LA, May 20-23, 2000.

Heit, J.A.; Silverstein, M.D.; Mohr, D.N.; Petterson, T.M.; O'Fallon, W.M. & Melton L.J. 3rd. (2000). Risk factors for deep vein thrombosis and pulmonary embolism: a population-based casecontrol study. *Arch Intern Med*, vol. 160, pp. 809-815, ISSN 0003-9926.

Heit, J.A.; O'Fallon, W.M.; Petterson, T.M.; Lohse, C.M.; Silverstein, M.D.; Mohr, D.N. & Melton, L.J. (2002). Relative impact of risk factors for deep vein thrombosis and pulmonary embolism - A population-based study. *Arch Intern Med*, vol. *162*, pp. 1245-1248, ISSN 0003-9926.

Icli, F.; Akbulut, H.; Utkan, G., et al. (2007). Low molecular weight heparin (LMWH) increases the efficacy of cisplatinum plus gemcitabine combination in advanced pancreatic cancer. *J Surg Oncol*, vol. 95, pp. 507-512. ISSN:0022-4790.

Kakkar, A.K.; Lemoine N.R.; Scully, M.F. et al. (1995). Tissue factor expression correlates with histological grade in human pancreatic cancer. *Br J Surg* vol.82, pp. 1101-1104, ISSN: 1365-2168.

Kaye, S.B. (1994). Gemcitabine: current status of phase I and II trials. *J Clin Oncol*, vol. 12, pp. 1527–1531, ISSN 2218-4333.

Karthaus, M.; Kretzschmar, A.; Kroning, H., et al. (2006). Dalteparin for prevention of catheter-related complications in cancer patients with central venous catheters: final results of a double-blind, placebo controlled phase III trial. *Ann Oncol*, vol. 17, pp. 289-296, ISSN 0923-7534.

Kirwan, C.C.; McDowell, G.; McCollum, C.N. & Byrne, G.J. (2011). Incidence of Venous Thromboembolism during Chemotherapy for Breast cancer_Impact on cancer outcome. *Anticancer Res*, vol. 31, no. 6, pp. 2383-2388, ISSN 0250-7005.

Klerk, C.P.; Smorenburg, S.M.; Otten, H.M.; Lensing, A.W.; Prins, M.H.; Piovella, F., et al. (2005). The effect of low molecular weight heparin on survival in patients with advanced malignancy. *J Clin Oncol*, vol. 23, pp. 2130-2135, ISSN 2218-4333.

Khorana, A.A. (2003). Malignancy, thrombosis and Trousseau: the case for an eponym. *J Thromb Haemost*, vol. 1, pp. 2463-2465, ISSN: 1538-7933.

Khorana, A.A, & Fine, R.L. (2004). Pancreatic cancer and thromboembolic disease. *Lancet Oncol*, vol. 5, pp. 655-663, ISSN 1470-2045.

Khorana, A.A.; Ahrendt S.A. & Ryan C.K. (2007). Tissue factor expression, angiogenesis and thrombosis in pancreatic cancer. *Clin Cancer Res* vol.13,no. 10, may 15, pp. 2870-2875, ISSN: 1078-0432.

Lee, A.Y.; Levine, M.N.; Baker, R.I., et al. (2003). Low molecular weight heparin versus a coumarin for the prevention of recurrent venous thromboembolism in patients with cancer. *N Engl J Med*, vol. 349, pp. 146-153, ISSN 0028-4793.

Levine, M.N. (1997). Prevention of thrombotic disorders in cancer patients undergoing chemotherapy. *Thromb Haemost*, vol. 78, pp. 133-136, ISSN: 0340-6245.

Levitan, N.; Dowlati, A.; Remick, S.C., et al. (1999). Rates of initial and recurrent thromboembolic disease among patients with malignancy versus those without malignancy. Risk analysis using Medicare claims data. *Medicine (Baltimore)*, vol. 78, pp. 285-291, ISSN: 0025-7974.

Liu, Y. & Mueller, B.M. (2006). Protease-activated receptor-2 regulates vascular endothelial growth factor expression in MDA-MB-231 cells via MAPK pathways. *Biochem Bioph Res*, vol. *344*, pp. 1263-1270, ISSN 0006-291X.

Lomberk, G. (2010). Angiogenesis. *Pancreatology*, vol. *10*, pp. 112-113, ISSN: 1424-3903.

Maraveyas, A.; Holmes, M.; Lofts, F., et al. (2007). Chemoanticoagulation versus chemotherapy in advanced pancreatic cancer: results of the interim analysis of the FRAGEM trial. Program and abstracts of the 43rd Annual Meeting of the American Society of Clinical Oncology; June 1-5, 2007; Chicago, Illinois. Abstract 4583. *J Clin Oncol*, vol. 25, pp. 4583, ISSN 2218-4333.

Mechtcheriakova, D.; Wlachos, A.; Holzmuller, H.; Binder, B.R. & Hofer, E. (1999). Vascular endothelial cell growth factor-induced tissue factor expression in endothelial cells is mediated by EGR-1. *Blood*, vol. 93,pp. 3811–3823, ISSN 0268-960X.

Meyer, G.; Marjanovic, Z.; Valcke, J., et al. (2002). Comparison of lowmolecular-weight heparin and warfarin for the secondary prevention of venous thromboembolism in patients with cancer: a randomized controlled study. *Arch Intern Med*, vol. 162, pp. 1729-1735, ISSN 0003-9926.

Milsom, C.C.; Yu, J.L.; Mackman, N.; Micallef, J.; Anderson, G.M.; Guha, A. & Rak, J.W. (2008). Tissue Factor Regulation by Epidermal Growth Factor Receptor and Epithelial-to-Mesenchymal Transitions: Effect on Tumor Initiation and Angiogenesis. *Cancer Res*, vol. *68*, pp. 10068-10076, ISSN: 0008-5472.

Nemerson, Y. (1988). Tissue factor and hemostasis. *Blood*, vol. *71*, pp. 1-8, ISSN 0268-960X.

Neoptolemos, J.P.; Dunn, J.A.; Stocken, D.D., et al. (2001). Adjuvant chemoradiotherapy and chemotherapy in respectable pancreatic cancer: a randomized controlled trial. *Lancet*, vol. 358, no. 9293, pp. 1576-1585, ISSN: 0140-6736.

Nitori, N.; Ino Y.; Nakanishi Y, et al. (2005). Prognostic significance of tissue factor in pancreatic ductal adenocarcinoma. *Clin Cancer Res*, vol. 11, pp. 2531-2539, ISSN: 1078-0432.

Offord, R.; Lloyd, A.C.; Anderson, P. & Bearne, A. (2004). Economic evaluation of enoxaparin for the prevention of venous thromboembolism in acutely ill medical patients. *Pharmacy World Sci*, vol. *26*, pp. 214-220, ISSN 0928-1231.

Palumbo, J.S.; Kombrinck, K.W.; Drew, A.F.; Grimes, T.S.; Kiser, J.H.; Degen, J.L. & Bugge,T.H. (2000). Fibrinogen is an important determinant of the metastatic potential of circulating tumor cells. *Blood*, vol. *96*, pp. 3302-3309, ISSN 0268-960X.

Pinzon, R.; Drewinko, B.; Trujillo, J.M. , et al. (1986). Pancreatic carcinoma and Trousseau's syndrome: experience at a large cancer center. *J Clin Oncol*, vol. 4, no. 4, pp. 509-514, ISSN 2218-4333.

Prandoni, P.; Lensing, A.W.; Piccioli, A., et al (2002). Recurrent venous thromboembolism and bleeding complications during anticoagulant treatment in patients with cancer and venous thrombosis. *Blood*, vol. 100, pp. 3484–3488, ISSN 0268-960X.

Price, L.H.; Nguyen M. B.; Picozzi V. J. & Kozarek R. A. (2010). Portal vein thrombosis in pancreatic cancer: Natural history, risk factors, and implications for patient management. Poster session Meeting: *2010 Gastrointestinal Cancers Symposium*, Orlando, Florida, USA, 22-24, January, 2010.

Rahr, H.B. & Sørensen, J.V. (1992). Venous thromboembolism and cancer. *Blood Coagul Fibrinolysis*, vol. 3, pp. 451-460, ISSN 09575235.

Rasmussen, M.S.; Wille-Jorgensen, P.; Jorgensen, L.N., et al. (2003). Prolongedthromboprophylaxis with low molecular weight heparin (dalteparin) following major abdominal surgery for malignancy [abstract]. *Blood*, vol. 102pp. 186, ISSN 0268-960X.

Reiss, H.; Pelzer, U.; Opitz, B., et al. (2010). A prospective, randomized trial of simultaneous pancreatic cancer treatemnet with enoxaparin and chemotherapy: Final results of the CONKO-004 trial. *J Clin Oncol*, vol. 28(15Suppl), pp. 4033, ISSN 2218-4333.

Rickles, F.R.; Patierno, S. & Fernandez, P.M. (2003).Tissue factor, thrombin, and cancer. *Chest*, vol. 124, pp. 58-68S, ISSN 0012-3692.

Ruf, W.; Fischer, E.G.; Huang, H.Y.; Miyagi, Y.; Ott, I.; Riewald, M. & Mueller, B.M. (2000). Diverse functions of protease receptor tissue factor in inflammation and metastasis. *Immunol Res*, vol. *21*, pp. 289-292, ISSN: 0923-2494 .

Sack, Jr G.H.; Levine, J. & Bel, W.R. (1977). Trousseau's syndrome and other manifestations of chronic disseminated coagulopathy in patients with neoplasms : clinical, pathophysiologic, and therapeutic features. *Medicine* (Baltimore), vol. 56, no. 1, pp. 1-37, ISSN: 0025-7974.

Sandset, P.R.; Bendz, B. & Hansen, J.B. (2000). Physiological function of tissue factor pathway inhibitor and interaction with heparins. *Haemostasis*, vol.30(suppl 2), pp. 48-56, ISSN: 0340-6245.

Shah, M.M. & Saif, M.W. (2010). Pancreatic cancer and thrombosis. Highlights from the "2010 ASCO Annual Meeting". Chicago, IL, USA. June 4-8, 2010. *JOP*; jul 5, vol.11, no. 4, pp. 331-333, ISSN 1590-8577.

Shen, Y.; Zhou, X.; Wang, Z.; Yang, G.; Jiang, Y.; Sun, C.; Wang, J.; Tong, Y. & Guo, H. (2011). Coagulation profiles and thromboembolic events of bortezomib plus thalidomide and dexamethasone therapy in newly diagnosed multiple myeloma. *Leuk Res*, vol. 35, no. 2, pp. 147-151, ISSN:0145-2126.

Sørensen, H.T.; Mellemkjaer, L.; Olsen, J.H., et al. (2000). Prognosis of cancers associated with venous thromboembolism. *N Engl J Med*, vol. 343, pp. 1846-1850, ISSN 0028-4793.

Sproul, E.E. (1938).Carcinoma and venous thrombosis: the frequency of association of carcinoma in the body or tail of the pancreas with multiple venous thromboses. *Am J Cancer*, vol. 34, pp. 566-573, ISSN: 1175-6357.

Tesselaar, M.E.T.; Romijn, F.; van der Linden, I.K.; Bertina, R.M. & Osanto, S. (2009). Microparticleassociated tissue factor activity in cancer patients with and without thrombosis. *J Thromb Haematol*, vol. *7*, pp. 1421-1423, ISSN 1740 3340.

Tilley, R.E.; Holscher, T.; Belani, R.; Nieva, J. & Mackman, N. (2008).Tissue factor activity is increased in a combined platelet and microparticle sample from cancer patients. *Thromb Res*, vol. *122*, pp. 604-609, ISSN: 0049-3848.

Traynelis, S.F.&Trejo, J. (2007). Protease-activated receptor signaling: New roles and regulatorymechanisms. *Cur Opin Hematol*, vol. *14*, pp. 230-235, ISSN: 1065-6251.

Trousseau, A. (1865). Plegmasia alba dolens. Lectures on clinical medicine, delivered at the Hotel-Dieu, Paris, vol. 5, pp. 281-332.

van den Belt, A.G.; Prins, M.H.; Lensing, A.W., et al. (2000). Fixed dose subcutaneous low molecular weight heparins versus adjusted dose unfractionated heparin for venous thromboembolism. *Cochrane Database Syst Rev*, CD001100, **ISSN**:1469-493X.

Varki, A. (2007). Trousseau's syndrome: multiple definitions and multiple mechanisms. *Blood*, vol.110, pp. 1723-1729, ISSN 0268-960X.

Verso, M. & Agnelli, G. (2003). Venous thromboembolism associated with long-term use of central venous catheters in cancer patients. *J Clin Oncol*, vol. 21, pp. 3665-3675.

Verso, M.; Agnelli, G.; Kamphuisen, P.W., et al. (2008). Risk factors for upper limb deep vein thrombosis associated with the use of central vein catheter in cancer patients. *Intern Emerg Med*, vol. 3, no.2, pp. 117-122, ISSN: 1828-0447.

Ueda, C.; Hirohata, Y.; Kihara, Y.; Nakamura, H.; Abe, B.; Akahane, K.; Okamoto, K.; Itoh, H. & Otsuki, M. (2001). Pancreatic cancer complicated bydisseminated intravascular coagulation associated with production of tissue factor. J Gastroenterol, vol. 36, no.12, pp. 848-850.

Wada, H.; Wakita, Y. & Shiku, H. (1995). Tissue factor expression in endothelial-cells in health anddisease. *Blood Coagul Fibrin*, *6*, S26-S31, ISSN 09575235.

Wall, J.G.; Weiss, R.B.; Norton, L.; Perloff, M.; Rice, M.A.; Korzun, A.H. & Wood, W.C. (1989). Arterial thrombosis associated with adjuvant chemotherapy for breast carcinoma-a cancer and leukemia group study. *Am J Med*, vol.*87*, pp. 501-504, ISSN: 0002-9343.

Yamanaka, Y.; Friess, H.; Kobrin, M.S.; Buchler, M.; Beger, H.G. & Korc, M. (1993). Coexpression of epidermal growth factor receptor and ligands in human pancreatic cancer is associated with enhanced tumor aggressiveness. *Anticancer Res*, vol.*13*, pp. 565-569, ISSN: 0250-7005.

Zacharski, L.R.; Henderson, W.G.; Rickles, F.R., et al. (1981). Effect of warfarin on survival in small cell carcinoma of the lung. *JAMA*, vol. 245, pp. 831-835, ISSN 00987484.

Zangari, M.; Fink, L.M.; Elice, F., et al (2009). Thrombotic Events in Patients with Cancer Receiving Antiangiogenesis Agents. *JCO* (October 10), vol. 27, no. 29, pp. 4865-4873, ISSN 0732-183X.

Zhang, Y.M.; Deng, Y.H.; Luther, T.; Muller, M.; Ziegler, R.; Waldherr, R.; Stern, D.M. & Nawroth, P.P. (1994). Tissue factor controls the balance of angiogenic and antiangiogenic properties of tumour-cells in mice. *J Clin Invest*, vol. *94*, pp. 1320-1327, ISSN 0021-9738.

Zwicker, J.I.; Kos, C.A.; Johnston, K.A.; Liebman, H.A.; Furie, B.C. & Furie, B. (2007). Tissue factor bearing microparticles is associated with an increased risk of venous thromboembolic events in cancer patients. *Thromb Res*, vol. *120*, pp. S143-S143, ISSN 0049-3848.

Clinical Implications of an Expandable Metallic Mesh Stent for Malignant Portal Vein Stenosis in Management of Unresectable or Recurrent Pancreatic Cancer

Yoshinori Nio
Nio Surgery Clinic,
Japan

1. Introduction

Pancreatic cancer (PC) remains one of the most lethal common malignancies. More than 80% of patients with PC cannot be cured by surgical resection (Li D et al., 2004); the actuarial 5-year survival rate after curative resection is approximately 20% (Crist et al., 1987), and the median survival time (MST) after surgical resection ranges between 11 and 24 months (Nitecki et al., 1995). In other words, most patients develop recurrent disease in the near future even after curative resection.

Advanced or recurrent PC frequently invades the surrounding organs or tissues, and the patients require substantial palliative interventions, especially against biliary obstruction, gastric or duodenal outlet obstruction, and severe abdominal or back pain. In addition, when the portal vein (PV) is invaded and occluded, the patient suffers from various portal hypertension (PH)-associated symptoms and liver dysfunction, including jaundice, ascites, and bleeding tendencies, which disturb chemotherapy (ChT) or radiotherapy (RT).

PC-associated portal obstruction is classified into two categories, intrahepatic obstruction and extrahepatic obstruction. In the case of intrahepatic or hilar PV stenosis, a wall-stent is usually applied (Tsukamoto et al., 2003); however, a wall-stent cannot be used for the extrahepatic PV stenosis, because it may occlude the splenic vein, which joins the extrahepatic PV, leading to serious complications. In patients with extrahepatic PV obstruction, we placed an expandable metallic mesh (EMM) stent into the PV *via* the ileocecal vein following a mini-laparotomy. A total of 14 patients with inoperable or recurrent PC were given an EMM-PV-stent and received subsequent ChT and/or RT, and the treatment results were retrospectively compared with patients without an EMM-PV-stent.

2. Patients and methods

2.1 Patients

We treated a total of 97 patients with inoperable or recurrent PC. Of 97 patients, 68 received ChT, 28 received RT using LINAC at 40 - 60Gy (2Gy × 20 - 30 times) and 14 were given an

EMM-PV-stent. All patients were treated in the Department of Surgery, Shimane University School of Medicine.

2.2 Methods

A Bird Luminex EMM-stent (6 - 12 mm in diameter and 4 - 8 cm in length) was used. The patients received a mini-laparotomy at the ileocecal region and the ileocecal vein was cut-down. Under guidance with image roentgenography, the stenotic portion of the PV was dilated by a balloon catheter and the EMM-stent was placed. In one case, 3 stents were placed, and in the other 13 cases, a single stent was placed. All patients were given heparin continuously at 5,000 U/day for 7 days, and then biaspirin or warfarin for 1 - 3 months.

2.3 Chemotherapy (ChT) and radiotherapy (RT)

The ChT included oral UFT (uracil and tegafur) at 300 - 400 mg/day daily, oral cyclophosphamide (CPA) at 50 mg/day every other day, and/or gemcitabine (GEM) at 200 - 400 mg/body weekly or biweekly in combination or singly. The regimens administered were decided according to the performance status with fully informed consent of the patients and/or their families. Six patients were given a UC (UFT and CPA) regimen orally in combination with GEM, and the other 7 patients received other regimens: 2 UC, 2 GEM alone, 1 UC + cisplatin + epirubicin, 1 UFT alone, and one GEM + TS-1. However, 1 patient died without receiving any ChT.

RT was performed using LINAC at 40 - 60Gy (2Gy × 20 - 30 fractions).

2.4 Evaluation of the objective response (OR) to the therapies

The OR of the tumor was assessed using roentgenography, computed tomography (CT), or ultrasonography (US) using the following standard criteria: i) a complete response (CR) indicated total disappearance of the tumor for at least 4 weeks, during which time the patient was free of all symptoms related to pancreatic cancer; ii) a partial response (PR) was defined as a 50% or greater reduction in the sum of the products of the two perpendicular diameters of all measurable tumor lesions as compared to their original size for at least 4 weeks. During this time, there must have been no increase of >25% in the size of any single lesion or the appearance of any new lesion; and iii) progressive disease (PD) was defined as a greater than a 25% increase in the sum of the products of the diameters of all measurable lesions, the appearance of any new lesion, or a deterioration in the clinical status that was consistent with disease progression; and iv) stable disease (SD) was indicated for those patients who failed to meet the criteria for a CR, PR or PD, and who remained in the study for at least 8 weeks. The duration of the response was measured from the first day of injection of the agents to the day of the increase in tumor size.

2.5 Evaluation of side-effects

The National Cancer Institute - Common Toxicity Criteria were used for evaluation of side-effects (NCI-CTC version 2.0). All of the patients were followed by physical examination, routine hematological and biochemical examinations, and serum tumor marker assays to evaluate side-effects.

2.6 Statistics

The effects of the therapies were evaluated with respect to the response rate (RR) of the tumor and the survival rate after therapy. The overall survival (OS) was calculated by the Kaplan-Meier method. Multivariate analysis of the maximum likelihood estimates using Cox's proportional hazard model was used to obtain the conditional risk of carcinoma-related death. All analyses were performed using StatView software (SAS Institute Inc., Cary, NC, USA) and a *p*-value less than 0.05 was considered statistically significant.

3. Treatment results

The effects of the EMM-PV-stent are summarized in **Table 1**. In 4 cases, the EMM-PV-stent was very effective, and the ascites and/or hemorrhagic tendency were improved. Furthermore, ChT and RT were also effective and 3 CRs and 3 PRs were observed: the overall RR (CR + PR) was 42.9%, and SDs were observed in 3 patients. However, in the 2 remaining cases, the EMM-PV-stent was not effective: one patient died of gastrointestinal bleeding and the other died of liver dysfunction and cachexia due to increased liver metastasis.

I. Objective response	
Complete response (CR)	3
Partial response (PR)	3
Stable disease (SD)	3
Progressive disease (PD)	5
Overall response rate (CR+PR)	42.9%(6/14)
II. Other clinical benefits	
Pain relief	2
Decrease or disappearance of ascites	2
Improvement in hyperglycemia	1
Improvement in thrombocytopenia	1

Table 1. Objective response and clinical benefits

The procedure for an EMM-PV-stent is shown in the treatment course of one representative case in **Figure 1 - 4.** The patient had a pancreatic head carcinoma causing obstructive jaundice, and the PC was diagnosed as inoperable because splenic metastasis and PV occlusion were observed (**Figure 1A,1B and 1C**).

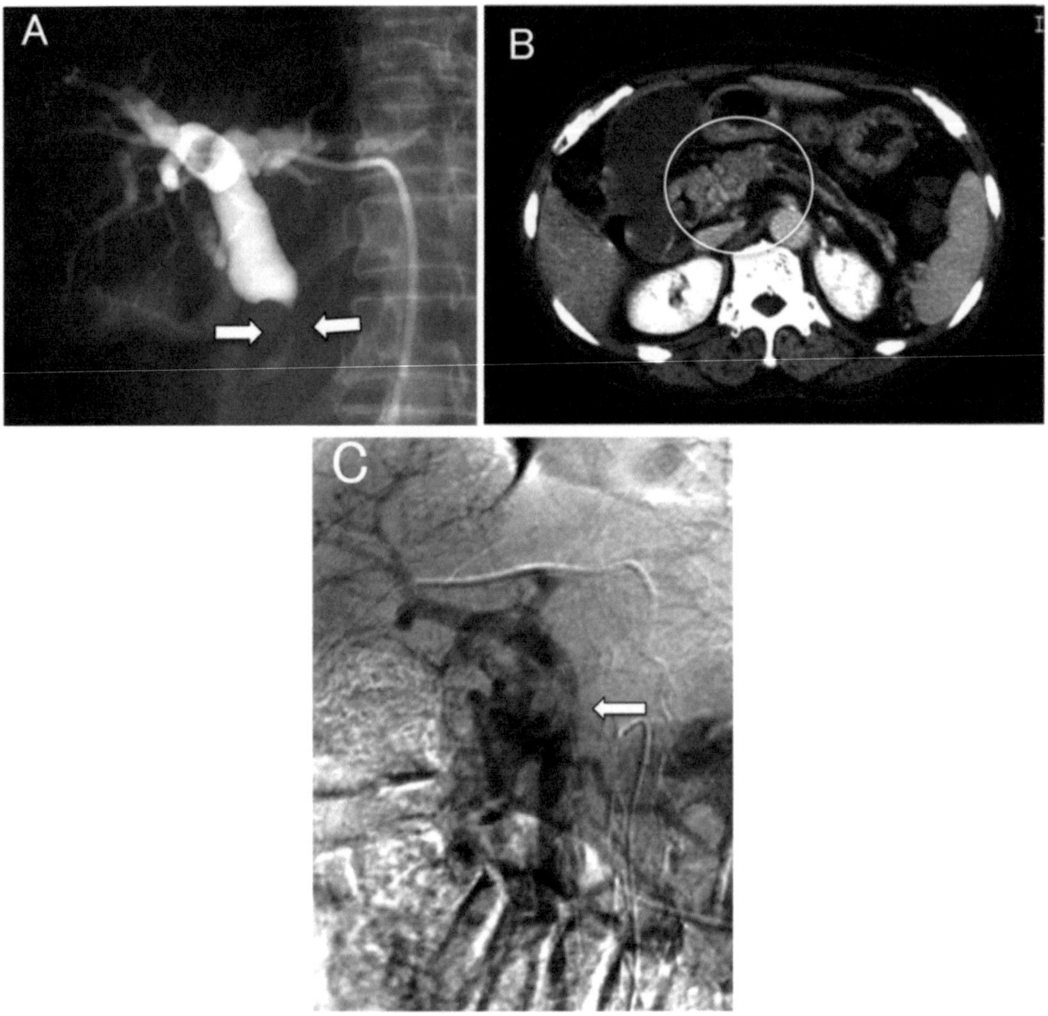

Fig. 1. A representative case with portal stenosis
A. Percutaneous transhepatic cholangiography. Arrows indicate stenosis.
B. CT. Circle indicates a pancreatic head cancer
C. Portography. Arrow indicates extrahepatic portal stenosis

The patient underwent a laparotomy, but peritoneal dissemination and malignant ascites were also seen. In order to release the obstruction of the bile duct and duodenum, the patient received bypass surgeries with a cholecysto-jejunostomy and a gastro-jejunostomy. In addition, she received placement of an EMM-PV-stent with three metallic stents, as shown in **Figure 2A,2B,2C,2D and 2E**.

After surgery, she was treated with ChT consisting of oral UFT plus CPA with intravenous GEM, and RT to a total of 50 Gy. The tumor responded well to the therapies, and the splenic metastasis and primary lesion disappeared completely 4 months after the surgery **(Figure 3)**. Finally, she died of malignant ascites 21 months after the initiation of treatment. **Figure 4** summarizes the treatment course.

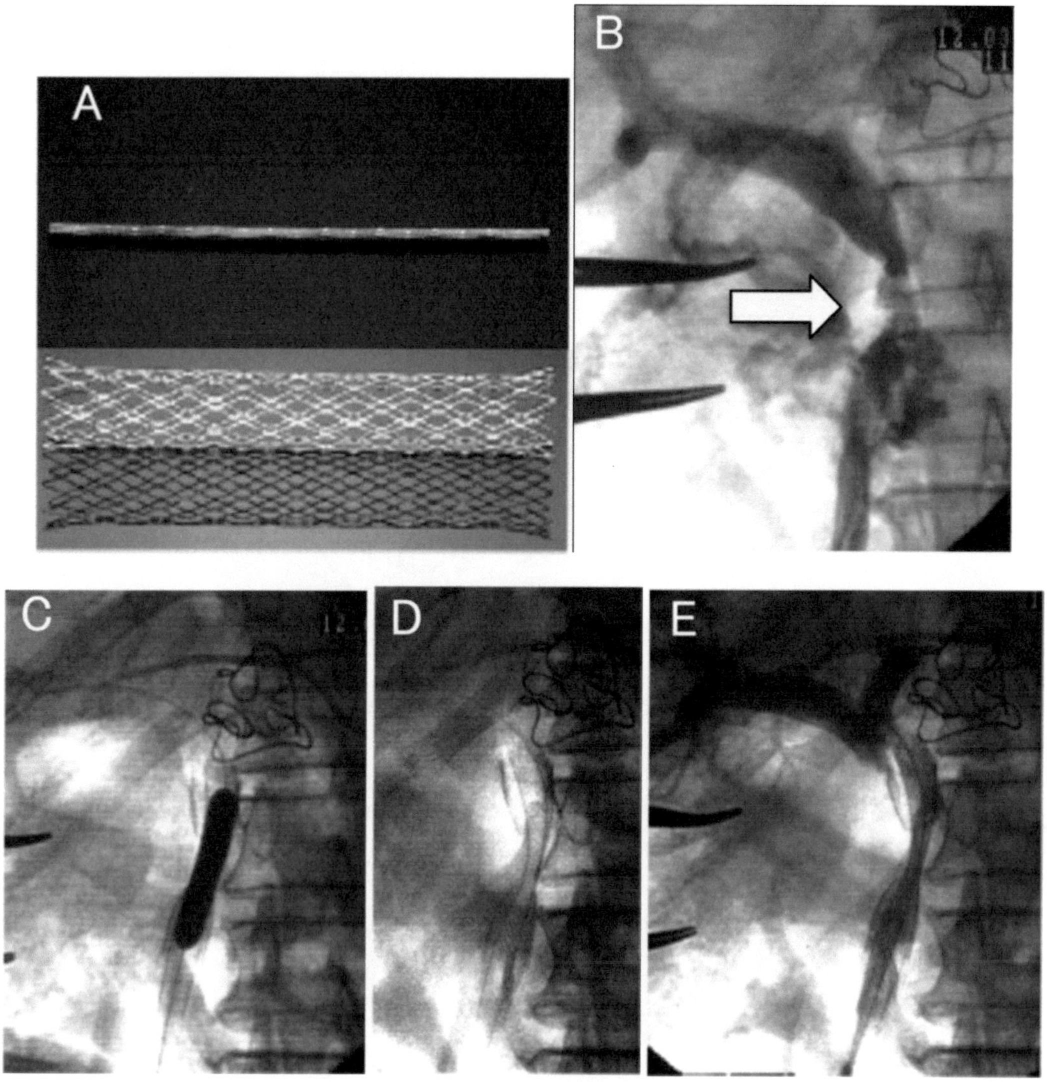

Fig. 2. Procedure of portal stent
A. An expandable metallic mesh stent (Bird Luminex)
B. Arrow indicates portal stenosis
C. Balloon dilatation
D. Insertion of three stents
E. Portography after portal stent

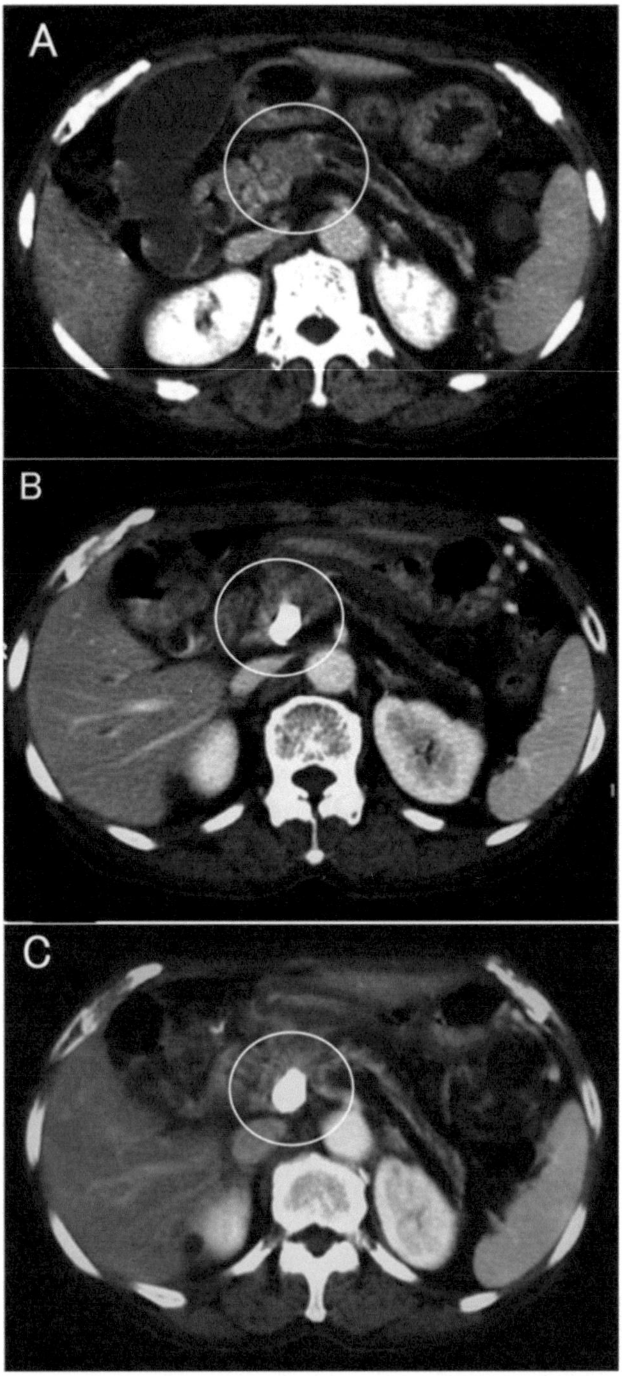

Fig. 3. Comparative CT before and after PV-stent
A. Before PV-stent
B. Two months after PV-stent
C. Six months after PV-stent

Circles indicate pancreas head and portal vein.

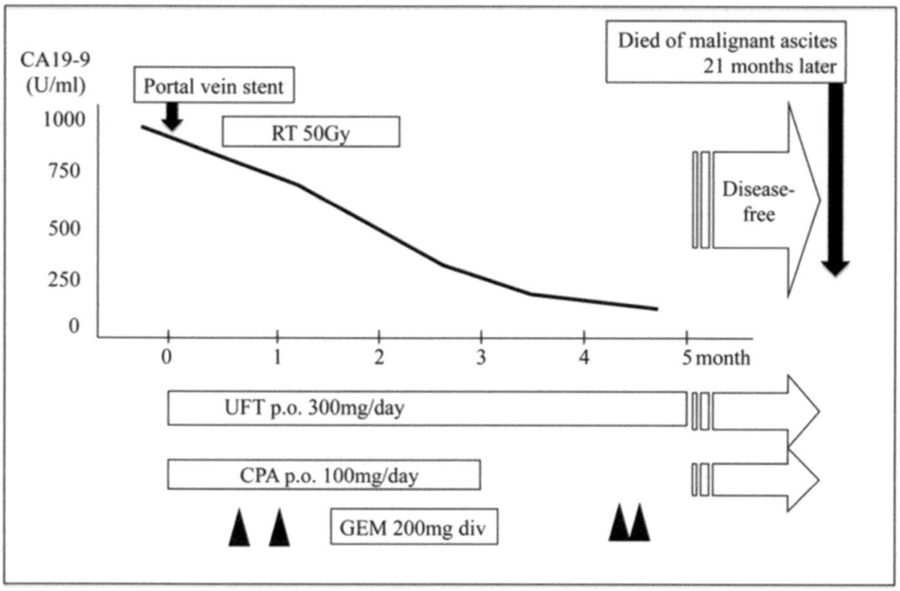

Fig. 4. Treatment course

The survival curves after the initiation of treatment and placement of the EMM-PV-stent are shown in **Figure 5**.

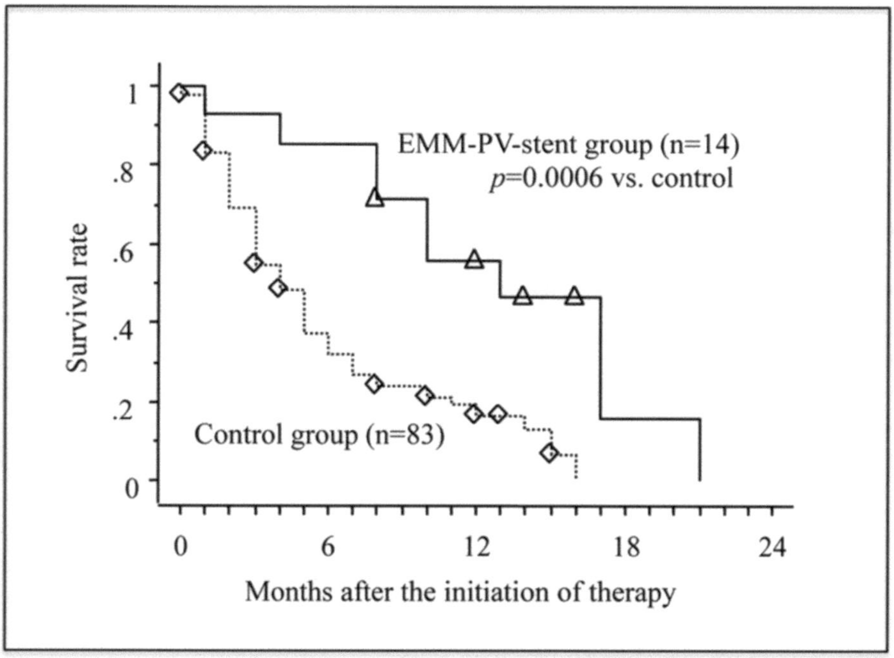

Fig. 5. Comparative survival curves.

The survival curve of the EMM-PV-stent group was significantly higher than that of the remaining patients (control group, n=83) (p=0.0006 by Cox-Mantel): the 6 months and 1-year survival rates were 85.7% and 54.5% for the EMM-PV-stent group vs. 32.0% and 16.2% for the control group, respectively, while the MSTs were 13.0 vs. 4.0 months, respectively (**Table 2**).

	Survival rate (%)		Median survival	
Group	6-month	1-year	(months)	*p*-value
Control	32.0	16.2	5.9	0.0006
EMM-PV-stent	85.7	54.5	12.7	

Table 2. Comparative survival between the control and EMM-PV-stent groups

The implications of EMM-PV-stenting in the treatment results were analyzed by multivariate analysis (**Table 3**), but this demonstrated that an EMM-PV-stent was not a significant factor, while RT and ChT were significant prognostic factors. This suggests that an EMM-PV-stent itself does not improve the patients' survival, but it is beneficial for improving the efficacy of ChT or RT by reducing the risk of liver failure or hemorrhagic tendency.

Variables	Conditional risk ratio (95% confidence limit)	*p*-value
Age	1.000 (0.978 – 1.022)	0.9718
Palliative surgery	0.830 (0.485 – 1.423)	0.4986
PV-stent	0.537 (0.195 – 1.481)	0.2298
Chemotherapy	0.349 (0.206 – 0.590)	<0.001
Radiotherapy	0.427 (0.220 – 0.830)	0.012

Table 3. Multivariate analysis by Cox's proportional hazard risk model

4. Discussion

In the present study, we used an EMM-stent as the PV-stent, although in general, for a vascular stent, a wall stent is used. The reason for using an EMM-stent is that a wall stent occludes the splenic vein, which is joined to the PV, and may lead to serious complications. In intrahepatic PV stenosis cases, a wall stent can be used, but pancreatic cancer usually causes extrahepatic PV stenosis. Furthermore, in intrahepatic PV stenosis, a percutaneous transhepatic procedure is usually applied to place the wall stent into the PV. However, we placed an EMM-stent into the PV via the ileocecal vein using laparotomy because it is very difficult to define the occlusive site from the distal PV under image roentgenography, and a percutaneous transhepatic procedure carries various risks such as intra-abdominal bleeding and perforation, which can be more easily managed by laparotomy.

One of the disadvantages of placing an EMM-stent is that the tumor frequently invades through the mesh into the lumen, resulting in re-obstruction. Accordingly, RT and/or ChT are essential to inhibit tumor invasion into the lumen.

The present study included 14 patients who received placement of an EMM-PV-stent and adjuvant ChT or RT, and the RR was 43%: the 1-year survival rate was 54.5% for the EMPVstent group vs. 16.2% for the control group, and the MSTs were 13.0 vs. 4.0 months, respectively (p=0.0006). These RR and survival rates are high and long for PC, as compared with previous reports, in which the RR of a combination regimen with 5-FU, GEM and their combinations ranged between 5% and 25%, while the MST ranged between 4 and 10 months (Van Cutsem et al., 2004; Okusaka & Kosuge, 2004; Pasetto et al., 2004; Heinemann, 2002; Novarino et al., 2004; Berlin et al., 2002), although the sample size of the present study was too small to draw any conclusive interpretations.

The present study also demonstrated that an EMM-PV-stent was not a significant prognostic factor, although the survival rate was significantly higher in the EMM-PV-stent group than the control group. However, ChT and RT were significant prognostic factors by multivariate analysis (p<0.001 and 0.0120, respectively). These results indicate that the EMM-PV-stent itself does not improve prognosis, but that ChT and RT may play important roles in regressing the tumor, and that an EMM-PV-stent helps to improve the efficacy of ChT and RT in patients with PH-associated complications that cause liver dysfunction and pancytopenia, especially thrombocytopenia and leucocytopenia (due to hypersplenism), and gastrointestinal bleeding. However, in order to achieve clinically beneficial treatment results, ChT and RT at a sufficient dose to regress the tumor are very important in patients with PH, as a dose of ChT or RT sufficient to regress the tumor cannot be administered. Since liver dysfunction and pancytopenia can easily be exacerbated by ChT and RT, there are major difficulties for the administration of a dose of ChT or RT sufficient to induce regression of PC. Therefore, placement of a PV-stent improves the efficacy of these adjuvant therapies by removing any PH-associated co-morbidities. Furthermore, in the present study, pain and other PH-associated symptoms such as ascites and hyperglycemia were also improved.

We administered UFT, CPA, and GEM as the ChT regimen in most patients. These regimens were unique to our team. GEM now plays a core role in ChT for advanced PC, and various combination regimens have been attempted. The present study used a low dose of GEM at 200 - 400 mg (almost equivalent to 150 - 300 mg/m^2), although most studies used standard doses of GEM at 800 - 1000 mg/m^2. However, this low dose was used in order to reduce the side-effects in combination with RT because our previous preliminary study on RT in combination with GEM at standard doses for inoperable PC resulted in serious myelosuppression, especially thrombocytopenia. Our previous study using this combination regimen with UFT, CPA and GEM at low doses resulted in a 27% RR and 23% clinical benefit response (CBR), and a 10.7 month MST (Nio et al., 2005.).

Here, we oral UFT instead of *iv* 5-fluorouracil (5-FU). In Japan, UFT has been used as a substitute for *iv* 5-FU for various malignancies such as gastric, colorectal, lung and breast cancer, and several studies in other countries have demonstrated that UFT was as effective as *iv* 5-FU, with a better toxicity profile (Sulkes et al., 1998; Van Cutsem & Peeters, 2000). Furthermore, the present ChT combined CPA in addition to GEM and UFT because previous reports including ours demonstrated that CPA augments the antitumor activity of fluoropyrimidines by modulating the activity of various enzymes, which are associated with pyrimidine metabolism, such as augmenting ribonucleotide reductase, inducing thymidine phosphorylase and inhibiting intratumoral activity of dihydropyrimidine dehydrogenase (Haga et al., 1999; Endo et al., 1999; Nio et al., 2007).

As discussed above, the treatment results of advanced or recurrent PC are not satisfactory, and the EMM-stent itself has no effect to regress the tumor; it only improves the PH-associated symptoms. Recently, various new agents have been introduced to the ChT for advanced PC, including TS-1, capecitabine, oxaliplatin, irinotecan, erlotinib, and taxanes, and these should help to improve the poor outcomes for patients with PC.

5. Conclusion

The placement of an EMM-PV-stent is very beneficial for managing PH-associated symptoms, as well as improving the efficacy of ChT and RT in pancreatic cancer with malignant PV stenosis or obstruction.

6. References

Berlin JD, et al.(2002). Phase III study of gemcitabine in combination with fluorouracil versus gemcitabine alone in patients with advanced pancreatic carcinoma: Eastern Cooperative Oncology Group trial E2297. J Clin Oncol *20*: 3270-3275.

Crist DW, et al.(1987). Improved hospital morbidity, mortality, and survival after the Whipple procedure. Ann Surg 206: 358-365.

Endo M, et al.(1999). Induction of thymidine phosphorylase expression and enhancement of efficacy of capecitabine or 5′-deoxy-5-fluorouridine by cyclophosphamide in mammary tumor models. Int J Cancer *83*: 127-134.

Haga S, et al.(1999). Antitumor efficacy of combination chemotherapy with UFT and cyclophosphamide against human breast cancer xenografts in nude mice. Anticancer Res *19 (3A)*: 1791-1796.

Heinemann V.(2002). Gemcitabine-based combination treatment of pancreatic cancer. Semin Oncol *29(1 Suppl 3)*: 25-35.

Li D, et al.(2004). Pancreatic Cancer. Lancet 363: 1049-1057.

NCI-CTC version 2.0. Common toxicity criteria, Notice of modifications. (http://ctep.info. nih.gov/).

Nio Y, et al.(2005). Phase II study on low-dose gemcitabine plus oral chemotherapy with uracil-tegafur and cyclophosphamide in combination with radiotherapy against recurrent and advanced pancreatic cancer. Oncol Rep *14*: 401-408.

Nio Y, et al.(2007). Cyclophosphamide augments the anti-tumor efficacy of uracil and tegafur by inhibiting dihydropyrimidine dehydrogenase. Oncol Rep 17(1): 153-159.

Nitecki SS, et al.(1995). Long-term survival after resection for ductal adenocarcinoma of the pancreas. Is it really improving? Ann Surg *221*: 59-66.

Novarino A, et al.(2004). Phase II study of cisplatin. gemcitabine and 5-fluorouracil in advanced pancreatic cancer. Ann Oncol *15*: 474-477.

Okusaka T and Kosuge T.(2004). Systemic chemotherapy for pancreatic cancer. Pancreas *28*: 301-304.

Pasetto LM, et al.(2004). Old and new drugs in systemic therapy of pancreatic cancer. Crit Rev Oncol Hematol *49*: 135-151.

Sulkes A, et al.(1998). Uracil-tegafur: An oral fluoropyrimidine active in colorectal cancer. J Clin Oncol *16*: 3461-3475.

Tsukamoto T, et al.(2003). Percutaneous transhepatic metallic stent placement for malignant portal vein stenosis. Hepatogastroenterol *50*: 453-455.

Van Cutsem E and Peeters M.(2000). Oral fluoropyrimidines in colorectal cancer. Semin Oncol *27 (Suppl 10)*: 91-95.

Van Cutsem E, et al.(2004). Systemic treatment of pancreatic cancer. Eur J Gastroenterol Hepatol *16*: 265-27.

17

Pancreatic Neuroendocrine Tumors: Emerging Management Paradigm

Syed F. Zafar and Bassel El-Rayes
Department of Hematology and Medical Oncology, Winship Cancer Institute of Emory University, Atlanta, USA

1. Introduction

Neuroendocrine tumors comprise a spectrum of slow growing neoplasm, characterized by storage and secretion of variable peptides and neuroamines (Massironi et al., 2008). Pancreatic neuroendocrine tumors (PNET) are relatively rare, with an estimated incidence of less than 1 per 1000,000 individuals (Metz and Jensen, 2008). A recent review of surveillance epidemiology and end results (SEER) (1950-2007) database reported the frequency of PNET to be around 7% among all identified neuroendocrine tumors (Lawrence et al., 2011a). Furthermore, they comprise 1-2% of all pancreatic neoplasms (Metz and Jensen, 2008). However, the incidence is considered to be increasing , perhaps in part due to improved diagnostic capabilities. Median overall survival in PNET ranges from more than 10 years in localized disease to approximately 2 years in metastatic disease (Yao et al., 2008a). Recently, considerable headway has been made in the realm of therapeutics. Therefore, it is imperative that oncologists today have a heightened awareness of this disease entity in order to provide effective care.

2. Diagnosis, staging and classification

PNETs have also been referred to as pancreatic endocrine or islet cell tumors. It is important to note that carcinoid and PNETs, although exhibiting identical characteristics histologically, should be considered separately. It is increasingly clear that these two tumor types are different in their biology and response to therapy. The clinical presentation of PNET is extremely variable which depends on the originating cell type and whether there is secretion of active hormones. Majority of patients remain asymptomatic, but a significant proportion present with clinical symptoms and hepatic metastases at the time of diagnosis (Modlin et al., 2008).

Most cases of PNET occur sporadically, however, approximately 10% of cases may be associated with multiple endocrine neoplasia type 1 (MEN1). MEN1 is an autosomal dominant syndrome associated with mutations in the tumor suppressor gene *menin* and characterized by multiple neuroendocrine tumors in the pancreas, parathyroid and pituitary glands (Agarwal et al., 2004). PNETs have also been associated with MEN2, Von Hippel-Lindau disease, Tuberous sclerosis and Neurofibromatosis (Kulke et al., 2011). Although the incidence of these inherited syndromes is low, it may be important to consider these syndromes in the diagnostic work up of patients with PNETs.

It is important to discern the diagnosis of PNET from the more common pancreatic adenocarcinoma. Grossly, PNETs are solitary well demarcated, tan soft tumors which can have a nodular appearance, when they exhibit fibrosis. The histological criteria for diagnosis are well established. These tumors can range from well differentiated ,low grade tumors to more poorly differentiated high grade types. Well differentiated tumors can exhibit various histological patterns, ranging from a common solid nesting, trabecular to tubular-acinar and mixed patterns .The cells are characterized by round to ovoid shape, with eosinophilic granular cytoplasm and prominent nucleoli. Unusual types can exhibit a spindle cell morphology which is referred to as the "rhabdoid" type. High grade malignancies with high mitotic rate usually encompass large cell and small cell carcinomas (Asa, 2011).

The usually employed classification schemes, although inconsistent in their criteria, reflect a basic separation between more indolent, well differentiated and aggressive poorly differentiated ones. While a number of histologic classification systems have been proposed for PNET, tumors with high mitotic count (>20/10 high power field) or a Ki-67 proliferation rate of >20%, generally represent highly aggressive malignancies and should be evaluated apart from the more classic well differentiated tumors such as classic carcinoid or islet cell type. These high grade malignancies are generally treated according to small cell carcinoma guidelines (Asa, 2011; Kloppel et al., 2004; Rindi and Kloppel, 2004). Table 1 outlines the histologic classification of neuroendocrine tumors.

Differentiation	Mitotic count	Grade	Ki-67 index (%)	General features	ENETS, WHO classification
Well differentiated	<2 per 10 HPF	Low Grade (G1)	≤2	Without local invasion (angioinvasion or perineural invasion). Traditionally include carcinoid and PNETs	Neuroendocrine tumor grade 1, WHO type 1.1 (pancreatic)
	2-20 per 10 HPF	Intermediate grade (G2)	3-20	With or without gross local invasion or metastases. Traditionally include carcinoid, atypical carcinoid and some PNET	Neuroendocrine tumor, Grade 2, WHO type 1.2 and 2 (pancreatic)
Poorly Differentiated	>20 per 10 HPF	High Grade (G3)	>20 %	Small cell or large cell carcinoma, often widely invasive or metastatic.	Neuroendocrine Carcinoma grade 3 (small cell or large cell), WHO type 3 (pancreatic)

ENETS: European Neuroendocrine Tumor Society; WHO: World Health Organization.

Table 1. Histologic classification of Neuroendocrine Tumors.

Several organizations, including the European Neuroendocrine Tumor Society (ENETS), and the American Joint Committee on Cancer (AJCC), have proposed staging systems for neuroendocrine tumors using the TNM notation (Edge and Compton, 2010). Although these two staging systems are similar for tumor arising in the luminal gut, they differ for earlier stage PNETs. The ENETS system incorporates tumor diameter in its assessment for T stage, whereas the AJCC incorporates factors determining resectability. However, both systems are nearly identical in defining stage IV disease. Because the AJCC system has been widely accepted and adopted in North America, this is preferably and more commonly used for classification by tumor stage.

3. Clinical manifestation

When functional, PNETs can be characterized by the type of hormone secreted leading to a specific clinical manifestation (Table 2). Specific details about some common tumors, based on the presentation are discussed below.

3.1 Insulinoma

Insulinomas are the most common PNET, comprising 30-40% of these tumors. Overall, they remain a rare entity with an incidence of approximately 0.4/100,000 patient years (Mathur et al., 2009).Classically, they present with "Whipple's Triad": a combination of symptoms of hypoglycemia, inappropriately high insulin level and associated blood glucose levels of <50 mg/dl with relief of symptoms on administration of glucose (Whipple and Frantz, 1935). In a 25-year Massachusetts General Hospital experience with insulinoma, the most common clinical symptoms in this series of 61 patients were confusion, visual disturbances and diaphoresis (Nikfarjam et al., 2008). Biochemical diagnosis requires confirmation of inappropriately elevated insulin, C-peptide and proinsulin levels in the presence of low serum glucose. Biochemical diagnosis is usually followed by radiological (CT or MRI) or endoscopic diagnosis. At early stages, the hypoglycemia can be managed with diazoxide and somatostatin analogues should be used cautiously as it can worsen hypoglycemia (Goode et al., 1986). Everolimus, an mTOR inhibitor, has been reported to be efficacious in cases of refractory hypoglycemia (Kulke et al., 2009a).

3.2 Gastrinoma

Gastrinoma and Zollinger-Ellison syndrome are suspected in a patient with recurrent or refractory peptic ulcer disease and unexplained secretory diarrhea. In such patients, fasting gastrin level >100 pg/ml is highly suspicious of this diagnosis (Jensen, 1996). Other common causes of gastric hypersecretion should be excluded, which includes treatment with proton pump inhibitors (PPI), atrophic gastritis and pernicious anemia. Approximately 25% of patients will present with diarrhea as primary manifestation without peptic ulcer disease (Perry and Vinik, 1995). Gastrinomas have a strong predilection for a "gastrinoma triangle" that includes the pancreatic head, first two-thirds of the duodenum and the porta hepatis (Howard et al., 1990). A significant proportion of gastrinomas are malignant, with up to one-third of patients presenting with liver metastases (Mittendorf et al., 2006). PPI therapy is highly effective for initial symptom management and somatostatin analogues have also shown effectiveness in controlling symptoms and concomitantly offering tumor stabilization (Lambers et al., 1984; Shojamanesh et al., 2002).

3.3 Glucagonoma

Majority of the patients with glucagonomas present with a dermatitis called necrolytic migratory erythema, causing pruritis and often becoming secondarily infected (Perry and Vinik, 1995). The clinical manifestation may also include diabetes, depression and deep vein thrombosis. Glucagonomas are frequently found in the pancreatic tail and have a malignant potential with a predilection for metastases. A serum glucagon level >500 pg/ml is highly suspicious of the diagnosis, whereas, a concentration of >10,000 pg/ml is virtually diagnostic (Chastain, 2001). However, a normal level does not exclude the diagnosis as secretion of glucagon may be episodic and a high concentration may be seen in other clinical syndromes such as sepsis, renal and hepatic failure. Initial management with somatostatin analogues are usually very effective in controlling symptoms however, such treatment may not have an effect on tumor growth. (Jockenhovel et al., 1994)

3.4 Somatostatinoma

Pancreatic somatostatinoma are usually malignant, and can present clinically with a syndrome of diabetes, steatorrhea and cholelithiasis (Warner, 2005). The diagnosis can be confirmed biochemically with marked elevation of serum somatostatin followed by imaging and endoscopic ultrasound, as with other pancreatic neuroendocrine tumors. Management with somatostatin analogues may be effective in symptomatic patients.

3.5 VIPoma

Verner and Morrison first described pancreatic endocrine tumors with a clinical syndrome of watery diarrhea, hypokalemia and achlorohydria (Verner and Morrison, 1958). This syndrome was subsequently found to be due to ectopic vasoactive intestinal peptide (VIP) secretion. Biochemical analysis assists in establishing a diagnosis when a marked elevation (>200 pg/dl) in the serum level of VIP is found (Smith et al., 1998). Symptomatic control of the diarrhea can be achieved with somatostatin analogues (Kraenzlin et al., 1985).

Tumor Type	Symptoms or signs	Incidence of metastases
Insulinoma	Hypoglycemia leading to confusion, visual disturbance, diaphoresis.	<15% (Vinik and Gonzales, 2011)
Gastrinoma (Zollinger-Ellison Syndrome)	Abdominal pain, diarrhea (secretory), recurrent peptic ulcer disease	50-85% (Batcher et al., 2011; Mittendorf et al., 2006)
Glucagonoma	Diabetes, necrotizing migratory erythema, cachexia, depression, deep vein thrombosis	75% (Batcher et al., 2011)
VIPoma, Verner-Morrison syndrome,WDHA syndrome	Watery diarrhea (secretory), hypokalemia	70-80% (Vinik and Gonzales, 2011)
Somatostatinoma	Cholelithiasis, steatorrhea, diabetes	80% (Vinik and Gonzales, 2011)
Non-functioning	Abdominal pain, weight loss, jaundice	60-85% (Vinik and Gonzales, 2011)

WDHA: Watery diarrhea, hypokalemia and achlorohydria

Table 2. Clinical manifestation of Pancreatic Neuroendocrine Tumors.

4. Biochemical testing in PNET

As majority of PNETs are non-functional, hormonal assays cannot be used for clinical assessment. Hence, serum chromogranin A (CgA) has come to represent a common denominator peptide with the putative ability to serve as a marker of disease activity, in both functional and non functional tumors. Granins are found as major components of the soluble core of dense secretory granules in neuroendocrine cells and are secreted in a physiologically regulated manner (Kim et al., 2001). Eight members have been identified including CgA, chromogranin B, chromogranin C, SgIII, SgIV, SgV, SgVI and VGF nerve growth factor-inducible. Granins have been proposed as playing important roles in secretory granule formation and development. CgA was the initial member identified, and originally detected in the chromaffin granules of the adrenal medulla (Blaschko et al., 1967). Although the definitive function of CgA remains unclear, CgA derived peptides mediate a number of biologic functions including regulation of parathyroid hormone secretion, carbohydrate metabolism, lipid metabolism and catecholamine secretion etc (Lawrence et al., 2011b).

Serum concentrations of CgA may decrease in patients responding to somatostatin analogs or other therapies. CgA should be used with caution as a marker of disease activity in patients treated with somatostatin analogs, because these agents significantly reduce plasma CgA levels which may falsely reflect any change in tumor size. Increased CgA concentrations assist in the clinical evaluation of PNETs but they are not specific for this kind of malignancy. Benign causes of CgA elevation should also be taken into consideration which include renal insufficiency, liver diseases and in patient taking proton pump inhibitors. Therefore, use of CgA as a diagnostic or screening test for PNET is discouraged.

5. Conventional imaging and Somatostatin Receptor Scintigraphy (SRS)

Although conventional imaging which include CT or MRI scans are usually employed in the initial diagnostic workup, they detect less than 50% of most PNETs that are less than 1 cm, therefore frequently missing small tumors (especially insulinomas, duodenal gastrinomas) and small liver metastases (Noone et al., 2005; Rockall and Reznek, 2007). Although, CT imaging with contrast is perhaps the most common initial imaging obtained, in certain clinical scenarios endoscopic ultrasound (EUS) paired with fine needle aspiration, remains the main endoscopic diagnostic technique. Several small studies reveal impressive diagnostic capability of this modality with reported sensitivity between 80% and 90% (De Angelis et al., 2011). EUS is much more effective for localizing intrapancreatic PNETs than extrapancreatic PNETs such as duodenal gastrinomas or somatostatinomas. Moreover, EUS is particularly helpful in localizing insulinomas, which are small, almost always intrapancreatic, and frequently missed by conventional imaging (Kulke et al., 2010a).

PNETs frequently overexpress somatostatin receptors and bind synthetic somatostatin analogues with high affinity. A number of radiolabeled analogues have been developed, with the most widely used worldwide and the only one available in the United States being ^{111}In-DTPA-octreotide (Octreoscan). SRS usually utilizes both planar imaging with either whole body scanning or multiple static acquisitions and single-photon computed tomography (SPECT). The latter modality can potentially improve the accuracy of SRS. This can allow SRS to detect up to 50% to 70% of primary PNETs and more than 90% of patients with metastatic disease. False-positive localizations can occur in up to 12% of patients, so it is important to interpret the results cautiously (Dabizzi et al., 2010; Kulke et al., 2010a) .

6. Role of surgery and liver directed therapy

The therapeutic plan of PNETs is based on the histologic classification and tumor stage. Surgery remains the cornerstone of treatment of early stage PNETs. Surgical resection of localized PNETs offers excellent prognosis and curative potential. Depending on the site and size, in the absence of distant metastases enucleation may be sufficient. This approach can easily be employed for many PNETs specially insulinomas, small non functioning PNETs (<2 cm) and small gastrinomas (Kulke et al., 2010a) . The long term survival in certain cases may exceed 90% (Service et al., 1991). Whipple pancreatoduodenectomy, left pancreatectomy or total pancreatectomy can offer a 5-year survival rates of 61%-79% even in some advanced cases (Dabizzi et al., 2010). The role of surgery in patients with MEN1 syndrome is complicated and remains controversial because the risk of additional neoplasms within the remaining pancreas and other sites (Demeure et al., 1991).

In patients with limited hepatic metastases, surgical hepatic resection may be feasible to debulk the tumor burden and help alleviate symptoms. Surgical resection of majority of the tumor is possible in only 5-15% of PNETs with hepatic metastases (Norton, 2005; Que et al., 2006). This approach can offer improvement in symptoms in over 90% of patients (Sarmiento and Que, 2003).Even though most of the evidence in this area is derived from uncontrolled studies, many agree that surgical resection should be attempted in malignant PNET with limited hepatic metastases if it is deemed possible that >90% of viable tumor can be removed (Kulke et al., 2010a).

In patients who are not candidates for surgical hepatic resection, hepatic arterial embolization remains a viable palliative approach. Important characteristics that are important for patient consideration is a preserved performance status , liver confined disease and a patent portal vein. Response rates are generally encouraging (>50%) as measured by either radiographic regression or hormonal secretion (Gupta et al., 2003; O'Toole and Ruszniewski, 2005; Toumpanakis et al., 2007). Although a number of techniques exist, including bland embolization, chemo-embolization or radioisotope-embolization, no data exist determining the superiority of one approach over another.

Other radiological approaches that can be employed in treating the hepatic metastases in malignant PNET, are radiofrequency ablation and cryoablation (Toumpanakis et al., 2007). These approaches may not be a feasible option in bulky hepatic disease and the benefit derived in small volume disease is also not clear. The advantage may be that these techniques seem to cause less morbidity. Therefore, careful patient selection is crucial to consider ablative techniques in order to avoid any unwarranted adverse effects.

7. Peptide Reception Radiation Technique (PRRT)

Majority of PNETs express somatostatin receptors, which provides a rationale for PRRT in selected cases. The most frequently used radionucleotides for PRRT are yttrium (^{90}Y) and lutetium (^{177}Lu), which have different physical and biological characteristics. One study reported encouraging results with 129 patients with malignant NETs treated with [^{177}Lu-DOTA-Tyr3]octreotate and resulted in a complete response in 2%, partial in 32%, and stabilization in 34% (Kwekkeboom et al., 2008). This form of treatment is generating widespread interest and more randomized studies are warranted in order to better explain its efficacy, role and toxicity.

8. Role of somatostatin analogs

The high expression of somatostatin receptors in PNETs also provides a rationale for utilizing somatostatin analogs for therapeutic purposes. In the PROMID study, which was a randomized, placebo-controlled, prospective trial in patients with midgut carcinoid, treatment with somatostatin analog octreotide was associated with improved time to progression over placebo (Rinke et al., 2009). Whether this hold true for PNETs, remains to be seen and is currently being explored in a number of ongoing studies. According to the National Comprehensive Cancer Network guidelines, somatostatin analogs should be considered in patients with hormone hypersecretion, although the authors do state that no randomized studies to date have demonstrated anti-tumor effect of somatostatin analogs in PNETs (Kulke, 2011). Octreotide 150-250 mcg subcutaneously three times a day or octreotide LAR 20-30 mg intramuscularly every 4 weeks can be considered for symptom control. Short acting octreotide can be added to octreotide LAR for treatment of breakthrough symptoms.

9. Cytotoxic chemotherapy

A number of chemotherapeutic agents have been tested in advanced metastatic PNETs, with encouraging results showing antitumor activity. Streptozocin was approved by the FDA in July, 1982 as a treatment for advanced PNET after initial studies showed sufficient antitumor effect and response rates. A number of studies by Moertel et al in the 1970's were crucial in this area. One trial randomized 84 patients to either streptozocin alone or streptozocin and fluorouracil. Based on non-standard criteria, 63% of patients were reported to have a response to therapy, with 33% complete responses in the combination arm (Moertel et al., 1980). Other combinations that have been evaluated are streptozocin/doxorubicin or streptozocin/doxorubicin/fluorouracil (Kulke et al., 2010a; Moertel et al., 1992). Treatment with streptozocin and doxorubicin was associated in a combined radiological and biochemical response rate of 69% with a median survival approaching 2 years (Moertel et al., 1992). Based on retrospective data, the 3-drug regimen of streptozocin, 5-fluorouracil, and doxorubicin is associated with an overall response rate of 39% and a median survival duration of 37 months (Kouvaraki et al., 2004) .The combination of 5-fluorouracil, Cisplatin and streptozocin was tested in a series of 82 patients with advanced neuroendocrine tumor, prospectively identified from a database .Sixty percent of patients in this series were identified to have a pancreatic primary. Although, limited by a number of weaknesses in the study, the investigators reported a response rate of 38% in PNETs (Turner et al., 2010). Patients with advanced poorly differentiated PNETs should be treated along the small cell carcinoma guidelines with therapy based on platinum regimens. This approach has been shown to result in a response rate of 40 to 70% (Kulke et al., 2010a). Although, these data support the antitumor activity of streptozocin based regimens, the acceptability of this approach has been limited because of a cumbersome administration schedule and toxicity profile.

Temozolomide has been combined with other biological agents such as thalidomide, bevacizumab and everolimus is phase II studies, yielding a response rate from 24-45% (Kulke et al., 2010b; Kulke et al., 2006a; Kulke et al., 2006b). Moreover, the combination of temozolomide and capecitabine has been reported to have an objective response rate of 70% (Strosberg et al., 2011) .There is also evidence to suggest that 0^6-methylguanine DNA methyltransferase (MGMT) deficiency can predict treatment responses to temozolomide in PNETs (Kulke et al., 2009b). Considering the available data, temozolomide based treatment has comparable efficacy to streptozocin based therapies with favorable toxicity profile. Further larger trials are warranted to further elaborate the role of temozolomide in the context of modern treatment paradigm in PNET.

10. Biologically targeted therapies

Recently, a number of studies have demonstrated activity in PNETs, targeting the vascular endothelial growth factor (VEGF) signaling and the mammalian target of rapamycin (mTOR) pathways. Although, obejective responses have been persistently low across studies, improvements in progression free survival have been encouraging.

10.1 Targeting VEGF pathway

PNETs are characterized by upregulation of VEGF and VEGF receptor (VEGFR). This correlates with increased angiogenesis, metastases and can potentially lead to decreased progression free survival (Zhang et al., 2007). Tyrosine kinase inhibitors with activity against VEGFR, such as pazopanib, sorafenib and sunitinib, have been evaluated in advanced PNET demonstrating encouraging results. Pazopanib was evaluated in a multi-instituion phase II study treating a total of 51 patients , 29 of which had PNET. Patients received pazopanib 800 mg daily, in addition to octerotide LAR. The response rate among patients with PNETs was reported to be 17%. Median PFS was reported to be 11.7 months. Grade 3/4 toxicities were relatively rare and included anemia, neutropenia, hypertriglyceridemia and liver function derangement (Phan et al., 2010). Another phase II trial is evaluating the role of pazopanib in patients with neuroendocrine tumors who may have had treatment with antiangiogenic and mTOR inhibitors. The trial is currently accruing and is expected to complete accrual in September 2011 (Capdevila et al., 2011). Sorafenib, another small molecule tyrosine kinase inhibitor, was evaluated in a phase II study that included 43 patients with PNET. Patients received sorafenib 400 mg twice daily. In a preliminary analysis, 10% of patients with PNET were observed to have a partial response (Hobday et al., 2007).

Sunitinib was evaluated in a multi-institutional phase II study that included 66 patients with PNET. Patients were treated with repeated 6 week cycles of oral sunitinib (50 mg/d) for 4 weeks followed by 2 weeks off treatment. Overall, objective response rate in PNET was observed to be 16.7% . One-year survival rate was reported to be 81% in the PNET group (Kulke et al., 2008). Based on encouraging results from this study, a phase III trial to confirm the activity of sunitinib was undertaken. Patients were randomized to receive once daily oral sunitinib at a dose of 37.5 mg or matching placebo. After enrollment of 171 patients, the data safety monitoring committee recommended the discontinuation of study and accrual was stopped before the preplanned efficacy analysis. The discontinuation of the study precluded definitive hypothesis testing for progression free survival difference between the two arms. An analysis of the enrolled patients, 86 of whom received sunitinib and 85 of whom received placebo, showed that the median progression free survival was significantly longer with sunitinib compared to placebo (11.4 months vs. 5.5 months ; hazard ratio= 0.42; $p < 0.001$). The objective response rate was 9.3% in the sunitinib group vs. 0% in the placebo group. At the data cut off point, the hazard ratio of death was 0.41 (95% CI, 0.19-0.89; P=0.02), with 10% of deaths reported in the sunitinib arm compared with 25% of deaths reported in the placebo arm (Raymond et al., 2011a). Grade 3/4 adverse events were uncommon in the treatment arm with the most common being neutropenia (12%) and hypertension (10%). Updated results, however, showed continued favorable trend for overall survival in the sunitinib arm but without statistical significance, with a hazard ratio of 0.737 (95% CI 0.465- 1.168; p=0.1926) (Raymond et al., 2011b). Based on this trial, FDA approved sunitinib for advanced PNET in May, 2011.

10.2 Targeting mTOR pathway

mTOR is an intracellular protein kinase which regulates cellular response to nutrients and energy in addition to mediating signaling through downstream growth factors such as insulin-like growth factor (IGF-1).Sporadic neuroendocrine tumors are known to co-express both IGF-1 and its receptor. There is in vitro evidence suggesting stimulation of mTOR pathway and inhibition of this pathway has demonstrated tumor regression in preclinical models (von Wichert et al., 2000; Yao, 2007). Temsirolimus and everolimus are rapamycin derivatives that have been tested in PNET. Temsirolimus was evaluated in a phase II clinical trial in advanced neuroendocrine tumors which included 15 patients with PNET. Partial response rate of 6.7% was observed in the PNET patient population (Duran et al., 2006). In an initial phase 2 study the combination of everolimus and octerotide was evaluated, reporting a partial response of 27% in patients with PNET (Yao et al., 2008b). The activity of everoliumus was subsequently evaluated in an international phase II multicenter trial (RADIANT-1). A total of 160 patients with advanced PNET were enrolled into the study. In this non randomized study, treatment with everolimus was associated with an overall response rate of 4.4% and progression free survival duration of 16.7 months in patients receiving concomitant octerotide. In patients not receiving octerotide, the response rate was 9.6% and progression free survival duration was 9.7 months (Yao et al., 2010a). This was followed by an international phase III randomized clinical trial (RADIANT 3) assigning 410 patients to receive treatment with everolimus or placebo. Everolimus was administered as 10 mg once daily, in conjunction with best supportive care. Octreotide was given at the discretion of the investigator. More than 80% of patients had well differentiated disease and more than 90% had metastases to liver. The median progression free survival as assessed by the local investigator was 11 months in the everolimus group as compared to 4.6 months in the placebo arm (hazard ratio 0.35; 95% CI 0.27-0.45; p<0.001). Grade 3/4 adverse events were rare in the treatment group which included anemia (6%) and hyperglycemia (5%). The overall tumor response rate associated with everolimus in this study was 5% (Yao et al., 2011). Based on this trial, the FDA approved everolimus for advanced PNET in May, 2011.

11. Combination strategies

Strategies to combine biological agents have begun in patients with advanced PNET. In a phase II trial, the combination of everolimus and bevacizumab was recently shown to be well tolerated and associated with an overall response rate of 26% in low to intermediate grade neuroendocrine tumors (Yao et al., 2010b). CALGB 80701 is currently randomizing patients with advanced PNET to receive either treatment with everolimus or everolimus + bevacizumab, to asses efficacy and toxicity. This trial will hopefully shed more light on the role for combination strategy in the treatment armamentarium for PNET.

12. Conclusions

PNETs are a heterogeneous group of rare tumors with a wide range of biological activity, manifestation and variable prognosis. Accurate clinical, pathologic and histologic diagnosis is an important first step in developing an appropriate management plan. PNETs should be considered separately from carcinoid tumors as they are dissimilar in clinical behavior, response to treatment and prognosis. Surgical resection remains the mainstay of treatment for early stage disease. Advanced PNET often requires a multidisciplinary approach. Options for advanced stage include liver directed therapies including surgery and radioembolization techniques. Systemic treatment option include somatostatin analogs for symptom control, cytotoxic chemotherapy (temozolomide or streptozocin based regimens) and molecularly targeted agents (sunitinib and everolimus). No specific treatment sequence currently exists. Future studies will provide more insight into combination strategies and expand our treatment options for patients with this disease.

13. References

Agarwal, S.K., Lee Burns, A., Sukhodolets, K.E., Kennedy, P.A., Obungu, V.H., Hickman, A.B., Mullendore, M.E., Whitten, I., Skarulis, M.C., Simonds, W.F., *et al.* (2004). Molecular pathology of the MEN1 gene. Ann N Y Acad Sci *1014*, 189-198.

Asa, S.L. (2011). Pancreatic endocrine tumors. Mod Pathol *24 Suppl 2*, S66-77.

Batcher, E., Madaj, P., and Gianoukakis, A.G. (2011). Pancreatic neuroendocrine tumors. Endocr Res *36*, 35-43.

Blaschko, H., Comline, R.S., Schneider, F.H., Silver, M., and Smith, A.D. (1967). Secretion of a chromaffin granule protein, chromogranin, from the adrenal gland after splanchnic stimulation. Nature *215*, 58-59.

Capdevila, J., Teule, A., Castellano, D.E., Sastre, J., Garcia-Carbonero, R., Sevilla, I., Duran, I., Escudero, P., Fuster, J., and Grande Pulido, E. (2011). PAZONET: A phase II trial of pazopanib in patients with metastatic neuroendocrine tumors (NETs) who may have previously received antiangiogenic or mTOR treatment. J Clin Oncol 29: 2011 (suppl; abstr TPS171).

Chastain, M.A. (2001). The glucagonoma syndrome: a review of its features and discussion of new perspectives. Am J Med Sci *321*, 306-320.

Dabizzi, E., Panossian, A., and Raimondo, M. (2010). Management of pancreatic neuroendocrine tumors. Minerva Gastroenterol Dietol *56*, 467-479.

De Angelis, C., Pellicano, R., Rizzetto, M., and Repici, A. (2011). Role of endoscopy in the management of gastroenteropancreatic neuroendocrine tumours. Minerva Gastroenterol Dietol *57*, 129-137.

Demeure, M.J., Klonoff, D.C., Karam, J.H., Duh, Q.Y., and Clark, O.H. (1991). Insulinomas associated with multiple endocrine neoplasia type I: the need for a different surgical approach. Surgery *110*, 998-1004; discussion 1004-1005.

Duran, I., Kortmansky, J., Singh, D., Hirte, H., Kocha, W., Goss, G., Le, L., Oza, A., Nicklee, T., Ho, J., *et al.* (2006). A phase II clinical and pharmacodynamic study of temsirolimus in advanced neuroendocrine carcinomas. Br J Cancer *95*, 1148-1154.

Edge, S.B., and Compton, C.C. (2010). The American Joint Committee on Cancer: the 7th edition of the AJCC cancer staging manual and the future of TNM. Ann Surg Oncol *17*, 1471-1474.

Goode, P.N., Farndon, J.R., Anderson, J., Johnston, I.D., and Morte, J.A. (1986). Diazoxide in the management of patients with insulinoma. World J Surg *10*, 586-592.

Gupta, S., Yao, J.C., Ahrar, K., Wallace, M.J., Morello, F.A., Madoff, D.C., Murthy, R., Hicks, M.E., and Ajani, J.A. (2003). Hepatic artery embolization and chemoembolization for treatment of patients with metastatic carcinoid tumors: the M.D. Anderson experience. Cancer J *9*, 261-267.

Hobday, T.J., Rubin, J., Holen, K., Picus, J., Donehower, R., Marschke, R., Maples, W., Lloyd, R., Mahoney, M., and C., E. (2007). MC044h, a phase II trial of sorafenib in patients (pts) with metastatic neuroendocrine tumors (NET): A Phase II Consortium (P2C) study. Journal of Clinical Oncology, 2007 ASCO Annual Meeting Proceedings Part I Vol 25, No 18S (June 20 Supplement), 2007: 4504.

Howard, T.J., Stabile, B.E., Zinner, M.J., Chang, S., Bhagavan, B.S., and Passaro, E., Jr. (1990). Anatomic distribution of pancreatic endocrine tumors. Am J Surg *159*, 258-264.

Jensen, R.T. (1996). Gastrointestinal endocrine tumours. Gastrinoma. Baillieres Clin Gastroenterol *10*, 603-643.

Jockenhovel, F., Lederbogen, S., Olbricht, T., Schmidt-Gayk, H., Krenning, E.P., Lamberts, S.W., and Reinwein, D. (1994). The long-acting somatostatin analogue octreotide alleviates symptoms by reducing posttranslational conversion of prepro-glucagon to glucagon in a patient with malignant glucagonoma, but does not prevent tumor growth. Clin Investig *72*, 127-133.

Kim, T., Tao-Cheng, J.H., Eiden, L.E., and Loh, Y.P. (2001). Chromogranin A, an "on/off" switch controlling dense-core secretory granule biogenesis. Cell *106*, 499-509.

Kloppel, G., Perren, A., and Heitz, P.U. (2004). The gastroenteropancreatic neuroendocrine cell system and its tumors: the WHO classification. Ann N Y Acad Sci *1014*, 13-27.

Kouvaraki, M.A., Ajani, J.A., Hoff, P., Wolff, R., Evans, D.B., Lozano, R., and Yao, J.C. (2004). Fluorouracil, doxorubicin, and streptozocin in the treatment of patients with locally advanced and metastatic pancreatic endocrine carcinomas. J Clin Oncol *22*, 4762-4771.

Kraenzlin, M.E., Ch'ng, J.L., Wood, S.M., Carr, D.H., and Bloom, S.R. (1985). Long-term treatment of a VIPoma with somatostatin analogue resulting in remission of symptoms and possible shrinkage of metastases. Gastroenterology *88*, 185-187.

Kulke, M.H. (2011). National Comprehensive Cancer Network guidelines: Neuroendocrine Tumors.

Kulke, M.H., Anthony, L.B., Bushnell, D.L., de Herder, W.W., Goldsmith, S.J., Klimstra, D.S., Marx, S.J., Pasieka, J.L., Pommier, R.F., Yao, J.C., *et al.* (2010a). NANETS treatment guidelines: well-differentiated neuroendocrine tumors of the stomach and pancreas. Pancreas *39*, 735-752.

Kulke, M.H., Bendell, J., Kvols, L., Picus, J., Pommier, R., and Yao, J. (2011). Evolving diagnostic and treatment strategies for pancreatic neuroendocrine tumors. J Hematol Oncol *4*, 29.

Kulke, M.H., Bergsland, E.K., and Yao, J.C. (2009a). Glycemic control in patients with insulinoma treated with everolimus. N Engl J Med *360*, 195-197.

Kulke, M.H., Blaszkowsky, L., Zhu, A., and al., e. (2010b). Phase I/II study of everolimus (RAD001) in combination with temozolomide (TMZ) in patients with advanced pancreatic neuroendocrine tumors. 2010 Gastrointestinal Cancer Symposium.

Kulke, M.H., Hornick, J.L., Frauenhoffer, C., Hooshmand, S., Ryan, D.P., Enzinger, P.C., Meyerhardt, J.A., Clark, J.W., Stuart, K., Fuchs, C.S., *et al.* (2009b). O6-methylguanine

DNA methyltransferase deficiency and response to temozolomide-based therapy in patients with neuroendocrine tumors. Clin Cancer Res *15*, 338-345.

Kulke, M.H., Lenz, H.J., Meropol, N.J., Posey, J., Ryan, D.P., Picus, J., Bergsland, E., Stuart, K., Tye, L., Huang, X., *et al.* (2008). Activity of sunitinib in patients with advanced neuroendocrine tumors. J Clin Oncol *26*, 3403-3410.

Kulke, M.H., Stuart, K., Earle, C., and al., e. (2006a). A phase II study of temozolomide and bevacizumab in patients with advanced neuroendocrine tumors. J Clin Oncol *24*, suppl; abstr 4044.

Kulke, M.H., Stuart, K., Enzinger, P.C., Ryan, D.P., Clark, J.W., Muzikansky, A., Vincitore, M., Michelini, A., and Fuchs, C.S. (2006b). Phase II study of temozolomide and thalidomide in patients with metastatic neuroendocrine tumors. J Clin Oncol *24*, 401-406.

Kwekkeboom, D.J., de Herder, W.W., Kam, B.L., van Eijck, C.H., van Essen, M., Kooij, P.P., Feelders, R.A., van Aken, M.O., and Krenning, E.P. (2008). Treatment with the radiolabeled somatostatin analog [177 Lu-DOTA 0,Tyr3]octreotate: toxicity, efficacy, and survival. J Clin Oncol *26*, 2124-2130.

Lambers, C.B., Lind, T., Moberg, S., Jansen, J.B., and Olbe, L. (1984). Omeprazole in Zollinger-Ellison syndrome. Effects of a single dose and of long-term treatment in patients resistant to histamine H2-receptor antagonists. N Engl J Med *310*, 758-761.

Lawrence, B., Gustafsson, B.I., Chan, A., Svejda, B., Kidd, M., and Modlin, I.M. (2011a). The epidemiology of gastroenteropancreatic neuroendocrine tumors. Endocrinol Metab Clin North Am *40*, 1-18, vii.

Lawrence, B., Gustafsson, B.I., Kidd, M., Pavel, M., Svejda, B., and Modlin, I.M. (2011b). The clinical relevance of chromogranin A as a biomarker for gastroenteropancreatic neuroendocrine tumors. Endocrinol Metab Clin North Am *40*, 111-134, viii.

Massironi, S., Sciola, V., Peracchi, M., Ciafardini, C., Spampatti, M.P., and Conte, D. (2008). Neuroendocrine tumors of the gastro-entero-pancreatic system. World J Gastroenterol *14*, 5377-5384.

Mathur, A., Gorden, P., and Libutti, S.K. (2009). Insulinoma. Surg Clin North Am *89*, 1105-1121.

Metz, D.C., and Jensen, R.T. (2008). Gastrointestinal neuroendocrine tumors: pancreatic endocrine tumors. Gastroenterology *135*, 1469-1492.

Mittendorf, E.A., Shifrin, A.L., Inabnet, W.B., Libutti, S.K., McHenry, C.R., and Demeure, M.J. (2006). Islet cell tumors. Curr Probl Surg *43*, 685-765.

Modlin, I.M., Oberg, K., Chung, D.C., Jensen, R.T., de Herder, W.W., Thakker, R.V., Caplin, M., Delle Fave, G., Kaltsas, G.A., Krenning, E.P., *et al.* (2008). Gastroenteropancreatic neuroendocrine tumours. Lancet Oncol *9*, 61-72.

Moertel, C.G., Hanley, J.A., and Johnson, L.A. (1980). Streptozocin alone compared with streptozocin plus fluorouracil in the treatment of advanced islet-cell carcinoma. N Engl J Med *303*, 1189-1194.

Moertel, C.G., Lefkopoulo, M., Lipsitz, S., Hahn, R.G., and Klaassen, D. (1992). Streptozocin-doxorubicin, streptozocin-fluorouracil or chlorozotocin in the treatment of advanced islet-cell carcinoma. N Engl J Med *326*, 519-523.

Nikfarjam, M., Warshaw, A.L., Axelrod, L., Deshpande, V., Thayer, S.P., Ferrone, C.R., and Fernandez-del Castillo, C. (2008). Improved contemporary surgical management of insulinomas: a 25-year experience at the Massachusetts General Hospital. Ann Surg *247*, 165-172.

Noone, T.C., Hosey, J., Firat, Z., and Semelka, R.C. (2005). Imaging and localization of islet-cell tumours of the pancreas on CT and MRI. Best Pract Res Clin Endocrinol Metab *19*, 195-211.

Norton, J.A. (2005). Endocrine tumours of the gastrointestinal tract. Surgical treatment of neuroendocrine metastases. Best Pract Res Clin Gastroenterol *19*, 577-583.

O'Toole, D., and Ruszniewski, P. (2005). Chemoembolization and other ablative therapies for liver metastases of gastrointestinal endocrine tumours. Best Pract Res Clin Gastroenterol *19*, 585-594.

Perry, R.R., and Vinik, A.I. (1995). Clinical review 72: diagnosis and management of functioning islet cell tumors. J Clin Endocrinol Metab *80*, 2273-2278.

Phan, A.T., Yao, J.C., Fogelman, D.R., Hess, K.R., Ng, C.S., Bullock, S.A., Malinowski, P., Regan, E., and M.H., K. (2010). A prospective, multi-institutional phase II study of GW786034 (pazopanib) and depot octreotide (sandostatin LAR) in advanced low-grade neuroendocrine carcinoma (LGNEC). J Clin Oncol 28:15s, 2010 (suppl; abstr 4001).

Que, F.G., Sarmiento, J.M., and Nagorney, D.M. (2006). Hepatic surgery for metastatic gastrointestinal neuroendocrine tumors. Adv Exp Med Biol *574*, 43-56.

Raymond, E., Dahan, L., Raoul, J.L., Bang, Y.J., Borbath, I., Lombard-Bohas, C., Valle, J., Metrakos, P., Smith, D., Vinik, A., *et al.* (2011a). Sunitinib malate for the treatment of pancreatic neuroendocrine tumors. N Engl J Med *364*, 501-513.

Raymond, E., Niccoli, P., Raoul, J., Bang, Y., Borbath, I., Lombard-Bohas, C., Valle, J.W., Metrakos, P., Smith, D., Vinik, A., *et al.* (2011b). Updated overall survival (OS) and progression-free survival (PFS) by blinded independent central review (BICR) of sunitinib (SU) versus placebo (PBO) for patients (Pts) with advanced unresectable pancreatic neuroendocrine tumors (NET). J Clin Oncol 29: 2011 (suppl; abstr 4008).

Rindi, G., and Kloppel, G. (2004). Endocrine tumors of the gut and pancreas tumor biology and classification. Neuroendocrinology *80 Suppl 1*, 12-15.

Rinke, A., Muller, H.H., Schade-Brittinger, C., Klose, K.J., Barth, P., Wied, M., Mayer, C., Aminossadati, B., Pape, U.F., Blaker, M., *et al.* (2009). Placebo-controlled, double-blind, prospective, randomized study on the effect of octreotide LAR in the control of tumor growth in patients with metastatic neuroendocrine midgut tumors: a report from the PROMID Study Group. J Clin Oncol *27*, 4656-4663.

Rockall, A.G., and Reznek, R.H. (2007). Imaging of neuroendocrine tumours (CT/MR/US). Best Pract Res Clin Endocrinol Metab *21*, 43-68.

Sarmiento, J.M., and Que, F.G. (2003). Hepatic surgery for metastases from neuroendocrine tumors. Surg Oncol Clin N Am *12*, 231-242.

Service, F.J., McMahon, M.M., O'Brien, P.C., and Ballard, D.J. (1991). Functioning insulinoma--incidence, recurrence, and long-term survival of patients: a 60-year study. Mayo Clin Proc *66*, 711-719.

Shojamanesh, H., Gibril, F., Louie, A., Ojeaburu, J.V., Bashir, S., Abou-Saif, A., and Jensen, R.T. (2002). Prospective study of the antitumor efficacy of long-term octreotide treatment in patients with progressive metastatic gastrinoma. Cancer *94*, 331-343.

Smith, S.L., Branton, S.A., Avino, A.J., Martin, J.K., Klingler, P.J., Thompson, G.B., Grant, C.S., and van Heerden, J.A. (1998). Vasoactive intestinal polypeptide secreting islet cell tumors: a 15-year experience and review of the literature. Surgery *124*, 1050-1055.

Strosberg, J.R., Fine, R.L., Choi, J., Nasir, A., Coppola, D., Chen, D.T., Helm, J., and Kvols, L. (2011). First-line chemotherapy with capecitabine and temozolomide in patients with metastatic pancreatic endocrine carcinomas. Cancer *117*, 268-275.

Toumpanakis, C., Meyer, T., and Caplin, M.E. (2007). Cytotoxic treatment including embolization/chemoembolization for neuroendocrine tumours. Best Pract Res Clin Endocrinol Metab *21,* 131-144.

Turner, N.C., Strauss, S.J., Sarker, D., Gillmore, R., Kirkwood, A., Hackshaw, A., Papadopoulou, A., Bell, J., Kayani, I., Toumpanakis, C., *et al.* (2010). Chemotherapy with 5-fluorouracil, cisplatin and streptozocin for neuroendocrine tumours. Br J Cancer *102,* 1106-1112.

Verner, J.V., and Morrison, A.B. (1958). Islet cell tumor and a syndrome of refractory watery diarrhea and hypokalemia. Am J Med *25,* 374-380.

Vinik, A.I., and Gonzales, M.R. (2011). New and emerging syndromes due to neuroendocrine tumors. Endocrinol Metab Clin North Am *40,* 19-63, vii.von Wichert, G., Jehle, P.M., Hoeflich, A., Koschnick, S., Dralle, H., Wolf, E., Wiedenmann, B., Boehm, B.O., Adler, G., and Seufferlein, T. (2000). Insulin-like growth factor-I is an autocrine regulator of chromogranin A secretion and growth in human neuroendocrine tumor cells. Cancer Res *60,* 4573-4581.

Warner, R.R. (2005). Enteroendocrine tumors other than carcinoid: a review of clinically significant advances. Gastroenterology *128,* 1668-1684.

Whipple, A.O., and Frantz, V.K. (1935). Adenoma of Islet Cells with Hyperinsulinism: A Review. Ann Surg *101,* 1299-1335.

Yao, J.C. (2007). Neuroendocrine tumors. Molecular targeted therapy for carcinoid and islet-cell carcinoma. Best Pract Res Clin Endocrinol Metab *21,* 163-172.

Yao, J.C., Hassan, M., Phan, A., Dagohoy, C., Leary, C., Mares, J.E., Abdalla, E.K., Fleming, J.B., Vauthey, J.N., Rashid, A., *et al.* (2008a). One hundred years after "carcinoid": epidemiology of and prognostic factors for neuroendocrine tumors in 35,825 cases in the United States. J Clin Oncol *26,* 3063-3072.

Yao, J.C., Lombard-Bohas, C., Baudin, E., Kvols, L.K., Rougier, P., Ruszniewski, P., Hoosen, S., St Peter, J., Haas, T., Lebwohl, D., *et al.* (2010a). Daily oral everolimus activity in patients with metastatic pancreatic neuroendocrine tumors after failure of cytotoxic chemotherapy: a phase II trial. J Clin Oncol *28,* 69-76.

Yao, J.C., Phan, A.T., Chang, D.Z., Wolff, R.A., Hess, K., Gupta, S., Jacobs, C., Mares, J.E., Landgraf, A.N., Rashid, A., *et al.* (2008b). Efficacy of RAD001 (everolimus) and octreotide LAR in advanced low- to intermediate-grade neuroendocrine tumors: results of a phase II study. J Clin Oncol *26,* 4311-4318.

Yao, J.C., Phan, A.T., Fogleman, D., Ng, C.S., Jacobs, C.B., C.D., D., Leary, C., and Hess, K.R. (2010b). Randomized run-in study of bevacizumab (B) and everolimus (E) in low- to intermediate-grade neuroendocrine tumors (LGNETs) using perfusion CT as functional biomarker. J Clin Oncol 28:15s, 2010 (suppl; abstr 4002).

Yao, J.C., Shah, M.H., Ito, T., Bohas, C.L., Wolin, E.M., Van Cutsem, E., Hobday, T.J., Okusaka, T., Capdevila, J., de Vries, E.G., *et al.* (2011). Everolimus for advanced pancreatic neuroendocrine tumors. N Engl J Med *364,* 514-523.

Zhang, J., Jia, Z., Li, Q., Wang, L., Rashid, A., Zhu, Z., Evans, D.B., Vauthey, J.N., Xie, K., and Yao, J.C. (2007). Elevated expression of vascular endothelial growth factor correlates with increased angiogenesis and decreased progression-free survival among patients with low-grade neuroendocrine tumors. Cancer *109,* 1478-1486.

18

Generation and Impact of Neural Invasion in Pancreatic Cancer

Ihsan Ekin Demir, Helmut Friess and Güralp O. Ceyhan
Department of Surgery, Klinikum rechts der Isar, Technische Universität München, Munich, Germany

1. Introduction

Pancreatic cancer (PCa) as one of the most aggressive malignancies of mankind has an unparallelled propensity to invade intrapancreatic nerves. This "neural invasion" is therefore one of the most frequent routes of spread in PCa in addition to lymphatic and vascular paths. The major clinical relevance of neural invasion (NI) has triggered intense research efforts to understand its pathomechanims, and the findings derived from all these studies show how multi-faceted this peculiar route of cancer invasion in PCa is. This chapter is devoted to a thorough description of the characteristics, the pathomechanism and the clinical impact of NI in PCa, with the discussion of the most important pathways which may be future targets for therapeutic intervention.

2. What is "neural invasion" in pancreatic cancer?

NI is a relatively new and more comprehensive term for the traditionally used description "perineural invasion". In several malignancies, e.g. in the prostate, head and neck, but also several gastrointestinal malignancies, cancer cells are commonly encountered around nerves (Liebig et al., 2009). The frequent presence of cancer cells along the perineurium, the protective sheet around neural fascicles, has hence made pathologists adopt the term "perineural invasion". Classically, cancer cells which penetrate through the epineurium come to lie between the epineurium and the underlying perineurium and "push" on the nerve fascicles within the constrained intraneural area. The earliest report on perineural invasion stems from Cruveilheir in 1835 where he noticed that cancer cells can actually extend along the invaded nerves (Demir et al., 2010). Interestingly, although pathologists frequently observed perineural invasion in several types of tumors, its role except for serving as an additional path of cancer spread has not been genuinely investigated and understood until 1990s. In his pioneering article on the ultrastructural features of perineural invasion in PCa, Dale Bockman from Augusta, Georgia, USA performed an electron microscopic analysis of invaded nerves in PCa (Bockman et al., 1994). There, he noted that, in contrast with the traditional assumption, PCa cells penetrate through the perineurium and become intimately associated with the interior of nerve fascicles, i.e. axons and Schwann cells (Bockman et al., 1994). These observations made by Bockman during mid-1990s laid the foundation for our understanding and the subsequent research on NI in PCa into the present time.

It should be noted that NI is often used to denote invasion of intrapancreatic nerves (Liu&Lu, 2002). However, it is at the same time a more comprehensive term for intra- as well as extrapancreatic nerve invasion (Bockman et al., 1994; Takahashi et al., 1997; Takahashi et al., 2001; Mitsunaga et al., 2007). In contrast with their European counterparts, several studies from the Far East were devoted to the study of extrapancreatic nerve invasion through collection of specimens from retro- and peripancreatic nerves during autopsy (Nakao et al., 1996; Takahashi et al., 1997; Hirai et al., 2002; Liu&Lu, 2002; Mitsunaga et al., 2007). In those studies, "extrapancreatic nerve invasion" is often used synonymously with NI (Nakao et al., 1996; Takahashi et al., 1997; Hirai et al., 2002; Liu&Lu, 2002; Mitsunaga et al., 2007).

3. What are the specific histological characteristics of NI in PCa?

A review of scientific literature on NI in PCa reveals that NI has mostly been perceived as the presence of PCa on and along the perineurium (Kayahara et al., 2007; Liebig et al., 2009). Recent studies, however, revealed that PCa cells are readily encountered in the endoneural area, i.e. between nerve fascicles, as originally observed by Bockman (Ceyhan et al., 2009). Consequently, subsequent studies applied a scoring system to describe the degree of penetration of PCa cells into intrapancreatic nerves, classifying NI into "no invasion" (score of 0/zero), "perineural invasion" (score of I/one) and "endoneural invasion" (score of II/two) (Ceyhan et al., 2006; Ceyhan et al., 2009; Ceyhan et al., 2011). Importantly, the presence of PCa cells in the interior of nerves should not necessarily be perceived as the invasion of the "endoneurium" which is the connective tissue within nerve fascicles of a nerve. Similarly, invasion around nerves does not directly imply invasion of the "perineurium" as the connective tissue layer encircling nerve fascicles. Rather, "endo-" and "perineural" stand for "between" or "around" nerve fascicles (Figure 1) (Ceyhan et al., 2009; Ceyhan et al., 2011).

Careful examination of PCa tissue specimens also reveals that the presence of NI is not independent of the localization of the nerves within the pancreatic tissue. Particularly, we could demonstrate that NI in ductal adenocarcinoma of the pancreas is detected more frequently in areas with severe desmoplasia (Ceyhan et al., 2009). The reasons for this association between desmoplasia and NI are so far not known. However, it is assumed that the extracellular matrix is a rich source of growth factors which may be trophic upon nerves (Zhu et al., 1999; Demir et al., 2010). Still, NI should not be assumed to be limited to desmoplastic areas. In a histopathological study on the normal pancreatic regions of PCa patients who underwent pancreatic resection, NI was also encountered in normal pancreatic areas which are distant from the actual tumor (Takahashi et al., 1997). In the original study, this type of NI termed "nex" was found in more than 50% of resected pancreatic specimens and correlated to the grade of intrapancreatic neural invasion or the presence of extrapancreatic neural plexus invasion (Takahashi et al., 1997). Moreover, its presence was also found to correlate to worse survival after removal of the tumor (Takahashi et al., 1997). Therefore, the presence of NI in the supposedly normal regions of the pancreas implies that NI is a rapidly progressive process where PCa cells grow very early along intrapancreatic nerves.

The different histological appearances of NI in PCa have also been employed to understand its pathomechanism and spread pattern. In a study by Kayahara et al. (Kayahara et al.,

2007), the investigators analyzed consecutive sections of surgically resected PCa specimens in order to elucidate the main patterns of cancer cell growth along nerves: (1) direct invasion of the nerves, (2) continuous tumor cells growth in the perineural space, (3) branching of the growing tumor mass along neural branches, (4) formation of a foremost growth cone of tumor cells, and (5) direct invasion of contiguous lymph nodes (Kayahara et al., 2007). Hence, the authors could provide an anatomical mechanism for the manifestation of NI and particularly extrapancreatic neural plexus invasion. Importantly, their study proved the continuous growth of PCa cells along intrapancreatic nerves towards the extrapancreatic neural plexus (Kayahara et al., 2007).

4. Why is neural invasion so deciding in the course of PCa?

There are several factors which make NI a crucial aspect of PCa and an attractive field of research. First, NI has an utmost high prevalence in PCa, varying between 88% to 100% (Takahashi et al., 2001; Liu&Lu, 2002). Interestingly, according to a study by Kayahara et al., NI in PCa is significantly more common than in cancers which originate from direct anatomical neighbours of the pancreas, e.g. cancers of the distal bile duct or carcinoma of the papilla of Vater (Kayahara et al., 1991; Kayahara et al., 1993; Kayahara et al., 1994; Kayahara et al., 1995; Kayahara et al., 1996). Unfortunately, intrapancreatic NI is nearly always accompanied by invasion to the extrapancreatic neural plexus: In their series, Nakao et al detected intrapancreatic NI in 116 out of 129 (90%) patients, of whom 80 (69%) showed extrapancreatic nerve plexus involvement (Nakao et al., 1996). Based on these findings, it seems that clinicians should assume the presence of NI in every patient with PCa even if the pathology report does not include a statement regarding this histopathological feature.

In the face of such a high prevalence, NI is at the same time one of the foremost reasons for local tumor recurrence after curative tumor resection (Kayahara et al., 1991; Nagakawa et al., 1991; Kayahara et al., 1995; Kayahara et al., 1996; Nagakawa et al., 1996; Ozaki et al., 1999). In a study by Kayahara et al., the investigators analyzed the mode of recurrence in 30 patients who had originally undergone macroscopically curative resection (Kayahara et al., 1993; Liu&Lu, 2002). They showed that the rate of local retroperitoneal recurrence, i.e. the prevalence of extrapancreatic NI was 80%, of hepatic metastasis 66%, of peritoneal dissemination 53%, and of lymph node recurrence 47%, an observation which was confirmed by further antemortem studies (Kayahara et al., 1993; Kayahara et al., 1995; Liu&Lu, 2002). Among the several parts of the extrapancreatic neural plexus which demonstrate local tumor recurrence, pancreatic head plexus and splenic plexus are the most common sites of tumor recurrence (Liu&Lu, 2002). Based on the frequency of NI towards retropancreatic neural plexus, several surgeons advocated routine extended resections (including celiac plexus) or at least more aggressive surgery in the surgical treatment of PCa (Hiraoka et al., 1986; Nagakawa et al., 1991; Nagakawa et al., 1996; Imamura et al., 1999). However, subsequent clinical studies confirmed that, while extended resection - even in combination with radiotherapy- can contribute to local tumor control, there is no survival benefit for patients due to the early spread pattern of PCa (Bachmann et al., 2006; Takamori et al., 2008; Yokoyama&Nagino, 2011). However, these studies mostly concentrated on more extensive lymphadenectomy rather than plexus resection as the actual measure to reduce NI. In further newer studies (Hirano et al., ; Sperti et al., ; Kondo et al., 2001; Hirano et al., 2007; Chakravarty et al., 2011), the feasibility and safety of an en bloc resection including celiac artery, plexus and ganglia was demonstrated, but the actual survival beneift from this

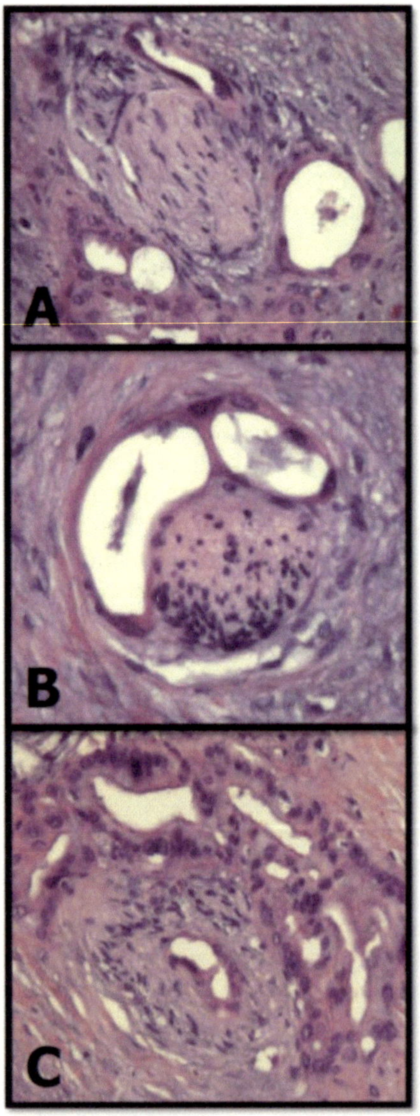

No neural invasion (score 0)

✓Intact epineurium
✓Cancer cells are often attached to the epineurium.
✓In several cases merely an „epineural association"

Perineural invasion (score I)

✓Epineural barrier not visible
✓Cancer cells are attached to the perineurium.
✓No contact of cancer cells with the endoneurium

Endoneural invasion (score II)

✓Cancer cells are encountered in the interior of the nerve, between nerve fascicles.
✓Neural integrity distorted

Fig. 1. Severity of neural invasion (NI) in pancreatic cancer (PCa). Examination of intrapancreatic nerves with NI reveals that PCa cells demonstrate varying degrees of interaction with the nerves. In many cases, PCa cells surround intrapancreatic nerves without breaching the epineural barrier (A, also termed epineural association). On the other hand, several nerves demonstrate a lack of the epineural barrier where pancreatic cancer cells surround the fascicles along their perineurium (B, perineural invasion). In most severe cases, PCa cells are encountered between nerve fascicles, along their endoneurium (C, endoneural invasion). There is a significant association between the severity of NI and the degree of pain sensation among PCa patients (please refer to the main text for the respective references). All images at 200x magnification.

radical operation remains to be demonstrated. Importantly, a common denominator of these studies on "en bloc" resection of retropancreatic neural plexus is the pronounced pain relief as a result of the resection of celiac plexus(Kondo et al., 2001; Hirano et al., 2007). This deciding association between extrapancreatic neural plexus and pain sensation builds up the link to the concept of "pancreatic neuropathy" in PCa which encompasses NI and several other neural alterations in PCa(Ceyhan et al., 2009), as explained in the following section.

5. Neural invasion as part of "pancreatic neuropathy" in PCa

The pancreas is one of the most densely innervated visceral organs(Bradley&Bem, 2003). The extrinsic component of its innervation is composed of nerve fibers running within the vagal and splanchnic nerves which originate from vagal nuclei or DRGs, respectively. Like the intestine, it also has an intrinsic innervation which is represented by intrapancreatic neurons. Importantly, enteric and intrapancreatic neurons are embryologically closely related: intrapancreatic neurons develop from a subgroup of neural crest-derived enteric nervous system (ENS) precursors and thus belong to the ENS (Kirchgessner&Gershon, 1990; Kirchgessner&Gershon, 1991). Moreover, there exists a direct innervation of the pancreas from the duodenum termed "entero-pancreatic innervations", as evidenced by the entrance of nerve fibers directly from the duodenal ENS into intrapancreatic ganglia (Kirchgessner&Gershon, 1990; Kirchgessner&Gershon, 1991).

In the currently most comprehensive systematic analysis of NI in PCa, our group aimed at the study of nerve morphology in 546 patients with different pancreatic tumors, including ductal adenocarcinoma, neuroendocrine tumors, intraductal papillary mucinous neoplasms (IPMN), serous and mucinous cystadenoma and other neoplasms of the pancreas (Ceyhan et al., 2009). In the mentioned study, we could demonstrate that ductal adenocarcinoma of the pancreas exhibits the highest degree of NI in comparison to all other pancreatic tumors (Ceyhan et al., 2009). Interestingly, ductal adenocarcinoma (PCa) also harbored an unparalleled degree of nerve alterations among all these tumors (Ceyhan et al., 2009). In particular, PCa was characterized by a prominently increased neural density, a pronounced neural hypertrophy and neural inflammatory cell infiltration ("pancreatic neuritis") (Ceyhan et al., 2006; Ceyhan et al., 2009). Moreover, we could also detect a key link between the severity of NI in PCa and the extent of intrapancreatic neuroplastic alterations: The more nerves and neural hypertrophy were present, the higher was the extent/severity of NI in PCa (Ceyhan et al., 2009).

This association between pancreatic neuroplasticity and NI gained a further dimension in a subsequent study where the pancreatic "innervation quality" in PCa was studied and compared to normal human pancreas (NP) (Ceyhan et al., 2009). Interestingly, not only had nerves in PCa tissue fewer sympathetic nerve fibers than in NP, but nerves with NI had at the same time reduced amounts of both sympathetic and cholinergic nerve fibers (Ceyhan et al., 2009). This "neural remodeling" in PCa implies that PCa cells may not be arbitrarily invading intrapancreatic nerves but also aiming at specific fiber qualities for so far unknown reasons. Overall, these neural alterations which seem to be specific for PCa, i.e. pancreatic neuroplasticity, neural remodeling and the high degree of NI, are the three hallmarks of so-called "pancreatic neuropathy" in PCa (Ceyhan et al., 2009).

While the mechanisms of these neuroplastic alterations are not completely understood, there is increasing evidence that these neuropathic alterations in PCa can in part be attributed to the neurotrophic character of the tumor microenvironment in PCa (Demir et al., 2010). In a novel *in vitro* neuroplasticity assay, we could demonstrate that tissue extracts of PCa, PCa cell supernatants and supernatants of human pancreatic stellate cells as main generators of desmoplasia can all induce axonal sprouting, increased neurite density and perikaryonal hypertrophy of neurons isolated from dorsal root ganglia or myenteric plecus under *in vitro* conditions (Demir et al., 2010). In a very recent study, Li et al. added a novel dimension to our understanding of neural alterations in PCa: In accordance with their former hypothesis (Li&Ma, 2008), patients with hyperglycemia demonstrate more pronounced neural hypertrophy and increased neural density than normoglycemic patients (Li et al., 2011). Hence, it is to be expected that research on pancreatic neuroplasticity and especially NI in PCa may take a direction towards increased investigation of the impact of impaired glucose metabolism upon pancreatic neuropathy in PCa.

6. The role of neural invasion in the pain due to PCa

Decreased survival and local tumor recurrence are undoubtedly among the leading factors which make NI into a highly relevant clinical subject. However, within the true clinical impact of NI, its role in *pain* sensation occupies a special place. It has long been accepted that the extension of PCa along the intrapancreatic nerves towards extrapancreatic neural plexus may be a causal factor in the generation of pain in advanced Pca (Kayahara et al., 1991; Nakao et al., 1996; Kayahara et al., 2007). Bockman also postulated a significant role for NI in pain generation in PCa(Bockman et al., 1994), but the actual pioneering study in this context came from Zhu et al. who for the first time demonstrated the correlation between the intrapancreatic expression of the nerve growth factor (NGF)(Zhu et al., 1999), the frequency of perineural invasion and the degree of pain sensation in PCa patients, an observation which was later also discovered for the expression of NGF receptor TrkA (Zhang et al., 2005; Dang et al., 2006). Owing to this study and its successors, it became increasingly clear that the extent of NI in the pancreas affects pain sensation, where nerve-derived molecules like NGF play a key role in both pain sensation and potentially in the attraction of PCa cell to nerves (Demir et al., 2010). The resulting interest in such nerve-derived mediators, especially in neurotrophic factors, have inaugurated the era of research on the molecular biological mechanisms of NI which last until the present time (Demir et al., 2010). Moreover, the identified cross-link between NI, pancreatic neuroplastic alterations and pain sensation by PCa patients revealed the potential involvement of "neuropathic" pain mechanisms in PCa (Ceyhan et al., 2009; Demir et al., 2010). Hence, researchers and clinicians have recently and increasingly understood that damage to nerves within the pancreas may be the actual pain-triggering mechanism in PCa (Ceyhan et al., 2009; Demir et al., 2010).

One can assume that the blockade of pain transmission via the damaged nerves from the pancreas may be of major benefit to treat pain due to PCa. As the celiac plexus contains a large portion of the afferent nerve fibers from the pancreas, several studies have tested the efficieny of celiac plexus blockade/neurolysis in the treatment of pain due to PCa. In all these studies, patients had significant pain relief (Wong et al., 2004; Stefaniak et al., 2005; Yan&Myers, 2007) following this intervention. While the efficiency of this "denervation" technique does not necessarily prove the neuropathic character of pain in PCa, it underlines the deciding contribution of nerves and the transmitted signals in the generation of the pain syndrome in PCa (Ceyhan et al., 2008) Considering the neuropathic character of pain in PCa, one can assume that neuropathic analgesics may be of benefit to treat PCa-associated pain. As of today, the impact of neuropathic analgesic regimens to treat of patients with advanced PCa has not yet been systematically investigated.

7. Why are pancreatic cancer cells attracted to nerves? Molecular mechanisms of neural invasion in PCa

7.1 In vitro models

Researchers and clinicians have long puzzled about why PCa cells are frequently encountered around intrapancreatic nerves. Early reports had claimed that PCa cells enter nerves through the perineurium at its weakest points, i.e. along neural lymph vessels(di Mola&di Sebastiano, 2008), which, however, could not be confirmed in later studies. In later studies, investigators suggested that PCa cells grow along the path of least resistance after entering nerves, which was thought to be the perineural space (Rodin et al., 1967; Bockman et al., 1994; di Mola&di Sebastiano, 2008). Indeed, a higher proliferative index and decreased apoptosis in the perineural space could previously be shown for prostate cancer cells invading nerves (Ayala et al., 2004). However, newer studies could demonstrate that limiting PCa cells' presence around nerves to the local physical circumstances may be an oversimplification of the utmost frequent NI in Pca (Demir et al., 2010). In particular, the development of novel in vitro research tools to study NI in PCa has enabled the discovery of a true cancer-nerve affinity as an important biological mechanism in Pca (Zhu et al., 1999; Zhu et al., 2002). Especially, we know today that peripheral nerves in the tumor microenvironment can serve a source of tumor-trophic factors and cancer-attracting molecules (Zhu et al., 1999; Ceyhan et al., 2008; Gil et al., 2010). This "biological cancer-nerve affinity" in PCa is today one of the cardinal pathomechanistic concepts in our understanding of NI in Pca (Zhu et al., 1999; Ceyhan et al., 2008; Demir et al., 2010; Gil et al., 2010).

This increased appreciation of cancer-nerve affinity in PCa was largely possible owing to increased efforts to develop novel advanced in vitro models of NI in PCa. These models generally employ heterotypic co-cultures of neurons and PCa cells as in of the earliest models by Dai et al (Dai et al., 2007). In their study, the investigators co-cultivated the human PCa cell line MiaPaCa-2 with neurons from mouse dorsal root ganglia (DRG). In accordance with the hypothesized trophic effect of nerves, PCa cells which were co-cultured with DRG exhibited stronger growth than non-co-cultured control PCa cells and over-expressed prosurvival genes like MALT1 and TRAF (Dai et al., 2007). As a frequent observation also made by other current models, also PCa cells supported the growth of the neurons, as evidenced by their increased neurite growth (Dai et al., 2007).

This mutual trophic effect gained a further dimension in a recent study by our group where we presented another in vitro model which allows a precise spatiotemporal monitoring of NI by PCa cells (Ceyhan et al., 2008). As shown in the original article, different PCa cell lines were co-cultured together with rat DRG or myenteric plexus (MP) cells in a three-dimensional (3D) extracellular matrix (ECM)-based migration assay (Ceyhan et al., 2008).

The presented assay offers several advantages: First, it initiates from a clear-cut physical separation of PCa cells and neurons, as it is the case under *in vivo* conditions. Therefore, the model allows exact monitoring of cell behavior from the very beginning. Second, the model includes a pre-defined migration path for PCa cells, i.e. defined ECM-bridges, which allows the generation of a chemical gradient for any chemotactic factor (Ceyhan et al., 2008). Using this novel assay, we could demonstrate that PCa cells react to the presence of neurons with a characteristic morphological alteration including cell flattening, grouping, colony formation and spike-like cellular polarization directed towards neurites. Following their targeted migration towards neurons, PCa cells established physical contact with neurites along which they were guided in their migration (Ceyhan et al., 2008). Similar to the findings by Dai et al., we also observed increased neurite growth from DRG neurons towards PCa cells when compared to non-co-cultured DRG neurons (Ceyhan et al., 2008). Moreover, the presented 3D-migration assay for the first time included a neuronal subtype which represents the intrinsic pancreatic neurons, i.e. neurons of the enteric nervous system (ENS). The key role of neurotrophins which was initially demonstrated by Zhu et al. for NGF could be confirmed by means of this novel assay where we monitored the quantitative alterations in the expression of neurotrophins, their receptors and the members of the glial-cell-derived neurotrophic factor (GDNF) family (Zhu et al., 1999; Ceyhan et al., 2008). As opposed to several members of the GDNF family, the nerve growth factor (NGF) increased continuously throughout the migration process of 120 hours (Ceyhan et al., 2008). Certainly, this novel 3D migration assays is at the same time a novel tool to investigate the contribution of numerous molecular factors from different cellular sources to NI in PCa. A very similar model, though without pre-defined paths for chemical gradient generation, has been recently reported by Gil et al. where the investigators could demonstrate a potent chemotactic effect of GDNF from DRG neurons upon PCa cells (Gil et al., 2010). In a further study, our group showed the potent enhancer effect of the neurotrophic factor artemin, a member of the GDNF family of neurotrophic factors, upon invasiveness of PCa cells (Ceyhan et al., 2006).

In the presence of an increasing number of studies on the role of neurotrophic factors in NI in PCa, there is only a limited of reports on the role of chemokines in NI in PCa (Marchesi et al., 2008; Marchesi et al., 2010; Marchesi et al., 2010). In one of the first studies where the potential role of chemokines was recognized, Marchesi et al could show that the neural immunoreactivity for the receptor of the chemokine fractalkine, i.e. CX3CR1, was significantly higher in perineural invasive lesions of PCa (Marchesi et al., 2008). By using CX3CR1-overexpressing PCa cells for an *in vivo* implantation model, they could also demonstrate that CX3CR1-overexpressing PCa cells exhibited a more pronounced infiltration of peripheral nerves (Marchesi et al., 2008). This study stands out in the literature due to the seminal investigation of chemokines in the generation of NI in PCa and pointed to the CX3CR1-CX3CL1 as a potential therapeutic target.

Interestingly, beyond molecules with chemoattractive potential, other nerve-derived molecules have also been the focus of recent research on NI in PCa. From these, in a mouse perineural invasion and orthotopic transplantation model, the stable knockdown of synuclein gamma (synuclein-γ) via by short hairpin RNA significantly reduced the incidence of perineural invasion and liver and lymph node metastasis (Hibi et al., 2009). In another study where the investigators provided a novel perspective on NI in PCa, Swanson et al. showed that Schwann cells of peripheral nerves express myelin-associated glycoprotein (MAG) which can serve as a receptor for the transmembrane mucin MUC1 on PCa cells (Swanson et al., 2007). Hence, based on this study, it seems that nerves in PCa tissue not only chemo-attract PCa cells but also can undergo direct physical contact, as initially observed by Bockman (Swanson et al., 2007; Demir et al., 2010).

It is conceivable that the presented *in vitro* models in the literature would enable the identification of a gene set which would reflect the differentially upregulated genes in NI in PCa. Accordingly, in a recent study, Abiatari et al. aimed at obtaining a transcriptome signature of NI in PCa by means of an *in vitro / ex vivo* model (Abiatari et al., 2009). Specifically, they confronted human PCa cell lines with explanted rat vagus nerves and quantified the differentially regulated genes in highly versus less nerve-invasive PCa cells (Abiatari et al., 2009). Interestingly, the differentially regulated genes which were identified by this study were primarily related to cell motility, including kinesin family member 14 (KIF14) and Rho-GDP dissociation inhibitor beta (ARHGDIbeta), a gene set which they could expand in a subsequent by two molecules, i.e., the microtubule-associated protein MAPRE2 and the nuclear protein YPEL2 (Abiatari et al., 2009; Abiatari et al., 2009; Abiatari et al., 2009). Based on these important observations, the investigators underlined the importance of increased PCa cell motility in the generation of NI in PCa as additional molecular biological mechanism (Abiatari et al., 2009; Abiatari et al., 2009).

7.2 In vivo models

The increasing number of efforts to elucidate the pathomechanism of NI in PCa necessitated the creation of *in vivo* models which better mimic NI in human PCa. The common characteristic of these models is that they involve implantation of PCa cells as xenograft tumors in one out of several locations, e.g. into the pancreas, under the skin or in the proximity of large-diameter peripheral nerves to allow NI by PCa cells. In the first one of these models, Eibl et al. aimed at creating a model to simulate the high rates of local recurrence and NI after curative resection (Eibl&Reber, 2005). For this purpose, they performed complete surgical resection of the tumor at 4, 6, and 8 weeks after orthotopic implantation of the PCa cell lines MiaPaCa-2 (undifferentiated) and Capan-2 (well-differentiated) in nude mice pancreas. Six weeks after tumor implantation, local tumor recurrence with extensive retroperitoneal nerve invasion and distant organ metastasis were observed in nude mice who had received MiaPaCa-2 cells (Eibl&Reber, 2005). Astonishingly, although the investigators achieved a successful simulation of the local recurrence and NI associated with PCa in this murine model, there has since been no application of this model to identify further pathomechanistic features of NI in PCa. Certainly, the model is probably not suitable to study the initial, early events leading to PCa, however, it can possibly be employed to examine the therapeutic potential of different agents on NI in PCa in an animal model of PCa. In another model, Koide et al. subcutaneously (s.c.) implanted different PCa cell lines with or without human peripheral nerves in nonobese diabetes/severe combined immunodeficient mice and analyzed the frequency of NI by these different cell lines (Koide et al., 2006). Furthermore, they performed an oligonucleotide microarray to obtain the expression profiles of high and low perineurally invasive cell lines. Interestingly, only two well-differentiated cell lines (Capan-1 and Capan-2) demonstrated invasion of mouse s.c. nerves. In these invasive cell lines, they identified over-expression of CD74 in the specifically perineural invasive cells, which they confirmed in human PCa tissue specimens (Koide et al., 2006). Despite the implantation of PCa cells under skin and not the actual organ of origin (i.e. the pancreas), this model sticks out owing to its uncomplicated performance. Still, it has to be underlined that none of these *in vivo* models has so far found widespread application.

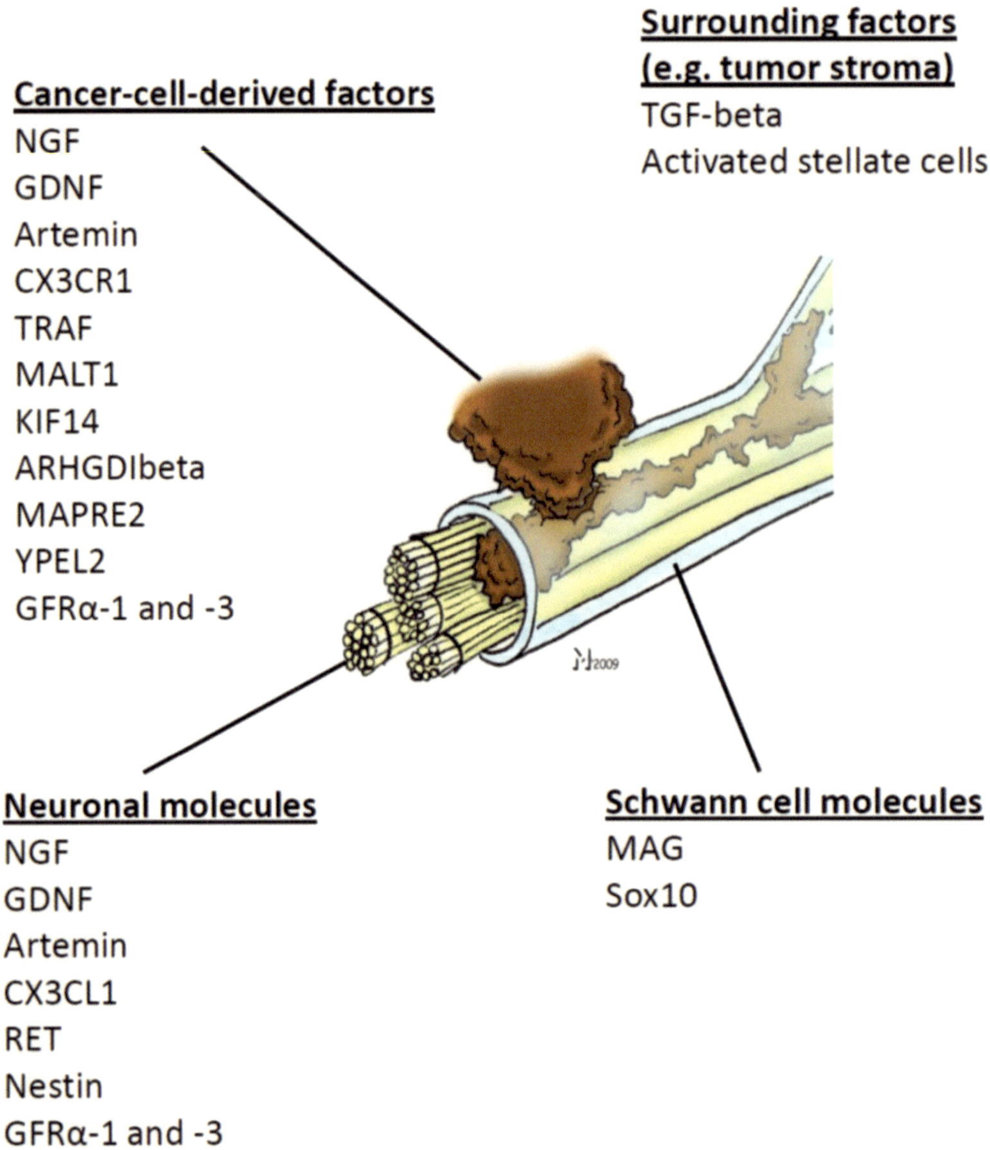

Fig. 2. Different sources of molecular actors in neural invasion (NI) in pancreatic cancer (PCa). Research from the past 15 years revealed that NI results from a complicated interplay of numerous molecular agents derived from different sources, e.g. PCa cells, neurons, Schwann cells and stromal cells. Please refer to the main text for the respective references

Investigator	Model characteristics	Advantages	Limitations
In Vitro Models			
Dai et al.	Matrigel-based heterotypic co-culture	One of the initial models Apt for studying expression changes	No pre-defined chemical gradient for chemo-attractants No remark on the initial cellular reactions Different species of confronted cells (murine neurons vs. human PCa cells)
Ceyhan et al.	ECM-based three-dimensional heterotypic migration assay	Initial physical separation of different cells Observation of initial cellular morphological reactions "Bridges" to enable chemical gradient generation Usage of myenteric neurons	Different species of confronted cells (murine neurons vs. human PCa cells)
Abiatari et al.	Ex vivo co-culture of rat nerves with PCa cells	Easy to perform	Confrontation with the "large-caliber" vagal nerve Different species of confronted cells (murine neurons vs. human PCa cells)
In Vivo Models			
Eibl et al.	Orthotopic PCa cell injection followed by tumor resection (murine)	Simulation of extrapancreatic NI	Lacking monitoring of initial pathophysiological events
Gil et al.	Tumor injection onto murine sciatic nerve	Easy to perform Therapeutic monitoring by observing degree of paralysis	Confrontation with the "large-caliber" sciatic nerve

Table 1. Experimental models of neural invasion (NI) in pancreatic cancer (PCa). The listed in vitro and in vivo models represent complicated heterotypic culture systems and possess several differences among each other. Their advantages, however, clearly overweigh their limitations. ECM: extracellular matrix. Please refer to the manuscript for the respective references.

8. Efforts of controlling neural invasion in PCa

Among all studies in the literature, there are so far two *in vivo* models of NI in PCa where a primarily therapeutic goal was pursued: In the first study, Gil et al. aimed at treating NI by means of an attenuated, replication-competent, oncolytic herpes simplex virus which inhabits nerves (Gil et al., 2007). After injection of PCa cell lines into the perineurium of the sciatic nerve of athymic mice, they monitored limb function for 9 days after injection. Excitingly, a single injection of the oncolytic herpes simplex virus 7 days after PCa cell injection effectively eradicated NI without compromising physiologic nerve function (Gil et al., 2007). The same group utilized this model in a subsequent study for intraoperative diagnosis of NI: By using enhanced green fluorescent protein (eGFP)-expressing oncolytic herpes virus, they could detect invaded nerves following intrasciatic implantation of PCa cell lines via intraoperative fluorescent stereoscopic imaging (Gil et al., 2008). Thereby, they proposed a novel tool for enhanced diagnosis and therapy of NI in PCa and for facilitated detection of invaded nerves in cases where an extended resection may be considered (Gil et al., 2008). In a third study, the group applied PCa cell injection onto mouse sciatic nerves and subsequently treated the mice with pyrazolopyrimidine-1, a tyrosine kinase inhibitor targeting the RET pathway (Gil et al., 2010). Strikingly, systemic therapy with this agent diminished nerve invasion toward the spinal cord and prevented limb paralysis (Gil et al., 2010). Still, the sensitivity and true effectiveness of their method remains to be confirmed in future studies.

9. Future directions in research on NI in PCa

Today, research on NI in PCa is in an era of "data collection" and "expansion of knowledge". The increasing number of *in vitro* and *in vivo* models, together with the rapidly growing scientific interest in NI, create the best possible conditions to learn and discover about this peculiar histopathological phenomenon. However, we are convinced that future studies should aim at the generation of models with an increasingly therapeutic intention, because there is urgent need to employ additional, novel tools to treat PCa. Furthermore, the main pathomechanistic hypothesis for the generation of NI, i.e. the neuro-affinity of PCa cells, has to be carefully reviewed. It should certainly be considered that PCa cells may not be responsible for every aspect of NI, but rather be reacting to the signals coming from the nerves. The increasing number of nerve-derived molecules like neurotrophic factors or neuronal chemokines which are continuously shown to contribute to NI should serve as a motivation to delve deeper into the involvement of neuronal molecules during NI.

While novel *in vitro* models of NI in PCa are being steadily developed, the currently available *in vivo* models still exhibit major deficits. In particular, these models lack:

1. Tumors that directly originate from the pancreas
2. Histopathological confirmation of the tumor phenotype as ductal adenocarcinoma
3. The confirmation of the presence of NI even at early stages of tumor development and progression
4. The specific extension of NI towards the extrapancreatic neural plexus
5. Accompanying neuropathic and desmoplastic alterations
6. Neuropathic pain sensation

Therefore, future *in vivo* models of NI in PCa should be superior to the current ones in the above-mentioned aspects, especially because they should increasingly be employed to deduce therapeutic targets and strategies.

10. Summary and conclusion

Neural invasion in PCa bears a unique importance in the biology of this disease due its impact on patient survival, local tumor reccurence and neuropathic pain sensation. Higher interest in NI has paved path for increased research on the biology of NI and accelarated the development of numerous experimental models. The discussed *in vitro* and *in vivo* models which shall help to eludicate the pathomechanisms of NI in PCa may provide novel tools to control and to reduce NI in this highly aggressive human malignancy. Considering the dismal average prognosis associated with PCa, one may wonder about the actual benefit of reducing the specific invasion of nerves in this tumor entity. Here, it should be underlined that reduction of NI can be regarded as one of several possibilities to control tumor growth, just as adjuvant therapy as an oncological therapy regimen aims at reaching microscopic tumor presence and reducing the systemic tumor burden. The control of NI, however, bears a further special importance since NI is not only the probably most common mode of spread for PCa, but also because nerves represent the most frequent site of local tumor recurrence in PCa. Moreover, limitation of NI is likely to have a considerable impact upon the neuropathic pain syndrome and thus quality of life of patients with PCa. Therefore, NI may find increased attention in the future as an additional therapeutic target for increased survival, enhanced postoperative outcome and improved quality of life among all patients with this dreadful malignancy.

11. Acknowledgements

The authors are grateful to Dr. Matthias Maak for his assistance with the figures.

12. References

Abiatari, I., DeOliveira, T., Kerkadze, V., Schwager, C., Esposito, I., Giese, N. A., Huber, P., Bergman, F., Abdollahi, A., Friess, H. & Kleeff, J. (2009). "Consensus transcriptome signature of perineural invasion in pancreatic carcinoma." *Mol Cancer Ther* 8(6): 1494-504.

Abiatari, I., Gillen, S., DeOliveira, T., Klose, T., Bo, K., Giese, N. A., Friess, H. & Kleeff, J. (2009). "The microtubule-associated protein MAPRE2 is involved in perineural invasion of pancreatic cancer cells." *Int J Oncol* 35(5): 1111-6.

Abiatari, I., Kiladze, M., Kerkadze, V., Friess, H. & Kleeff, J. (2009). "Expression of YPEL1 in pancreatic cancer cell lines and tissues." *Georgian Med News*(175): 60-2.

Ayala, G. E., Dai, H., Ittmann, M., Li, R., Powell, M., Frolov, A., Wheeler, T. M., Thompson, T. C. & Rowley, D. (2004). "Growth and survival mechanisms associated with perineural invasion in prostate cancer." *Cancer Res* 64(17): 6082-90.

Bachmann, J., Michalski, C. W., Martignoni, M. E., Buchler, M. W. & Friess, H. (2006). "Pancreatic resection for pancreatic cancer." *HPB (Oxford)* 8(5): 346-51.

Bockman, D. E., Buchler, M. & Beger, H. G. (1994). "Interaction of pancreatic ductal carcinoma with nerves leads to nerve damage." *Gastroenterology* 107(1): 219-30.

Bradley, E. L., 3rd & Bem, J. (2003). "Nerve blocks and neuroablative surgery for chronic pancreatitis." *World J Surg* 27(11): 1241-8.

Ceyhan, G. O., Bergmann, F., Kadihasanoglu, M., Altintas, B., Demir, I. E., Hinz, U., Muller, M. W., Giese, T., Buchler, M. W., Giese, N. A. & Friess, H. (2009). "Pancreatic neuropathy and neuropathic pain--a comprehensive pathomorphological study of 546 cases." *Gastroenterology* 136(1): 177-186 e1.

Ceyhan, G. O., Demir, I. E., Altintas, B., Rauch, U., Thiel, G., Muller, M. W., Giese, N. A., Friess, H. & Schafer, K. H. (2008). "Neural invasion in pancreatic cancer: a mutual tropism between neurons and cancer cells." *Biochem Biophys Res Commun* 374(3): 442-7.

Ceyhan, G. O., Demir, I. E., Rauch, U., Bergmann, F., Muller, M. W., Buchler, M. W., Friess, H. & Schafer, K. H. (2009). "Pancreatic neuropathy results in "neural remodeling" and altered pancreatic innervation in chronic pancreatitis and pancreatic cancer." *Am J Gastroenterol* 104(10): 2555-65.

Ceyhan, G. O., Giese, N. A., Erkan, M., Kerscher, A. G., Wente, M. N., Giese, T., Buchler, M. W. & Friess, H. (2006). "The neurotrophic factor artemin promotes pancreatic cancer invasion." *Ann Surg* 244(2): 274-81.

Ceyhan, G. O., Liebl, F., Maak, M., Schuster, T., Becker, K., Langer, R., Demir, I. E., Hartel, M., Friess, H. & Rosenberg, R. (2011). "The severity of neural invasion is a crucial prognostic factor in rectal cancer independent of neoadjuvant radiochemotherapy." *Ann Surg* 252(5): 797-804.

Ceyhan, G. O., Michalski, C. W., Demir, I. E., Muller, M. W. & Friess, H. (2008). "Pancreatic pain." *Best Pract Res Clin Gastroenterol* 22(1): 31-44.

Chakravarty, K. D., Hsu, J. T., Liu, K. H., Yeh, C. N., Yeh, T. S., Hwang, T. L., Jan, Y. Y. & Chen, M. F. (2011). "Prognosis and feasibility of en-bloc vascular resection in stage II pancreatic adenocarcinoma." *World J Gastroenterol* 16(8): 997-1002.

Dai, H., Li, R., Wheeler, T., Ozen, M., Ittmann, M., Anderson, M., Wang, Y., Rowley, D., Younes, M. & Ayala, G. E. (2007). "Enhanced survival in perineural invasion of pancreatic cancer: an in vitro approach." *Hum Pathol* 38(2): 299-307.

Dang, C., Zhang, Y., Ma, Q. & Shimahara, Y. (2006). "Expression of nerve growth factor receptors is correlated with progression and prognosis of human pancreatic cancer." *J Gastroenterol Hepatol* 21(5): 850-8.

Demir, I. E., Ceyhan, G. O., Liebl, F., J.G., D. H., Maak, M. & Friess, H. (2010). "Neural Invasion in Pancreatic Cancer: The Past, Present and Future." *Cancers* 2(3): 1513-1527.

Demir, I. E., Ceyhan, G. O., Rauch, U., Altintas, B., Klotz, M., Muller, M. W., Buchler, M. W., Friess, H. & Schafer, K. H. (2010). "The microenvironment in chronic pancreatitis and pancreatic cancer induces neuronal plasticity." *Neurogastroenterol Motil* 22(4): 480-90, e112-3.

di Mola, F. F. & di Sebastiano, P. (2008). "Pain and pain generation in pancreatic cancer." *Langenbecks Arch Surg* 393(6): 919-22.

Eibl, G. & Reber, H. A. (2005). "A xenograft nude mouse model for perineural invasion and recurrence in pancreatic cancer." *Pancreas* 31(3): 258-62.

Gil, Z., Cavel, O., Kelly, K., Brader, P., Rein, A., Gao, S. P., Carlson, D. L., Shah, J. P., Fong, Y. & Wong, R. J. (2010). "Paracrine regulation of pancreatic cancer cell invasion by peripheral nerves." *J Natl Cancer Inst* 102(2): 107-18.

Gil, Z., Kelly, K. J., Brader, P., Shah, J. P., Fong, Y. & Wong, R. J. (2008). "Utility of a herpes oncolytic virus for the detection of neural invasion by cancer." *Neoplasia* 10(4): 347-53.

Gil, Z., Rein, A., Brader, P., Li, S., Shah, J. P., Fong, Y. & Wong, R. J. (2007). "Nerve-sparing therapy with oncolytic herpes virus for cancers with neural invasion." *Clin Cancer Res* 13(21): 6479-85.

Hibi, T., Mori, T., Fukuma, M., Yamazaki, K., Hashiguchi, A., Yamada, T., Tanabe, M., Aiura, K., Kawakami, T., Ogiwara, A., Kosuge, T., Kitajima, M., Kitagawa, Y. & Sakamoto, M. (2009). "Synuclein-gamma is closely involved in perineural invasion and distant metastasis in mouse models and is a novel prognostic factor in pancreatic cancer." *Clin Cancer Res* 15(8): 2864-71.

Hirai, I., Kimura, W., Ozawa, K., Kudo, S., Suto, K., Kuzu, H. & Fuse, A. (2002). "Perineural invasion in pancreatic cancer." *Pancreas* 24(1): 15-25.

Hirano, S., Kondo, S., Hara, T., Ambo, Y., Tanaka, E., Shichinohe, T., Suzuki, O. & Hazama, K. (2007). "Distal pancreatectomy with en bloc celiac axis resection for locally advanced pancreatic body cancer: long-term results." *Ann Surg* 246(1): 46-51.

Hirano, S., Kondo, S., Tanaka, E., Shichinohe, T., Tsuchikawa, T., Kato, K. & Matsumoto, J. "Postoperative bowel function and nutritional status following distal pancreatectomy with en-bloc celiac axis resection." *Dig Surg* 27(3): 212-6.

Hiraoka, T., Watanabe, E., Katoh, T., Hayashida, N., Mizutani, J., Kanemitsu, K. & Miyauchi, Y. (1986). "A new surgical approach for control of pain in chronic pancreatitis: complete denervation of the pancreas." *Am J Surg* 152(5): 549-51.

Imamura, M., Hosotani, R. & Kogire, M. (1999). "Rationale of the so-called extended resection for pancreatic invasive ductal carcinoma." *Digestion* 60 Suppl 1: 126-9.

Kayahara, M., Nagakawa, T., Futagami, F., Kitagawa, H., Ohta, T. & Miyazaki, I. (1996). "Lymphatic flow and neural plexus invasion associated with carcinoma of the body and tail of the pancreas." *Cancer* 78(12): 2485-91.

Kayahara, M., Nagakawa, T., Konishi, I., Ueno, K., Ohta, T. & Miyazaki, I. (1991). "Clinicopathological study of pancreatic carcinoma with particular reference to the invasion of the extrapancreatic neural plexus." *Int J Pancreatol* 10(2): 105-11.

Kayahara, M., Nagakawa, T., Tsukioka, Y., Ohta, T., Ueno, K. & Miyazaki, I. (1994). "Neural invasion and nodal involvement in distal bile duct cancer." *Hepatogastroenterology* 41(2): 190-4.

Kayahara, M., Nagakawa, T., Ueno, K., Ohta, T., Takeda, T. & Miyazaki, I. (1993). "An evaluation of radical resection for pancreatic cancer based on the mode of recurrence as determined by autopsy and diagnostic imaging." *Cancer* 72(7): 2118-23.

Kayahara, M., Nagakawa, T., Ueno, K., Ohta, T., Tsukioka, Y. & Miyazaki, I. (1995). "Surgical strategy for carcinoma of the pancreas head area based on clinicopathologic analysis of nodal involvement and plexus invasion." *Surgery* 117(6): 616-23.

Kayahara, M., Nakagawara, H., Kitagawa, H. & Ohta, T. (2007). "The nature of neural invasion by pancreatic cancer." *Pancreas* 35(3): 218-23.

Kirchgessner, A. L. & Gershon, M. D. (1990). "Innervation of the pancreas by neurons in the gut." *J Neurosci* 10(5): 1626-42.

Kirchgessner, A. L. & Gershon, M. D. (1991). "Innervation and regulation of the pancreas by neurons in the gut." *Z Gastroenterol Verh* 26: 230-3.

Koide, N., Yamada, T., Shibata, R., Mori, T., Fukuma, M., Yamazaki, K., Aiura, K., Shimazu, M., Hirohashi, S., Nimura, Y. & Sakamoto, M. (2006). "Establishment of perineural invasion models and analysis of gene expression revealed an invariant chain (CD74) as a possible molecule involved in perineural invasion in pancreatic cancer." *Clin Cancer Res* 12(8): 2419-26.

Kondo, S., Katoh, H., Omi, M., Hirano, S., Ambo, Y., Tanaka, E., Okushiba, S., Morikawa, T., Kanai, M. & Yano, T. (2001). "Radical distal pancreatectomy with en bloc resection of the celiac artery, plexus, and ganglions for advanced cancer of the pancreatic body: a preliminary report on perfect pain relief." *Jop* 2(3): 93-7.

Li, J. & Ma, Q. (2008). "Hyperglycemia promotes the perineural invasion in pancreatic cancer." *Med Hypotheses* 71(3): 386-9.

Li, J., Ma, Q., Liu, H., Guo, K., Li, F., Li, W., Han, L., Wang, F. & Wu, E. (2011). "Relationship between neural alteration and perineural invasion in pancreatic cancer patients with hyperglycemia." *PLoS One* 6(2): e17385.

Liebig, C., Ayala, G., Wilks, J. A., Berger, D. H. & Albo, D. (2009). "Perineural invasion in cancer: a review of the literature." *Cancer* 115(15): 3379-91.

Liu, B. & Lu, K. Y. (2002). "Neural invasion in pancreatic carcinoma." *Hepatobiliary Pancreat Dis Int* 1(3): 469-76.

Marchesi, F., Locatelli, M., Solinas, G., Erreni, M., Allavena, P. & Mantovani, A. (2010). "Role of CX3CR1/CX3CL1 axis in primary and secondary involvement of the nervous system by cancer." *J Neuroimmunol* 224(1-2): 39-44.

Marchesi, F., Piemonti, L., Fedele, G., Destro, A., Roncalli, M., Albarello, L., Doglioni, C., Anselmo, A., Doni, A., Bianchi, P., Laghi, L., Malesci, A., Cervo, L., Malosio, M., Reni, M., Zerbi, A., Di Carlo, V., Mantovani, A. & Allavena, P. (2008). "The chemokine receptor CX3CR1 is involved in the neural tropism and malignant behavior of pancreatic ductal adenocarcinoma." *Cancer Res* 68(21): 9060-9.

Marchesi, F., Piemonti, L., Mantovani, A. & Allavena, P. (2010). "Molecular mechanisms of perineural invasion, a forgotten pathway of dissemination and metastasis." *Cytokine Growth Factor Rev* 21(1): 77-82.

Mitsunaga, S., Hasebe, T., Kinoshita, T., Konishi, M., Takahashi, S., Gotohda, N., Nakagohri, T. & Ochiai, A. (2007). "Detail histologic analysis of nerve plexus invasion in invasive ductal carcinoma of the pancreas and its prognostic impact." *Am J Surg Pathol* 31(11): 1636-44.

Nagakawa, T., Konishi, I., Ueno, K., Ohta, T., Akiyama, T., Kayahara, M. & Miyazaki, I. (1991). "Surgical treatment of pancreatic cancer. The Japanese experience." *Int J Pancreatol* 9: 135-43.

Nagakawa, T., Nagamori, M., Futakami, F., Tsukioka, Y., Kayahara, M., Ohta, T., Ueno, K. & Miyazaki, I. (1996). "Results of extensive surgery for pancreatic carcinoma." *Cancer* 77(4): 640-5.

Nakao, A., Harada, A., Nonami, T., Kaneko, T. & Takagi, H. (1996). "Clinical significance of carcinoma invasion of the extrapancreatic nerve plexus in pancreatic cancer." *Pancreas* 12(4): 357-61.

Ozaki, H., Hiraoka, T., Mizumoto, R., Matsuno, S., Matsumoto, Y., Nakayama, T., Tsunoda, T., Suzuki, T., Monden, M., Saitoh, Y., Yamauchi, H. & Ogata, Y. (1999). "The prognostic significance of lymph node metastasis and intrapancreatic perineural invasion in pancreatic cancer after curative resection." *Surg Today* 29(1): 16-22.

Rodin, A. E., Larson, D. L. & Roberts, D. K. (1967). "Nature of the perineural space invaded by prostatic carcinoma." *Cancer* 20(10): 1772-9.

Sperti, C., Berselli, M. & Pedrazzoli, S. "Distal pancreatectomy for body-tail pancreatic cancer: is there a role for celiac axis resection?" *Pancreatology* 10(4): 491-8.

Stefaniak, T., Basinski, A., Vingerhoets, A., Makarewicz, W., Connor, S., Kaska, L., Stanek, A., Kwiecinska, B., Lachinski, A. J. & Sledzinski, Z. (2005). "A comparison of two invasive techniques in the management of intractable pain due to inoperable pancreatic cancer: neurolytic celiac plexus block and videothoracoscopic splanchnicectomy." *Eur J Surg Oncol* 31(7): 768-73.

Swanson, B. J., McDermott, K. M., Singh, P. K., Eggers, J. P., Crocker, P. R. & Hollingsworth, M. A. (2007). "MUC1 is a counter-receptor for myelin-associated glycoprotein (Siglec-4a) and their interaction contributes to adhesion in pancreatic cancer perineural invasion." *Cancer Res* 67(21): 10222-9.

Takahashi, S., Hasebe, T., Oda, T., Sasaki, S., Kinoshita, T., Konishi, M., Ueda, T., Ochiai, T. & Ochiai, A. (2001). "Extra-tumor perineural invasion predicts postoperative development of peritoneal dissemination in pancreatic ductal adenocarcinoma." *Anticancer Res* 21(2B): 1407-12.

Takahashi, T., Ishikura, H., Motohara, T., Okushiba, S., Dohke, M. & Katoh, H. (1997). "Perineural invasion by ductal adenocarcinoma of the pancreas." *J Surg Oncol* 65(3): 164-70.

Takamori, H., Hiraoka, T., Kanemitsu, K., Tsuji, T., Tanaka, H., Chikamoto, A., Horino, K., Beppu, T., Hirota, M. & Baba, H. (2008). "Long-term outcomes of extended radical resection combined with intraoperative radiation therapy for pancreatic cancer." *J Hepatobiliary Pancreat Surg* 15(6): 603-7.

Wong, G. Y., Schroeder, D. R., Carns, P. E., Wilson, J. L., Martin, D. P., Kinney, M. O., Mantilla, C. B. & Warner, D. O. (2004). "Effect of neurolytic celiac plexus block on pain relief, quality of life, and survival in patients with unresectable pancreatic cancer: a randomized controlled trial." *Jama* 291(9): 1092-9.

Yan, B. M. & Myers, R. P. (2007). "Neurolytic celiac plexus block for pain control in unresectable pancreatic cancer." *Am J Gastroenterol* 102(2): 430-8.

Yokoyama, Y. & Nagino, M. (2011). "Role of extended surgery for pancreatic cancer: critical review of the four major RCTs comparing standard and extended surgery." *J Hepatobiliary Pancreat Sci.*

Zhang, Y., Dang, C., Ma, Q. & Shimahara, Y. (2005). "Expression of nerve growth factor receptors and their prognostic value in human pancreatic cancer." *Oncol Rep* 14(1): 161-71.

Zhu, Z., Friess, H., diMola, F. F., Zimmermann, A., Graber, H. U., Korc, M. & Buchler, M. W. (1999). "Nerve growth factor expression correlates with perineural invasion and pain in human pancreatic cancer." *J Clin Oncol* 17(8): 2419-28.

Zhu, Z., Kleeff, J., Kayed, H., Wang, L., Korc, M., Buchler, M. W. & Friess, H. (2002). "Nerve growth factor and enhancement of proliferation, invasion, and tumorigenicity of pancreatic cancer cells." *Mol Carcinog* 35(3): 138-47.